AF127334

Targeting Inflammation and Inflammatory-Related Diseases with Natural Bioactives

Targeting Inflammation and Inflammatory-Related Diseases with Natural Bioactives

Editor

Francesco Maione

MDPI • Basel • Beijing • Wuhan • Barcelona • Belgrade • Manchester • Tokyo • Cluj • Tianjin

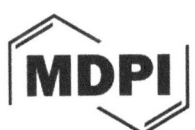

Editor
Francesco Maione
Pharmacy
Federico II
Naples
Italy

Editorial Office
MDPI
St. Alban-Anlage 66
4052 Basel, Switzerland

This is a reprint of articles from the Special Issue published online in the open access journal *Molecules* (ISSN 1420-3049) (available at: www.mdpi.com/journal/molecules/special_issues/molecules_inflammation).

For citation purposes, cite each article independently as indicated on the article page online and as indicated below:

LastName, A.A.; LastName, B.B.; LastName, C.C. Article Title. *Journal Name* **Year**, *Volume Number*, Page Range.

ISBN 978-3-0365-7297-0 (Hbk)
ISBN 978-3-0365-7296-3 (PDF)

© 2023 by the authors. Articles in this book are Open Access and distributed under the Creative Commons Attribution (CC BY) license, which allows users to download, copy and build upon published articles, as long as the author and publisher are properly credited, which ensures maximum dissemination and a wider impact of our publications.

The book as a whole is distributed by MDPI under the terms and conditions of the Creative Commons license CC BY-NC-ND.

Contents

About the Editor vii

Preface to "Targeting Inflammation and Inflammatory-Related Diseases with Natural Bioactives" ix

Anella Saviano, Federica Raucci, Gian Marco Casillo, Chiara Indolfi, Alessia Pernice and Carmen Foreste et al.
Present Status and Future Trends of Natural-Derived Compounds Targeting T Helper (Th) 17 and Microsomal Prostaglandin E Synthase-1 (mPGES-1) as Alternative Therapies for Autoimmune and Inflammatory-Based Diseases
Reprinted from: *Molecules* **2020**, *25*, 6016, doi:10.3390/molecules25246016 1

Hassan Rakhshandeh, Hamed Rajabi Khasevan, Anella Saviano, Mohammad Reza Mahdinezhad, Vafa Baradaran Rahimi and Sajjad Ehtiati et al.
Protective Effect of *Portulaca oleracea* on Streptozotocin-Induced Type I Diabetes-Associated Reproductive System Dysfunction and Inflammation
Reprinted from: *Molecules* **2022**, *27*, 6075, doi:10.3390/molecules27186075 15

Stefano Pieretti, Anella Saviano, Adriano Mollica, Azzurra Stefanucci, Anna Maria Aloisi and Marcello Nicoletti
Calceolarioside A, a Phenylpropanoid Glycoside from *Calceolaria* spp., Displays Antinociceptive and Anti-Inflammatory Properties
Reprinted from: *Molecules* **2022**, *27*, 2183, doi:10.3390/molecules27072183 33

Hammad Ullah, Alessandro Di Minno, Cristina Santarcangelo, Ariyawan Tantipongpiradet, Marco Dacrema and Rita di Matteo et al.
In Vitro Bioaccessibility and Anti-Inflammatory Activity of a Chemically Characterized *Allium cepa* L. Extract Rich in Quercetin Derivatives Optimized by the Design of Experiments
Reprinted from: *Molecules* **2022**, *27*, 9065, doi:10.3390/molecules27249065 45

Sherihan El-Sayed, Sally Freeman and Richard A. Bryce
A Selective Review and Virtual Screening Analysis of Natural Product Inhibitors of the NLRP3 Inflammasome
Reprinted from: *Molecules* **2022**, *27*, 6213, doi:10.3390/molecules27196213 61

Christina Barda, Konstantina Anastasiou, Ariadni Tzara, Maria-Eleni Grafakou, Eleftherios Kalpoutzakis and Joerg Heilmann et al.
A Bio-Guided Screening for Antioxidant, Anti-Inflammatory and Hypolipidemic Potential Supported by Non-Targeted Metabolomic Analysis of *Crepis* spp.
Reprinted from: *Molecules* **2022**, *27*, 6173, doi:10.3390/molecules27196173 75

Hyun-Su Lee, Eun-Nam Kim and Gil-Saeng Jeong
Ameliorative Effect of Citropten Isolated from *Citrus aurantifolia* Peel Extract as a Modulator of T Cell and Intestinal Epithelial Cell Activity in DSS-Induced Colitis
Reprinted from: *Molecules* **2022**, *27*, 4633, doi:10.3390/molecules27144633 93

Jiacheng Zhang, Zhaoran Zhang, Jianfeng Xu, Chun Ye, Shulin Fu and Chien-An Andy Hu et al.
Protective Effects of Baicalin on Peritoneal Tight Junctions in Piglets Challenged with *Glaesserella parasuis*
Reprinted from: *Molecules* **2021**, *26*, 1268, doi:10.3390/molecules26051268 109

Tingting Luo, Xiazhou Fu, Yaoli Liu, Yaoting Ji and Zhengjun Shang
Sulforaphane Inhibits Osteoclastogenesis via Suppression of the Autophagic Pathway
Reprinted from: *Molecules* **2021**, *26*, 347, doi:10.3390/molecules26020347 . . . . **125**

Thilina U. Jayawardena, K. K. Asanka Sanjeewa, Lei Wang, Won-Suk Kim, Tae-Ki Lee and Yong-Tae Kim et al.
Alginic Acid from *Padina boryana* Abate Particulate Matter-Induced Inflammatory Responses in Keratinocytes and Dermal Fibroblasts
Reprinted from: *Molecules* **2020**, *25*, 5746, doi:10.3390/molecules25235746 . . . . **141**

About the Editor

Francesco Maione

Francesco Maione graduated in Pharmacy in 2005 from the University of Naples Federico II and trained in Pharmacology in the Department of Experimental Pharmacology of the Faculty of Pharmacy. Whilst obtaining his PhD in Pharmacology (2005–2008), he studied the role of N-formyl-peptides (fMLF and FTM) in different models of pain and inflammation. During these studies, Dr. Francesco Maione demonstrated that these endogenous (fMLF) and synthetic peptides (FTM) have remarkable in vivo inflammatory and painful activity. Dr. Maione extended this research path after beginning his post-doctoral training in the laboratory of Prof. Mauro Perretti and Prof. Fulvio D'acquisto, at William Harvey Research Institute, Queen Mary University of London (2008–2010). During this time, he expanded his knowledge on inflammation by focusing on immune-mediated inflammatory diseases and investigated the role of Annexin-1 (ANX-1) and interleukin-17A (IL-17A) in different models of inflammation. Since 2010, he has been a member of Prof. Nicola Mascolo's laboratory where he has re-established his long-term interest in natural compound biology, charting an unexplored path in the role of natural molecules in the inflammatory response and cardiovascular system. In 2013, Dr. Francesco Maione obtained a Specialization in Clinical Pharmacy at the University of Naples Federico II. Moreover, Francesco Maione is an Associate Professor in Pharmacology and is the Head of the ImmunoPharmaLab (certified ISO9001 for preclinical studies in immunopharmacology) in the Department of Pharmacy, the University of Naples Federico II.

Preface to "Targeting Inflammation and Inflammatory-Related Diseases with Natural Bioactives"

Inflammation is a complex biological response to injury as a result of different stimuli such as pathogens, damaged cells, or irritants. Inflammatory injuries induce the release of a variety of systemic mediators, cytokines, and chemokines that orchestrate cellular infiltration, consequentially bringing about the resolution of inflammatory responses and the restoration of tissue integrity. However, persistent inflammatory stimuli or the disregulation of the mechanisms of the resolution phase can lead to chronic inflammation and inflammatory-based diseases. Nowadays, commercially approved anti-inflammatory drugs are represented by nonsteroidal anti-inflammatory drugs (NSAID); glucocorticoids (SAID); and, in some cases, immunosuppressant and/or biological drugs. These agents are effective for the relief of the main inflammatory symptoms. However, they induce severe side effects, and most of them are inadequate for chronic use. Starting from these premises, the demand for new, effective, and safe anti-inflammatory drugs has led research in new therapeutic directions. The recent and emerging scientific community slant is oriented towards natural products/compounds that could represent a boon for the discovery of new active molecules and for the development of new drugs and potentially useful therapeutic agents in different inflammatory-related diseases.

Francesco Maione
Editor

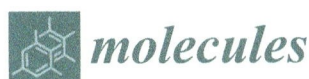

Opinion

Present Status and Future Trends of Natural-Derived Compounds Targeting T Helper (Th) 17 and Microsomal Prostaglandin E Synthase-1 (mPGES-1) as Alternative Therapies for Autoimmune and Inflammatory-Based Diseases

Anella Saviano [1], Federica Raucci [1], Gian Marco Casillo [1], Chiara Indolfi [1], Alessia Pernice [1], Carmen Foreste [1], Asif Jilani Iqbal [1,2], Nicola Mascolo [1,*] and Francesco Maione [1,*]

1. ImmunoPharmaLab, Department of Pharmacy, School of Medicine and Surgery, University of Naples Federico II, Via Domenico Montesano 49, 80131 Naples, Italy; nella.1993@hotmail.it (A.S.); federica.raucci@unina.it (F.R.); gianmarcocasillo@virgilio.it (G.M.C.); chiara_indolfi@hotmail.it (C.I.); alessiapernice.ap@gmail.com (A.P.); carmenforeste@gmail.com (C.F.); A.J.Iqbal@bham.ac.uk (A.J.I.)
2. Institute of Cardiovascular Sciences (ICVS), College of Medical and Dental Sciences, University of Birmingham, Birmingham B15 2TT, UK
* Correspondence: nicola.mascolo@unina.it (N.M.); francesco.maione@unina.it (F.M.); Tel.: +39-081-678-412 (N.M.); +39-081-678-429 (F.M.)

Academic Editors: Karel Šmejkal and Bruno Botta
Received: 1 November 2020; Accepted: 17 December 2020; Published: 18 December 2020

Abstract: Several natural-based compounds and products are reported to possess anti-inflammatory and immunomodulatory activity both in vitro and in vivo. The primary target for these activities is the inhibition of eicosanoid-generating enzymes, including phospholipase A2, cyclooxygenases (COXs), and lipoxygenases, leading to reduced prostanoids and leukotrienes. Other mechanisms include modulation of protein kinases and activation of transcriptases. However, only a limited number of studies and reviews highlight the potential modulation of the coupling enzymatic pathway COX-2/mPGES-1 and Th17/Treg circulating cells. Here, we provide a brief overview of natural products/compounds, currently included in the Italian list of botanicals and the BELFRIT, in different fields of interest such as inflammation and immunity. In this context, we focus our opinion on novel therapeutic targets such as COX-2/mPGES-1 coupling enzymes and Th17/Treg circulating repertoire. This paper is dedicated to the scientific career of Professor Nicola Mascolo for his profound dedication to the study of natural compounds.

Keywords: BELFRIT; immunity; mPGES-1; natural compounds; Th17

1. Introduction

The Belgian decree on botanicals, published 20 years ago, was the prototype of legislation and regulatory practice used in several European countries. In 1997, Belgium was one of the first countries to introduce a notification procedure and scientific risk evaluation by an Advisory Commission. Contextually, the authorities of Belgium, France, and Italy, each assisted by renowned scientific experts, decided to develop a common approach to evaluating botanicals [1]. As a first step, the three parties drafted a standard list of traditionally used plants safe to use in food supplements, commonly known as the BELFRIT project or BELFRIT list [2,3]. This evolved with the support of the European Commission and Member States and now guarantees the safety, quality, and effectiveness to health promoting prosperities of food supplements. Most other Member States acknowledge the importance of European Union (EU) harmonization in this "self-growing" area [4–6].

Modern medicine makes use of many plant-derived products/compounds as the basis for pharmaceutical drugs [7]; and quite often it applies modern standards of effectiveness testing to herbs and medicines derived from natural sources, performs high-quality clinical trials and uses standards for purity or dosage [8]. In this scenario, many botanicals are used in both food supplements and nutraceuticals, and yet a precise, unique, and standardized definition/s and procedure/s are still missing.

In this opinion paper, we provide a current state of the art about the anti-inflammatory and immunomodulatory properties of natural-derived compounds (including nutraceuticals, functional food, and dietary supplements) targeting microsomal prostaglandin E synthase-1 (mPGES-1) and the T helper 17 cells (Th17) and regulatory T-cells (Treg) axis, in order to provide a scientific rationale for their potential therapeutic use. Further investigation, in both pre-clinical and clinical fields, are required to provide in-depth evaluation of these botanicals and their bioactive components in the context of autoimmune and inflammatory-based diseases for health-promoting and disease-preventing purposes.

Nutraceuticals, functional foods, and dietary supplements have been known to exert beneficial effects against a variety of disease conditions [9–11]. Several medicinal plants and their isolated components have also been identified to possess health-promoting properties [12]. Moreover, a varied diet containing certain phytochemicals or introduced through supplementation have shown potential antioxidant, anti-inflammatory, and immunomodulatory benefit [13,14]. Therefore, the role of natural products and food is essential in maintaining and/or improving immune function [15,16]. Functional foods are those enriched or enhanced that provide health benefits beyond essential nutrients when consumed at efficacious levels as part of a varied diet. These mainly include berries, fermented dairy products, green tea, garlic, citrus fruits, and other herbal formulations [17–19]. In contrast the term "dietary supplement" describes a broad and different category of products (mainly containing vitamin C, vitamin D, minerals, omega-3 fatty acid, docosahexaenoic acid, etc.) that we eat or drink to support good health and supplement the diet. While nutraceuticals are food components, such as polyphenols, flavonoids, carotenoids, saponins, sulfides, which are derived from food sources with extra health benefits in addition to fundamental nutritional value [20–24].

These products could work both at the cellular and molecular level by triggering immune cells, up-regulating immune-related genes, and manipulating the systemic immune system, thereby providing natural immunotherapeutic options. These cellular and molecular mechanisms of natural products are essential to define the possible molecular and cellular targets, which could pave the way for discovering novel natural products/compounds exerting the immune-boosting effects [25,26].

2. Selected Studies and Inclusion and Exclusion Criteria

All studies were selected through a Medline–PubMed search using different combination of terms or keywords such as Th17, COX-2, mPGES-1, medicinal plants, and natural compounds/products. We have identified only original articles in English that evaluated pre-clinical studies, in vivo rodents models, and isolated and/or well-characterized compounds/extracts from all articles. Studies that analyzed natural substances purchased commercially were not excluded in this work. The next selection was to consider reports in which the method adopted used a natural compound in a well-established disease. The final selection criteria was choosing medicinal plants according to their presence in the Italian list of botanicals and the BELFRIT list.

3. Natural Compounds Targeting COX-2/mPGES-1/PGE$_2$ Cascade in Inflammatory-Based Diseases

Inflammation is a complex protective mechanism against noxious stimuli of chemical, physical, and/or biological origin, characterized by molecular and cellular defensive responses aimed at resolution of ongoing inflammation and restoration of tissue integrity [27–29]. However, the persistence of inflammatory inducers and the alteration of processes directed to homeostasis restoration can lead to the onset of chronic inflammation [30,31]. Inflammatory processes are generally associated with the innate immune system, but scientific evidence has shown that innate and adaptive immune cells collectively orchestrate the inflammatory response and that adaptive immune components are also involved in the production of memory cells that can sustain the chronic nature of inflammation-driven by the innate arm [32]. During the past decade, considerable progress has been made in understanding the cellular and molecular events in the acute inflammatory response and the role primary mediators have in infection and tissue injury [33]. Every early immunity "battle" begins with neutrophils, quickly recruited to sites of inflammation for an early response against the noxious stimulus under close control of several endogenous mediators [34]. This phlogistic scenario correlates with a transient increase of pro-inflammatory factors including (i) cytokines such as the interleukin (IL)-1 family (IL-1α/β), IL-6, and tumor necrosis factor-α (TNF-α) that are involved in the early stages of inflammatory and immune processes and warn the host to induce an inflammatory reaction against pathogens [35]; (ii) chemokines for the control of leukocyte extravasation and chemotaxis towards the affected tissues; (iii) the complement fragments (C3a, C4a, and C5a also known as anaphylatoxins) that promote granulocyte and monocytes recruitment and induce mast-cell degranulation [36]; and (iv) prostaglandins (PGs), in particular PGE$_2$, one of the principal lipid mediators of the Arachidonic acid cascade [37]. The first sign of recovery is the switch from PGs (pro-inflammatory lipid mediators) to lipoxins and resolvins (anti-inflammatory lipid mediators); indeed, it inhibits the recruitment of neutrophils and promotes the recruitment of monocytes, restoring homeostatic conditions [38,39].

In the last few years, in the context of acute inflammation, the scientific community has focused the spotlight on mPGES-1 enzyme that acts as a crucial regulator in the terminal steps of PGE$_2$ production from intermediate PGH$_2$ [40]. The baseline expression of mPGES-1 in different tissues is low, but in response to inflammatory stimuli and cytokines such as lipopolysaccharide (LPS), IL-1β, TNF-α, and IL-17A, mPGES-1 is up-regulated and functionally coupled with COX-2 to mediate pro-inflammatory PGE$_2$ production [41–44]. This elevation in lipid mediators is implicated in the pathogenesis of several inflammatory diseases such as gouty arthritis, rheumatoid arthritis (RA), and atherosclerosis [45–47].

Selective inhibition of downstream mPGES-1 [48] for a specific reduction in PGE$_2$ production is proposed as a safer alternative compared with nonsteroidal anti-inflammatory drugs (NSAIDs) [49,50]. A variety of compounds which target mPGES-1 have been described in the literature and are summarized in Figure 1 [51–54]. Of particular interest is baicalin, a bioactive flavone extracted from the root of *Scutellaria baicalensis* Georgi. It has been reported that baicalin and, its aglycone baicalein not only suppress the overexpression of pro-inflammatory mediators such as nitric oxide (NO), PGE$_2$, TNF-α, IL-1β, and IL-6 [55,56] but also inhibit the expression of inducible enzymes COX-2 and inducible nitric oxide synthase (iNOS) [57]. Similarly, the main component of turmeric *Curcuma longa* has been reported as an efficacious agent against both PGE$_2$ production, COX-2 expression [58], and Matrix Metalloproteinase (MMPs) secretion [59].

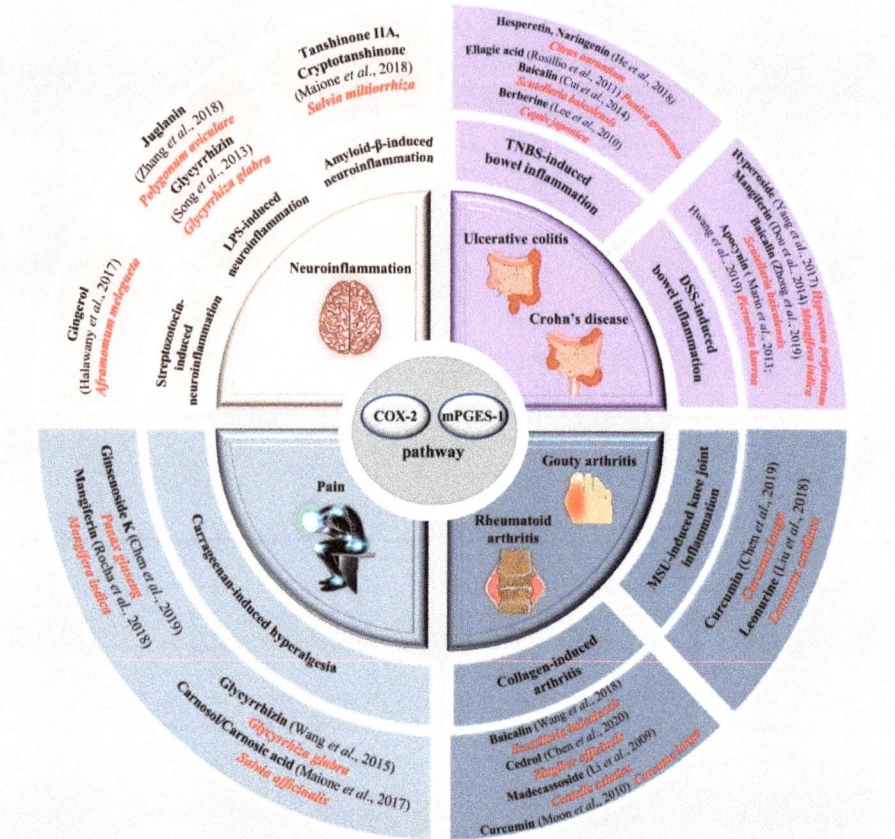

Figure 1. Schematic representation of natural compounds (black bold), by different botanical sources (in red) targeting COX-2/mPGES-1 pathway as alternative therapies for different inflammatory-related diseases. The figure, also, shows the pre-clinical models (black bold), where these active components have been tested with related bibliographic references.

Furthermore, polyphenols, such as naringenin and hesperetin from *Citrus aurantium* [60], ellagic acid from *Punica granatum* [61], apocynin from *Picrorhiza kurroa* [62,63], hyperoside from *Hypericum perfoaratum* [64], mangiferin from *Mangifera indica* [65], and alkaloids as berberine (from *Coptis japonica*) are all capable of attenuating the severity and extension of intestinal-inflammatory injuries via inhibition of neutrophil infiltration, pro-inflammatory proteins COX-2, iNOS, and nuclear factor kappa-light-chain-enhancer of activated B cells (NF-κB) activation [66]. Notably, mangiferin also presents analgesic properties due to its ability to reduce pain via PGE_2 reduction [67].

A series of in vivo studies found that cedrol, from *Zingiber officinale* [68], leonurine from *Leonurus cardiaca* [69], and madecassoside, triterpenoid isolated from *Centella asiatica* [70], can effectively alleviate inflammatory response through the inhibition of inflammatory pathway COX-2/mPGES-1/5-Lipoxigenase (5-LO) and the up-regulation of anti-inflammatory molecule IL-10.

Moreover, recent work examining the actions of glycyrrhizin (from *Glycyrrhiza glabra*) [71,72], cryptotanshinone and tanshinone IIA (from *Salvia miltiorrhiza* Bunge) [73], juglanin (a natural compound derived from the crude *Polygonum aviculare*) [74], and gingerol (from *Aframomum melegueta*) [75], in neuroinflammation and nociception, indicate that these natural compounds are potential therapeutic agents in neurodegenerative diseases and painful conditions.

Finally, the anti-inflammatory and analgesic properties of carnosol, carnosic acid (diterpenoids isolated from *Salvia Officinalis*) [76] and ginsenoside K (saponins from *Panax ginseng*) [77] have been intensively described for their ability to modulate pathways involved in inflammation and painful syndromes, including COX-2, mPGES-1 and 5-LO.

These findings pave the way for the use of these botanical-derived compounds as novel anti-inflammatory and analgesic agents targeting COX-2/mPGES-1 pathway.

4. Natural Compounds Targeting Th17/Treg Axis in Immune-Mediated Inflammatory Diseases

Considering inflammation from a "cellular point of view", although neutrophils and macrophages have traditionally been looked upon as dominant cell types during the resolution phase, accessory cells such as Th17 and Treg have more recently emerged as important players during resolution. They may link innate and adaptive immune systems [78]. CD4 T cells regulate several immune answers in order to fight against different disease-causing noxious stimuli. The binding of T cell receptor (TCR) to the peptide–major histocompatibility complex (MHC) activates naïve CD4 T cells that differentiate into effectors cells, including Th17 and Treg [79,80]. Th17, which express the transcription factor retinoic acid receptor-related orphan receptor γt (RORγt), arbitrate immune responses against extracellular bacteria, fungi, and viruses [81]. They produce IL-17, IL-22, and IL-23, stimulate many cell types to recruit neutrophils, and promote inflammation at the site of infection [82]. Consequentially, therapeutic strategies directed to neutralizing these cytokines utilizing monoclonal antibodies have shown encouraging results [46,83–87]. By contrast, Tregs express the transcription factor forehead box P3 (Foxp3) and produce anti-inflammatory cytokines like IL-10 and transforming growth factor-β (TGF-β) which inhibit immune responses to control immune homeostasis. These two classes of T cells subsets have opposing roles during inflammatory and immune responses: Th17 can cause, while Treg suppress autoimmune and inflammatory-based diseases [88]. Moreover, Th17 and Treg share a common signaling pathway mediated by TGF-β, but the external milieu present during activation determines these cells' polarisation [89–91]. Considering the "plasticity" of the differentiation process and since in inflammatory states each cell type can convert to the other, it is not unexpected that the equilibrium between Th17/Treg is critical for pathogenesis, prognosis, and therapy of several autoimmune diseases [92–94].

Indeed, the Th17/Treg ratio is increased in patients with psoriasis, inflammatory bowel disease (IBD), RA [95], and multiple sclerosis (MS) [96].

In Figure 2, we have summarized the broad panel of natural compounds which could potentially modulate Th17/Treg function and prove potentially useful in preventing and/or treating different immune-mediated inflammatory diseases [78,93,97].

In vivo pre-clinical studies suggest that green tea and its active ingredient, epi-gallocatechin gallate (EGCG), may effectively improve the symptoms and inflammatory conditions of autoimmune diseases [98,99]. EGCG is also viewed as an anti-inflammatory agent [100] due to its inhibitory effect on the release of IL-6 and IL-17 [101] and the regulation of the Th17/Treg balance [102].

Baicalin, from *Scutellaria baicalensis*, has been shown to effectively reduced inflammation and tissue damage in colitis, and modulate Th17/Treg imbalance in the colon, ameliorating colorectal inflammation [103]. On the other hand, baicalin downregulated the levels of Th17-related cytokines (IL-17 and IL-6), that provoked chronic inhibition of autophagy and induction of claudin-2 expression, leading to apoptosis and dysregulated epithelial barrier function with subsequent gut dysbiosis and intestinal diseases [104]. These findings highlight a novel immunomodulatory role of baicalin not only in bowel inflammation [105] but also in asthma [106,107] and arthritis [108].

In addition, glycyrrhizin (or glycyrrhizic acid), from *Glycyrrhiza glabra*, with a corticosteroid-like structure, has been shown to possess several beneficial pharmacological activities, including anti-asthmatic effects [109] and anti-inflammatory activity [110], acting on the Th17/Treg balance and regulating the immune response in different models of chronic inflammation. Noteworthy are mangiferin [111] and neomangiferin [112], main active constituents of *Mangifera indica*, that decreased the proportion of Th17 and the levels of IL-17A, while increasing the balance of Treg and the expression of anti-inflammatory IL-10.

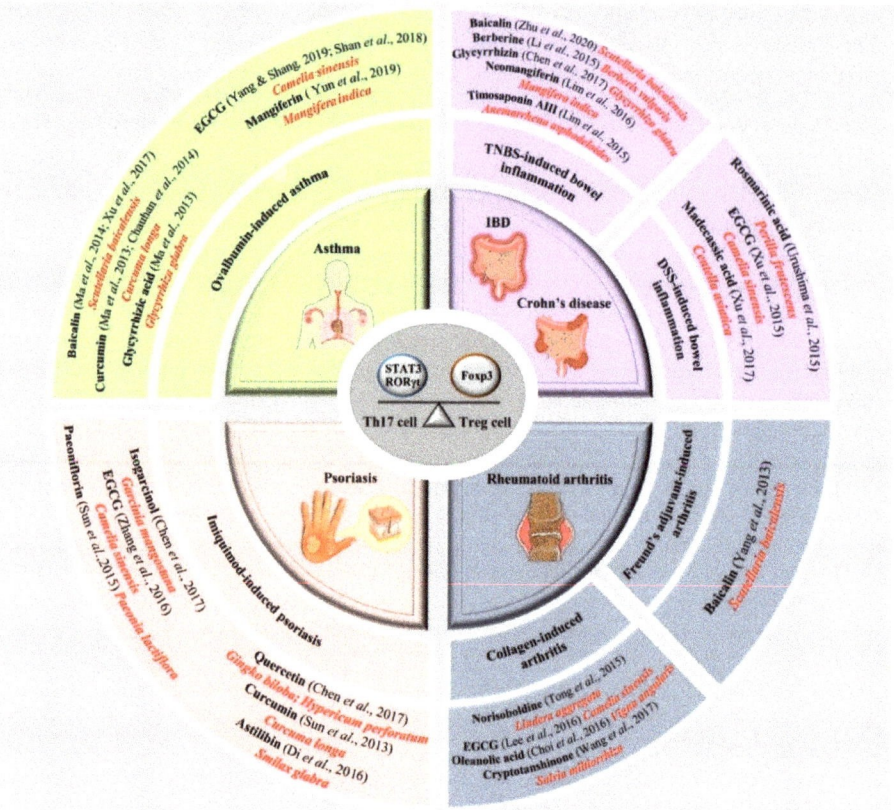

Figure 2. Schematic representation of natural compounds (black bold), by different botanical sources (in red) targeting Th17/Treg ratio as alternative therapies for different autoimmune-based diseases. The figure, also, shows the pre-clinical models (black bold), where these active components have been tested with related bibliographic references.

Th17 and Treg populations are also affected by other polyphenols: curcumin (from *Curcuma longa*) [113] and quercetin (from *Gingko biloba* and *Hypericum perforatum*) attenuatelevels of TNF-α, IL-6 [114] and IL-17 [115], associated with the downregulation of NF-κB [116].

Additionally, cryptotanshinone from *Salvia miltiorrhiza* [117], oleanolic acid isolated from *Vigna angularis* [118] and norisoboldine, the main active ingredient of the dry root of *Lindera aggregata* [119], were proven to have anti-arthritic effects, decreasing inflammation and joint destruction.

Taken together, these findings, in addition to the other medicinal plants and their active components such as berberine (from *Breberis vulgaris*) [120], rosmarinic acid (from *Perilla frutescens*) [121], timosaponin AIII (from *Anemarrhena asphodeloides*) [122], madecassic acid (from *Centella asiatica*) [123], isogarcinol (from *Garcinia mangostana*) [124], astilbin (from Smilax Glabra) [125] and paeoniflorin (from *Paeonia lactiflora*) [126], shown in Figure 2, highlight the important role natural compounds could play in the treatment of the most common autoimmune diseases, through their ability to act on Th17/Treg ratio.

5. Conclusions and Future Prospect

European legislation for food supplements and nutraceuticals is not fully harmonized and not adapted to meet current challenges. In this context, the Belgian, French, and Italian authorities have decided to develop a common approach for evaluating botanicals in the BELFRIT project providing harmonization in terms of identification and classification of medicinal plants used in food supplement and/or nutraceuticals. However, in the BELFRIT list, there are only a few and fragmented pieces of information regarding the natural products and compounds targeting COX-2/mPGES-1 coupling enzymes and Th17/Treg repertoire. In this regard, the information reported here (in particular for those secondary plant's metabolites targeting both pathways, Figure 3) highlights the need for further detailed studies, including mechanism exploration, safety profile, and clinical trials to discover clinically useful drugs and therapeutic targets in widespread pathologies related to inflammatory-based and autoimmune-related diseases.

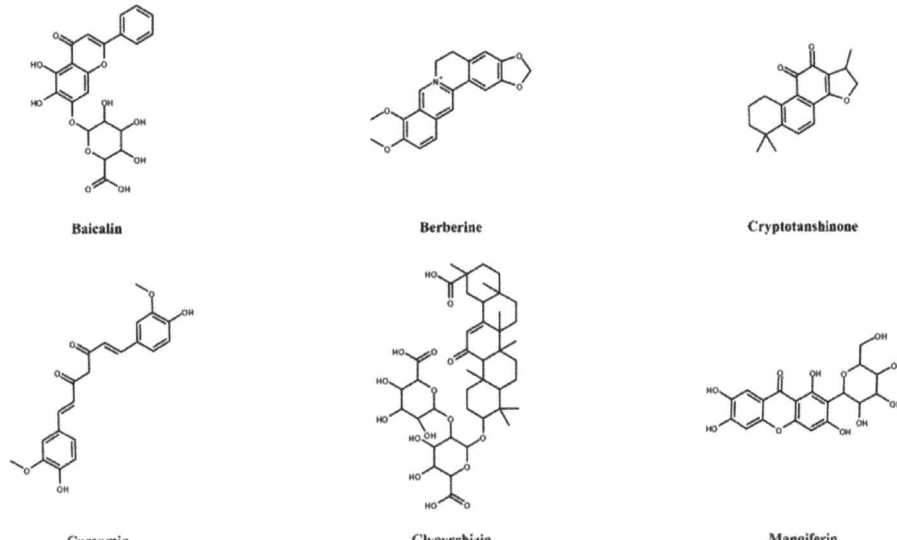

Figure 3. Chemical structures of most significant secondary metabolites targeting both COX-2/mPGES-1 pathway and Th17/Treg axis.

Author Contributions: A.S., F.R., G.M.C., C.I., A.P., and C.F. drafted the manuscript and figures. A.J.I., N.M., and F.M. wrote and revised the manuscript. All authors have read and agreed to the published version of the manuscript.

Funding: This research was funded by MIUR (PRIN 2017; 2017A95NCJ/2017A95NCJ_002, "Stolen molecules-Stealing natural products from the depot and reselling them as new drug candidates"). A.S. and F.R. are supported by University of Naples Federico II PhD scholarship. A.J.I. is supported by a Birmingham Fellowship.

Conflicts of Interest: This article has been conducted and written in the absence of any commercial or financial relationships that could be construed as a potential conflict of interest.

References

1. Cousyn, G.; Dalfrà, S.; Scarpa, B.; Geelen, J.; Anton, R.; Serafini, M.; Delmulle, L. Project BELFRIT: Harmonizing the Use of Plants in Food Supplements in the European Union: Belgium, France and Italy–A First Step. *Eur. Food Feed Law* **2013**, *8*, 187–196.
2. *Regulation (EC) No 258/97 of the European Parliament and of the Council of 27 January 1997 Concerning Novel Foods and Novel Food Ingredients*; EC: Brussels, Belgium, 1997; pp. 1–6.

3. *2008/558/EC: Commission Decision of 27 June 2008 Authorising the Placing on the Market of Refined Echium Oil as Novel Food Ingredient under Regulation (EC) No 258/97 of the European Parliament and of the Council*; EC: Brussels, Belgium, 2008; pp. 17–19.
4. *Commission Decision 2000/196/EC of 22 February 2000 Refusing the Placing on the Market of Stevia Rebaudiana Bertoni: Plants and Dried Leaves' as a Novel Food or Novel Food Ingredient under Regulation No 258/97*; EC: Brussels, Belgium, 2000; p. 14.
5. *Directive 2002/46/EC of the European Parliament and of the Council of 10 June 2002 on the Approximation of the Laws of the Member States Relating to Food Supplements*; EC: Brussels, Belgium, 2002; pp. 51–57.
6. Committee on Herbal Medicinal Products (HMPC) European Union Herbal Monograph on Hedera Helix L., Folium; 24 November 2015EMA/HMPC/586888/2014. Available online: http://www.ema.europa.eu/docs/en_GB/document_library/HerbalHerbal_monograph/2016/01/WC500199890.pdf (accessed on 18 December 2020).
7. Maione, F.; Russo, R.; Kha, H.; Mascolo, N. Medicinal plants with anti-inflammatory activities. *Nat. Prod. Res.* **2016**, *12*, 1343–1352. [CrossRef] [PubMed]
8. Izzo, A.A.; Teixeira, M.; Alexander, S.P.H.; Cirino, G.; Docherty, J.R.; George, C.H.; Insel, P.A.; Ji, Y.; Kendall, D.A.; Panattieri, R.A.; et al. A practical guide for transparent reporting of research on natural products in the British Journal of Pharmacology: Reproducibility of natural product research. *Br. J. Pharmacol.* **2020**, *10*, 2169–2178. [CrossRef] [PubMed]
9. López-Varela, S.; González-Gross, M.; Marcos, A. Functional foods and the immune system: A review. *Eur. J. Clin. Nutr.* **2002**, *56*, S29–S33. [CrossRef] [PubMed]
10. Granado-Lorencio, F.; Hernández-Alvarez, E. Functional Foods and Health Effects: A Nutritional Biochemistry Perspective. *Curr. Med. Chem.* **2016**, *23*, 2929–2957. [CrossRef]
11. Gul, K.; Singh, A.K.; Jabeen, R. Nutraceuticals and Functional Foods: The Foods for the Future World. *Crit. Rev. Food Sci. Nutr.* **2016**, *16*, 2617–2627. [CrossRef]
12. Thomford, N.E.; Senthebane, D.A.; Rowe, A.; Munro, D.; Seele, P.; Maroyi, A.; Dzobo, K. Natural Products for Drug Discovery in the 21st Century: Innovations for Novel Drug Discovery. *Int. J. Mol. Sci.* **2018**, *19*, 1578. [CrossRef]
13. Hoyles, L.; Vulevic, J. Diet, immunity and functional foods. *Adv. Exp. Med. Biol.* **2008**, *635*, 79–92. [CrossRef]
14. Sattigere, V.D.; Kumar, P.R.; Prakash, V. Science-based regulatory approach for safe nutraceuticals. *J. Sci. Food Agric.* **2020**, *14*, 5079–5082. [CrossRef]
15. Mora, J.R.; Iwata, M.; von Andrian, U.H. Vitamin effects on the immune system: Vitamins A and D take centre stage. *Nat. Rev. Immunol.* **2008**, *9*, 685–698. [CrossRef]
16. Ding, S.; Jiang, H.; Fang, J. Regulation of Immune Function by Polyphenols. *J. Immunol. Res.* **2018**, *2018*, 1264074. [CrossRef] [PubMed]
17. Jones, P.J.; Varady, K.A. Are functional foods redefining nutritional requirements? *Appl. Physiol. Nutr. Metab.* **2008**, *1*, 118–123. [CrossRef] [PubMed]
18. Eussen, S.R.; Verhagen, H.; Klungel, O.H.; Garssen, J.; van Loveren, H.; van Kranen, H.J.; Rompelberg, C.J. Functional foods and dietary supplements: Products at the interface between pharma and nutrition. *Eur. J. Pharmacol.* **2011**, *668*, S2–S9. [CrossRef] [PubMed]
19. Domínguez, D.L.; Fernández-Ruiz, V.; Cámara, M. The frontier between nutrition and pharma: The international regulatory framework of functional foods, food supplements and nutraceuticals. *Food Sci. Nutr.* **2020**, *10*, 1738–1746. [CrossRef]
20. Aronson, J.K. Defining 'nutraceuticals': Neither nutritious nor pharmaceutical. *Br. J. Clin. Pharmacol.* **2017**, *1*, 8–19. [CrossRef]
21. Santini, A.; Novellino, E. To Nutraceuticals and Back: Rethinking a Concept. *Foods* **2017**, *6*, 74. [CrossRef]
22. Adefegha, S.A. Functional Foods and Nutraceuticals as Dietary Intervention in Chronic Diseases; Novel Perspectives for Health Promotion and Disease Prevention. *J. Diet. Suppl.* **2018**, *6*, 977–1009. [CrossRef]
23. Santini, A.; Cammarata, S.M.; Capone, G.; Ianaro, A.; Tenore, G.C.; Pani, L.; Novellino, E. Nutraceuticals: Opening the debate for a regulatory framework. *Br. J. Clin. Pharmacol.* **2018**, *4*, 659–672. [CrossRef]
24. Daliu, P.; Santini, A.; Novellino, E. From pharmaceuticals to nutraceuticals: Bridging disease prevention and management. *Expert. Rev. Clin. Pharmacol.* **2019**, *12*, 1–7. [CrossRef]

25. Sultan, M.T.; Butt, M.S.; Qayyum, M.M.; Suleria, H.A. Immunity: Plants as effective mediators. *Food Sci. Nutr.* **2014**, *10*, 1298–1308. [CrossRef]
26. Wu, D.; Lewis, E.D.; Pae, M.; Meydani, S.N. Nutritional Modulation of Immune Function: Analysis of Evidence, Mechanisms, and Clinical Relevance. *Front. Immunol.* **2019**, *15*, 3160. [CrossRef] [PubMed]
27. Soehnlein, O.; Lindbom, L. Phagocyte partnership during the onset and resolution of inflammation. *Nat. Rev. Immunol.* **2010**, *6*, 427–439. [CrossRef] [PubMed]
28. Sun, S.; Ji, Y.; Kersten, S.; Qi, L. Mechanisms of inflammatory responses in obese adipose tissue. *Annu. Rev. Nutr.* **2012**, *32*, 261–286. [CrossRef] [PubMed]
29. Sugimoto, M.A.; Sousa, L.P.; Pinho, V.; Perretti, M.; Teixeira, M.M. Resolution of Inflammation: What Controls Its Onset? *Front. Immunol.* **2016**, *7*, 160. [CrossRef] [PubMed]
30. Perretti, M.; D'Acquisto, F. Annexin A1 and glucocorticoids as effectors of the resolution of inflammation. *Nat. Rev. Immunol.* **2009**, *9*, 62–70. [CrossRef] [PubMed]
31. D'Acquisto, F.; Maione, F.; Pederzoli-Ribeil, M. From IL-15 to IL-33: The never-ending list of new players in inflammation. Is it time to forget the humble aspirin and move ahead? *Biochem. Pharmacol.* **2010**, *79*, 525–534. [CrossRef] [PubMed]
32. Cooper, M.D.; Alder, M.N. The evolution of adaptive immune systems. *Cell* **2006**, *124*, 815–822. [CrossRef]
33. Varela, M.L.; Mogildea, M.; Moreno, I.; Lopes, A. Acute Inflammation and Metabolism. *Inflammation* **2018**, *4*, 1115–1127. [CrossRef]
34. Perretti, M.; Cooper, D.; Dalli, J.; Norling, L.V. Immune resolution mechanisms in inflammatory arthritis. *Nat. Rev. Rheumatol.* **2017**, *13*, 87–99. [CrossRef]
35. Ge, Y.; Huang, M.; Yao, Y.M. Autophagy and Proinflammatory Cytokines: Interactions and Clinical Implications. *Cytokine Growth Factor Rev.* **2018**, *43*, 38–46. [CrossRef]
36. Medzhitov, R. Origin and Physiological Roles of Inflammation. *Nature* **2008**, *7203*, 428–435. [CrossRef] [PubMed]
37. Higgs, G.A.; Moncada, S.; Vane, J.R. Eicosanoids in inflammation. *Ann. Clin. Res.* **1984**, *16*, 287–299. [PubMed]
38. Serhan, C.N. Pro-resolving lipid mediators are leads for resolution physiology. *Nature* **2014**, *510*, 92–101. [CrossRef] [PubMed]
39. Serhan, C.N.; Chiang, N.; Dalli, J. The resolution code of acute inflammation: Novel pro-resolving lipid mediators in resolution. *Semin. Immunol.* **2015**, *3*, 200–215. [CrossRef] [PubMed]
40. Murakami, M.; Naraba, H.; Tanioka, T.; Semmyo, N.; Nakatani, Y.; Kojima, F.; Ikeda, T.; Fueki, M.; Ueno, A.; Oh, S. Regulation of prostaglandin E2 biosynthesis by inducible membrane-associated prostaglandin E2 synthase that acts in concert with cyclooxygenase-2. *J. Biol. Chem.* **2000**, 32783–33279. [CrossRef]
41. Stichtenoth, D.O.; Thorén, S.; Bian, H.; Peters-Golden, M.; Jakobsson, P.J.; Crofford, L.J. Microsomal prostaglandin E synthase is regulated by proinflammatory cytokines and glucocorticoids in primary rheumatoid synovial cells. *J. Immunol.* **2001**, *167*, 469–474. [CrossRef]
42. Saegusa, M.; Murakami, M.; Nakatani, Y.; Yamakawa, K.; Katagiri, M.; Matsuda, K.; Kawaguchi, H. Contribution of membrane-associated prostaglandin E2 synthase to bone resorption. *J. Cell. Physiol.* **2003**, *197*, 348–356. [CrossRef]
43. Li, X.; Afif, H.; Cheng, S.; Martel-Pelletier, J.; Pelletier, J.P.; Ranger, P.; Fahmi, H. Expression and regulation of microsomal prostaglandin E synthase-1 in human osteoarthritic cartilage and chondrocytes. *J. Rheumatol.* **2005**, *32*, 887–895.
44. Samuelsson, B.; Morgenstern, R.; Jakobsson, P.J. Membrane prostaglandin E synthase-1: A novel therapeutic target. *Pharmacol. Rev.* **2007**, *3*, 207–224. [CrossRef]
45. Koeberle, A.; Werz, O. Perspective of microsomal prostaglandin E2 synthase-1 as drug target in inflammation-related disorders. *Biochem. Pharmacol.* **2015**, *1*, 1–15. [CrossRef]
46. Raucci, F.; Iqbal, A.J.; Saviano, A.; Minosi, P.; Piccolo, M.; Irace, C.; Caso, F.; Scarpa, R.; Pieretti, S.; Mascolo, N.; et al. IL-17A neutralizing antibody regulates monosodium urate crystal-induced gouty inflammation. *Pharmacol. Res.* **2019**, *147*, 104351. [CrossRef] [PubMed]
47. Maione, F.; Casillo, G.M.; Raucci, F.; Iqbal, A.J.; Mascolo, N. The functional link between microsomal prostaglandin E synthase-1 (mPGES-1) and peroxisome proliferator-activated receptor γ (PPARγ) in the onset of inflammation. *Pharmacol. Res.* **2020**, *157*, 104807. [CrossRef] [PubMed]

48. Chang, H.H.; Meuillet, E.J. Identification and development of mPGES-1 inhibitors: Where we are at? *Future Med. Chem.* **2011**, *15*, 1909–1934. [CrossRef]
49. Koeberle, A.; Werz, O. Inhibitors of the microsomal prostaglandin E (2) synthase-1 as alternative to non steroidal anti-inflammatory drugs (NSAIDs)—A critical review. *Curr. Med. Chem.* **2009**, *32*, 4274–4496. [CrossRef] [PubMed]
50. Bergqvist, F.; Morgenstern, R.; Jakobsson, P.J. A review on mPGES-1 inhibitors: From preclinical studies to clinical applications. *Prostaglandins Other Lipid Mediat.* **2020**, *147*, 106383. [CrossRef] [PubMed]
51. Koeberle, A.; Bauer, J.; Verhoff, M.; Hoffmann, M.; Northoff, H.; Werz, O. Green tea epigallocatechin-3-gallate inhibits microsomal prostaglandin E(2) synthase-1. *Biochem. Biophys. Res. Comm.* **2009**, *2*, 350–354. [CrossRef]
52. Koeberle, A.; Northoff, H.; Werz, O. Curcumin blocks prostaglandin E2 biosynthesis through direct inhibition of the microsomal prostaglandin E2 synthase-1. *Mol. Cancer Ther.* **2009**, *8*, 2348–2355. [CrossRef]
53. Siemoneit, U.; Koeberle, A.; Rossi, A.; Dehm, F.; Verhoff, M.; Reckel, S.; Maier, T.J.; Jauch, J.; Northoff, H.; Bernhard, F.; et al. Inhibition of microsomal prostaglandin E2 synthase-1 as a molecular basis for the anti-inflammatory actions of boswellic acids from frankincense. *Br. J. Pharmacol.* **2011**, *162*, 147–162. [CrossRef]
54. Yahfoufi, N.; Alsadi, N.; Jambi, M.; Matar, C. The Immunomodulatory and Anti-Inflammatory Role of Polyphenols. *Nutrients* **2018**, *11*, 1618. [CrossRef]
55. Cui, L.; Feng, L.; Zhang, Z.H.; Jia, X.B. The anti-inflammation effect of baicalin on experimental colitis through inhibiting TLR4/NF-κB pathway activation. *Int. Immunopharmacol.* **2014**, *23*, 294–303. [CrossRef]
56. Wang, C.; Song, Y.; Wang, X.; Mao, R.; Song, L. Baicalin Ameliorates Collagen-Induced Arthritis through the Suppression of Janus Kinase 1 (JAK1)/Signal Transducer and Activator of Transcription 3 (STAT3) Signaling in Mice. *Med. Sci. Monit.* **2018**, *24*, 9213–9222. [CrossRef] [PubMed]
57. Zhong, X.; Surh, Y.J.; Do, S.G.; Shin, E.; Shim, K.S.; Lee, C.K.; Na, H.K.J. Baicalein Inhibits Dextran Sulfate Sodium-induced Mouse Colitis. *Cancer Prev.* **2019**, *24*, 129–138. [CrossRef] [PubMed]
58. Chen, B.; Li, H.; Ou, G.; Ren, L.; Yang, X.; Zeng, M. Curcumin attenuates MSU crystal-induced inflammation by inhibiting the degradation of IκBα and blocking mitochondrial damage. *Arthritis Res. Ther.* **2019**, *2*, 193. [CrossRef] [PubMed]
59. Moon, D.O.; Kim, M.O.; Choi, Y.H.; Park, Y.M.; Kim, G.Y. Curcumin attenuates inflammatory response in IL-1beta-induced human synovial fibroblasts and collagen-induced arthritis in mouse model. *Int. Immunopharmacol.* **2010**, *10*, 605–610. [CrossRef]
60. He, W.; Li, Y.; Liu, M.; Yu, H.; Chen, Q.; Chen, Y.; Ruan, J.; Ding, Z.; Zhang, Y.; Wang, T. *Citrus aurantium* L. and Its Flavonoids Regulate TNBS-Induced Inflammatory Bowel Disease through Anti-Inflammation and Suppressing Isolated Jejunum Contraction. *Int. J. Mol. Sci.* **2018**, *19*, 3057. [CrossRef]
61. Rosillo, M.A.; Sanchez-Hidalgo, M.; Cárdeno, A.; de la Lastra, C.A. Protective effect of ellagic acid, a natural polyphenolic compound, in a murine model of Crohn's disease. *Biochem. Pharmacol.* **2011**, *82*, 737–745. [CrossRef]
62. Marín, M.; Giner, R.M.; Ríos, J.L.; Recio Mdel, C. Protective effect of apocynin in a mouse model of chemically-induced colitis. *Planta Med.* **2013**, *79*, 1392–1400. [CrossRef]
63. Hwang, Y.J.; Nam, S.J.; Chun, W.; Kim, S.I.; Park, S.C.; Kang, C.D.; Lee, S.J. Anti-inflammatory effects of apocynin on dextran sulfate sodium-induced mouse colitis model. *PLoS ONE* **2019**, *14*, e0217642. [CrossRef]
64. Yang, L.; Shen, L.; Li, Y.; Li, Y.; Yu, S.; Wang, S. Hyperoside attenuates dextran sulfate sodium-induced colitis in mice possibly via activation of the Nrf2 signalling pathway. *J. Inflamm.* **2017**, *14*, 25. [CrossRef]
65. Dou, W.; Zhang, J.; Ren, G.; Ding, L.; Sun, A.; Deng, C.; Wu, X.; Wei, X.; Mani, S.; Wang, Z. Mangiferin attenuates the symptoms of dextran sulfate sodium-induced colitis in mice via NF-κB and MAPK signaling inactivation. *Int. Immunopharmacol.* **2014**, *23*, 170–178. [CrossRef]
66. Lee, I.A.; Hyun, Y.J.; Kim, D.H. Berberine ameliorates TNBS-induced colitis by inhibiting lipid peroxidation, enterobacterial growth and NF-κB activation. *Eur. J. Pharmacol.* **2010**, *648*, 162–170. [CrossRef] [PubMed]
67. Rocha, L.W.; Bonet, I.J.M.; Tambeli, C.H.; de-Faria, F.M.; Parada, C.A. Local administration of mangiferin prevents experimental inflammatory mechanical hyperalgesia through CINC-1/epinephrine/PKA pathway and TNF-α inhibition. *Eur. J. Pharmacol.* **2018**, *830*, 87–94. [CrossRef] [PubMed]
68. Chen, X.; Shen, J.; Zhao, J.M.; Guan, J.; Li, W.; Xie, Q.M.; Zhao, Y.Q. Cedrol attenuates collagen-induced arthritis in mice and modulates the inflammatory response in LPS-mediated fibroblast-like synoviocytes. *Food Funct.* **2020**, *11*, 4752–4764. [CrossRef] [PubMed]

69. Liu, Y.; Duan, C.; Chen, H.; Wang, C.; Liu, X.; Qiu, M.; Tang, H.; Zhang, F.; Zhou, X.; Yang, J. Inhibition of COX-2/mPGES-1 and 5-LOX in macrophages by leonurine ameliorates monosodium urate crystal-induced inflammation. *Toxicol. Appl. Pharmacol.* **2018**, *351*, 1–11. [CrossRef]
70. Li, H.; Gong, X.; Zhang, L.; Zhang, Z.; Luo, F.; Zhou, Q.; Chen, J.; Wan, J. Madecassoside attenuates inflammatory response on collagen-induced arthritis in DBA/1 mice. *Phytomedicine* **2009**, *16*, 538–546. [CrossRef]
71. Song, J.H.; Lee, J.W.; Shim, B.; Lee, C.Y.; Choi, S.; Kang, C.; Sohn, N.W.; Shin, J.W. Glycyrrhizin alleviates neuroinflammation and memory deficit induced by systemic lipopolysaccharide treatment in mice. *Molecules* **2013**, *18*, 15788–15803. [CrossRef]
72. Wang, H.L.; Li, Y.X.; Niu, Y.T.; Zheng, J.; Wu, J.; Shi, G.J.; Ma, L.; Niu, Y.; Sun, T.; Yu, J.Q. Observing Anti-inflammatory and Anti-nociceptive Activities of Glycyrrhizin Through Regulating COX-2 and Pro-inflammatory Cytokines Expressions in Mice. *Inflammation* **2015**, *38*, 2269–2278. [CrossRef]
73. Maione, F.; Piccolo, M.; De Vita, S.; Chini, M.G.; Cristiano, C.; De Caro, C.; Lippiello, P.; Miniaci, M.C.; Santamaria, R.; Irace, C.; et al. Down regulation of pro-inflammatory pathways by tanshinone IIA and cryptotanshinone in a non-genetic mouse model of Alzheimer's disease. *Pharmacol. Res.* **2018**, *129*, 482–490. [CrossRef]
74. Zhang, F.X.; Xu, R.S. Juglanin ameliorates LPS-induced neuroinflammation in animal models of Parkinson's disease and cell culture via inactivating TLR4/NF-κB pathway. *Biomed. Pharmacother.* **2018**, *97*, 1011–1019. [CrossRef]
75. Halawany, A.M.E.; Sayed, N.S.E.; Abdallah, H.M.; Dine, R.S.E. Protective effects of gingerol on streptozotocin-induced sporadic Alzheimer's disease: Emphasis on inhibition of β-amyloid, COX-2, alpha-, beta-secretases and APH1a. *Sci. Rep.* **2017**, *7*, 2902. [CrossRef]
76. Maione, F.; Cantone, V.; Pace, S.; Chini, M.G.; Bisio, A.; Romussi, G.; Pieretti, S.; Werz, O.; Koeberle, A.; Mascolo, N.; et al. Anti-inflammatory and analgesic activity of carnosol and carnosic acid in vivo and in vitro and in silico analysis of their target interactions. *Br. J. Pharmacol.* **2017**, *174*, 1497–1508. [CrossRef]
77. Chen, J.; Si, M.; Wang, Y.; Liu, L.; Zhang, Y.; Zhou, A.; Wei, W. Ginsenoside metabolite compound K exerts anti-inflammatory and analgesic effects via downregulating COX2. *Inflammopharmacology* **2019**, *27*, 157–166. [CrossRef] [PubMed]
78. Noack, M.; Miossec, P. Th17 and regulatory T cell balance in autoimmune and inflammatory diseases. *Autoimmun. Rev.* **2014**, *13*, 668–677. [CrossRef]
79. Zhu, J.; Paul, W.E. Peripheral CD4+ T-cell differentiation regulated by networks of cytokines and transcription factors. *Immunol. Rev.* **2010**, *1*, 247–262. [CrossRef] [PubMed]
80. Li, M.O.; Rudensky, A.Y. T cell receptor signalling in the control of regulatory T cell differentiation and function. *Nat. Rev. Immunol.* **2016**, *4*, 220–233. [CrossRef] [PubMed]
81. Ivanov, I.I.; McKenzie, B.S.; Zhou, L.; Tadokoro, C.E.; Lepelley, A.; Lafaille, J.J.; Cua, D.J.; Littman, D.R. The orphan nuclear receptor ROR gammat directs the differentiation program of proinflammatory IL-17+ T helper cells. *Cell* **2006**, *6*, 1121–1133. [CrossRef]
82. Bettelli, E.; Korn, T.; Oukka, M.; Kuchroo, V.K. Induction and effector functions of Th17 cells. *Nature* **2008**, *453*, 1051–1057. [CrossRef] [PubMed]
83. Samson, M.; Audia, S.; Janikashvili, N.; Ciudad, M.; Trad, M.; Fraszczak, J.; Ornetti, P.; Maillefert, J.F.; Miossec, P.; Bonnotte, B. Brief report: Inhibition of interleukin-6 function corrects Th17/Treg cell imbalance in patients with rheumatoid arthritis. *Arthritis Rheum.* **2012**, *64*, 2499–2503. [CrossRef]
84. Li, S.; Wu, Z.; Li, L.; Liu, X. Interleukin-6 IL-6 receptor antagonist protects against rheumatoid arthritis. *Int. Med. J. Exp. Clin. Res.* **2016**, *22*, 2113–2118. [CrossRef]
85. Fasching, P.; Stradner, M.; Graninger, W.; Dejaco, C.; Fessler, J. Therapeutic potential of targeting the Th17/Treg axis in autoimmune disorders. *Molecules* **2017**, *22*, 134. [CrossRef]
86. Cristiano, C.; Volpicelli, F.; Lippiello, P.; Buono, B.; Raucci, F.; Piccolo, M.; Iqbal, A.J.; Irace, C.; Miniaci, M.C.; Perrone Capano, C.; et al. Neutralization of IL-17 rescues amyloid-β-induced neuroinflammation and memory impairment. *Br. J. Pharmacol.* **2019**, *18*, 3544–3557. [CrossRef] [PubMed]
87. Raucci, F.; Iqbal, A.J.; Saviano, A.; Casillo, G.M.; Russo, M.; Lezama, D.; Mascolo, N.; Maione, F. In-depth immunophenotyping data relating to IL-17Ab modulation of circulating Treg/Th17 cells and of in situ infiltrated inflammatory monocytes in the onset of gouty inflammation. *Data Brief.* **2019**, *25*, 104381. [CrossRef] [PubMed]

88. Littman, D.R.; Rudensky, A.Y. Th17 and regulatory T cells in mediating and restraining inflammation. *Cell* **2010**, *6*, 845–858. [CrossRef] [PubMed]
89. Bettelli, E.; Carrier, Y.; Gao, W.; Korn, T.; Strom, T.B.; Oukka, M.; Weiner, H.L.; Kuchroo, V.K. Reciprocal developmental pathways for the generation of pathogenic effector TH17 and regulatory T cells. *Nature* **2006**, *7090*, 235–238. [CrossRef]
90. Mangan, P.R.; Harrington, L.E.; O'Quinn, D.B.; Helms, W.S.; Bullard, D.C.; Elson, C.O.; Hatton, R.D.; Wahl, S.M.; Schoeb, T.R.; Weaver, C.T. Transforming growth factor-beta induces development of the T(H)17 lineage. *Nature* **2006**, *7090*, 231–234. [CrossRef]
91. Ivanov, I.I.; Zhou, L.; Littman, D.R. Transcriptional regulation of Th17 cell differentiation. *Semin. Immunol.* **2007**, *6*, 409–417. [CrossRef]
92. Zhou, L.; Chong, M.M.; Littman, D.R. Plasticity of CD4+ T cell lineage differentiation. *Immunity* **2009**, *30*, 646–655. [CrossRef]
93. Komatsu, N.; Okamoto, K.; Sawa, S.; Nakashima, T.; Oh-hora, M.; Kodama, T.; Tanaka, S.; Bluestone, J.A.; Takayanagi, H. Pathogenic conversion of Foxp3+ T cells into TH17 cells in autoimmune arthritis. *Nat. Med.* **2014**, *20*, 62–68. [CrossRef]
94. Gagliani, N.; Amezcua Vesely, M.C.; Iseppon, A.; Brockmann, L.; Xu, H.; Palm, N.W.; de Zoete, M.R.; Licona-Limon, P.; Paiva, R.S.; Ching, T.; et al. Th17 cells transdifferentiate into regulatory T cells during resolution of inflammation. *Nature* **2015**, *523*, 221–225. [CrossRef]
95. Boissier, M.C.; Assier, E.; Biton, J.; Denys, A.; Falgarone, G.; Bessis, N. Regulatory T Cells (Treg) in Rheumatoid Arthritis. *J. Bone Spine.* **2009**, *76*, 10–14. [CrossRef]
96. Chabaud, M.; Durand, J.M.; Buchs, N.; Fossiez, F.; Page, G.; Frappart, L.; Miossec, P. Human interleukin-17: A T cell-derived proinflammatory cytokine produced by the rheumatoid synovium. *Arthritis Rheum.* **1999**, *42*, 963–970. [CrossRef]
97. Wehrens, E.J.; Prakken, B.J.; van Wijk, F. T cells out of control—Impaired immune regulation in the inflamed joint. *Nat. Rev. Rheumatol.* **2013**, *9*, 34–42. [CrossRef] [PubMed]
98. Lee, S.Y.; Jung, Y.O.; Ryu, J.G.; Oh, H.J.; Son, H.J.; Lee, S.H.; Kwon, J.E.; Kim, E.K.; Park, M.K.; Park, S.H.; et al. Epigallocatechin-3-gallate ameliorates autoimmune arthritis by reciprocal regulation of T helper-17 regulatory T cells and inhibition of osteoclastogenesis by inhibiting STAT3 signaling. *J. Leukoc. Biol.* **2016**, *3*, 559–568. [CrossRef] [PubMed]
99. Zhang, S.; Liu, X.; Mei, L.; Wang, H.; Fang, F. Epigallocatechin-3-gallate (EGCG) inhibits imiquimod-induced psoriasis-like inflammation of BALB/c mice. *BMC Complement. Altern. Med.* **2016**, *1*, 334. [CrossRef] [PubMed]
100. Shan, L.; Kang, X.; Liu, F.; Cai, X.; Han, X.; Shang, Y. Epigallocatechin gallate improves airway inflammation through TGF-β1 signaling pathway in asthmatic mice. *Mol. Med. Rep.* **2018**, *18*, 2088–2096. [CrossRef] [PubMed]
101. Xu, Z.; Wei, C.; Zhang, R.U.; Yao, J.; Zhang, D.; Wang, L. Epigallocatechin-3-gallate-induced inhibition of interleukin-6 release and adjustment of the regulatory T/T helper 17 cell balance in the treatment of colitis in mice. *Exp. Ther. Med.* **2015**, *6*, 2231–2238. [CrossRef]
102. Yang, N.; Shang, Y.X. Epigallocatechin gallate ameliorates airway inflammation by regulating Treg/Th17 imbalance in an asthmatic mouse model. *Int. Immunopharmacol.* **2019**, *72*, 422–428. [CrossRef]
103. Zou, Y.; Dai, S.X.; Chi, H.G.; Li, T.; He, Z.W.; Wang, J.; Ye, C.; Huang, G.L.; Zhao, B.; Li, W.Y.; et al. Baicalin attenuates TNBS-induced colitis in rats by modulating the Th17/Treg paradigm. *Arch. Pharm. Res.* **2015**, *10*, 1873–1887. [CrossRef]
104. Hu, C.A.; Hou, Y.; Yi, D.; Qiu, Y.; Wu, G.; Kong, X.; Yin, Y. Autophagy and tight junction proteins in the intestine and intestinal diseases. *Anim. Nutr.* **2015**, *1*, 123–127. [CrossRef]
105. Zhu, L.; Xu, L.Z.; Zhao, S.; Shen, Z.F.; Shen, H.; Zhan, L.B. Protective effect of baicalin on the regulation of Treg/Th17 balance, gut microbiota and short-chain fatty acids in rats with ulcerative colitis. *Appl. Microbiol. Biotechnol.* **2020**, *104*, 5449–5460. [CrossRef]
106. Ma, C.; Ma, Z.; Fu, Q.; Ma, S. Anti-asthmatic effects of baicalin in a mouse model of allergic asthma. *Phytother. Res.* **2014**, *28*, 231–237. [CrossRef] [PubMed]

107. Xu, L.; Li, J.; Zhang, Y.; Zhao, P.; Zhang, X.J. Regulatory effect of baicalin on the imbalance of Th17/Treg responses in mice with allergic asthma. *J. Ethnopharmacol.* **2017**, *208*, 199–206. [CrossRef] [PubMed]
108. Yang, X.; Yang, J.; Zou, H. Baicalin inhibits IL-17-mediated joint inflammation in murine adjuvant-induced arthritis. *Clin. Dev. Immunol.* **2013**, *2013*, 268065. [CrossRef] [PubMed]
109. Ma, C.; Ma, Z.; Liao, X.L.; Liu, J.; Fu, Q.; Ma, S.J. Immunoregulatory effects of glycyrrhizic acid exerts anti-asthmatic effects via modulation of Th1/Th2 cytokines and enhancement of CD4(+)CD25(+)Foxp3+ regulatory T cells in ovalbumin-sensitized mice. *J. Ethnopharmacol.* **2013**, *3*, 755–762. [CrossRef]
110. Chen, X.; Fang, D.; Li, L.; Chen, L.; Li, Q.; Gong, F.; Fang, M. Glycyrrhizin ameliorates experimental colitis through attenuating interleukin-17-producing T cell responses via regulating antigen-presenting cells. *Immunol. Res.* **2017**, *3*, 666–680. [CrossRef]
111. Yun, C.; Chang, M.; Hou, G.; Lan, T.; Yuan, H.; Su, Z.; Zhu, D.; Liang, W.; Li, Q.; Zhu, H.; et al. Mangiferin suppresses allergic asthma symptoms by decreased Th9 and Th17 responses and increased Treg response. *Mol. Immunol.* **2019**, *114*, 233–242. [CrossRef]
112. Lim, S.M.; Kang, G.D.; Jeong, J.J.; Choi, H.S.; Kim, D.H. Neomangiferin modulates the Th17/Treg balance and ameliorates colitis in mice. *Phytomedicine* **2016**, *23*, 131–140. [CrossRef]
113. Chauhan, P.S.; Dash, D.; Singh, R. Intranasal curcumin attenuates airway remodeling in murine model of chronic asthma. *Int. Immunopharmacol.* **2014**, *21*, 63–75. [CrossRef]
114. Sun, J.; Zhao, Y.; Hu, J. Curcumin inhibits imiquimod-induced psoriasis-like inflammation by inhibiting IL-1beta and IL-6 production in mice. *PLoS ONE* **2013**, *8*, e67078. [CrossRef]
115. Ma, C.; Ma, Z.; Fu, Q.; Ma, S. Curcumin attenuates allergic airway inflammation by regulation of CD4+CD25+ regulatory T cells (Tregs)/Th17 balance in ovalbumin-sensitized mice. *Fitoterapia* **2013**, *87*, 57–64. [CrossRef]
116. Chen, H.; Lu, C.; Liu, H.; Wang, M.; Zhao, H.; Yan, Y.; Han, L. Quercetin ameliorates imiquimod-induced psoriasis-like skin inflammation in mice via the NF-κB pathway. *Int. Immunopharmacol.* **2017**, *48*, 110–117. [CrossRef] [PubMed]
117. Wang, Y.; Zhou, C.; Gao, H.; Li, C.; Li, D.; Liu, P.; Huang, M.; Shen, X.; Liu, L. Therapeutic effect of Cryptotanshinone on experimental rheumatoid arthritis through downregulating p300 mediated-STAT3 acetylation. *Biochem. Pharmacol.* **2017**, *138*, 119–129. [CrossRef] [PubMed]
118. Choi, J.K.; Kim, S.W.; Kim, D.S.; Lee, J.Y.; Lee, S.; Oh, H.M.; Ha, Y.S.; Yoo, J.; Park, P.H.; Shin, T.Y.; et al. Oleanolic acid acetate inhibits rheumatoid arthritis by modulating T cell immune responses and matrix-degrading enzymes. *Toxicol. Appl. Pharmacol.* **2016**, *290*, 1–9. [CrossRef] [PubMed]
119. Tong, B.; Dou, Y.; Wang, T.; Yu, J.; Wu, X.; Lu, Q.; Chou, G.; Wang, Z.; Kong, L.; Dai, Y.; et al. Norisoboldine ameliorates collagen-induced arthritis through regulating the balance between Th17 and regulatory T cells in gut-associated lymphoid tissues. *Toxicol. Appl. Pharmacol.* **2015**, *28*, 90–99. [CrossRef]
120. Li, C.; Xi, Y.; Li, S.; Zhao, Q.; Cheng, W.; Wang, Z.; Zhong, J.; Niu, X.; Chen, G. Berberine ameliorates TNBS induced colitis by inhibiting inflammatory responses and Th1/Th17 differentiation. *Mol. Immunol.* **2015**, *67*, 444–454. [CrossRef]
121. Urushima, H.; Nishimura, J.; Mizushima, T.; Hayashi, N.; Maeda, K.; Ito, T. Perilla frutescens extract ameliorates DSS-induced colitis by suppressing proinflammatory cytokines and inducing anti-inflammatory cytokines. *Am. J. Physiol. Gastrointest. Liver Physiol.* **2015**, *308*, G32–G41. [CrossRef]
122. Lim, S.M.; Jeong, J.J.; Kang, G.D.; Kim, K.A.; Choi, H.S.; Kim, D.H. Timosaponin AIII and its metabolite sarsasapogenin ameliorate colitis in mice by inhibiting NF-κB and MAPK activation and restoring Th17/Treg cell balance. *Int. Immunopharmacol.* **2015**, *25*, 493–503. [CrossRef]
123. Xu, X.; Wang, Y.; Wei, Z.; Wei, W.; Zhao, P.; Tong, B.; Xia, Y.; Dai, Y. Madecassic acid, the contributor to the anti-colitis effect of madecassoside, enhances the shift of Th17 toward Treg cells via the PPARγ/AMPK/ACC1 pathway. *Cell Death Dis.* **2017**, *8*, e2723. [CrossRef]
124. Chen, S.; Han, K.; Li, H.; Cen, J.; Yang, Y.; Wu, H.; Wei, Q.J. Isogarcinol Extracted from Garcinia mangostana L. Ameliorates Imiquimod-Induced Psoriasis-like Skin Lesions in Mice. *Agric. Food Chem.* **2017**, *65*, 846–857. [CrossRef]
125. Di, T.T.; Ruan, Z.T.; Zhao, J.X.; Wang, Y.; Liu, X.; Wang, Y.; Li, P. Astilbin inhibits Th17 cell differentiation and ameliorates imiquimod-induced psoriasis-like skin lesions in BALB/c mice via Jak3/Stat3 signaling pathway. *Int. Immunopharmacol.* **2016**, *32*, 32–38. [CrossRef]

126. Sun, Y.; Zhang, J.; Huo, R.; Zhai, T.; Li, H.; Wu, P.; Zhu, X.; Zhou, Z.; Shen, B.; Li, N. Paeoniflorin inhibits skin lesions in imiquimod-induced psoriasis-like mice by downregulating inflammation. *Int. Immunopharmacol.* **2015**, *24*, 392–399. [CrossRef] [PubMed]

Publisher's Note: MDPI stays neutral with regard to jurisdictional claims in published maps and institutional affiliations.

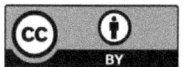

© 2020 by the authors. Licensee MDPI, Basel, Switzerland. This article is an open access article distributed under the terms and conditions of the Creative Commons Attribution (CC BY) license (http://creativecommons.org/licenses/by/4.0/).

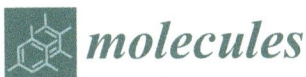

Article

Protective Effect of *Portulaca oleracea* on Streptozotocin-Induced Type I Diabetes-Associated Reproductive System Dysfunction and Inflammation

Hassan Rakhshandeh [1,†], Hamed Rajabi Khasevan [1,†], Anella Saviano [2], Mohammad Reza Mahdinezhad [3], Vafa Baradaran Rahimi [4], Sajjad Ehtiati [1,3], Leila Etemad [5,6], Alireza Ebrahimzadeh-bideskan [7,8], Francesco Maione [2,*] and Vahid Reza Askari [2,8,9,10,*]

1. Pharmacological Research Center of Medicinal Plants, Mashhad University of Medical Sciences, Mashhad 9177948564, Iran
2. ImmunoPharmaLab, Department of Pharmacy, School of Medicine and Surgery, University of Naples Federico II, Via Domenico Montesano 49, 80131 Naples, Italy
3. Department of Clinical Biochemistry, Faculty of Medicine, Mashhad University of Medical Sciences, Mashhad 9177948564, Iran
4. Department of Cardiovascular Diseases, Faculty of Medicine, Mashhad University of Medical Sciences, Mashhad 9177948564, Iran
5. Pharmaceutical Research Center, Pharmaceutical Technology Institute, Mashhad University of Medical Sciences, Mashhad 9177948564, Iran
6. Department of Drug Control, School of Pharmacy, Mashhad University of Medical Sciences, Mashhad 9177948564, Iran
7. Department of Anatomy and Cell Biology, Faculty of Medicine, Mashhad University of Medical Sciences, Pardis Campus, Azadi Square, Mashhad 9177948564, Iran
8. Applied Biomedical Research Center, Mashhad University of Medical Sciences, Mashhad 9177948564, Iran
9. Department of Pharmaceutical Sciences in Persian Medicine, School of Persian and Complementary Medicine, Mashhad University of Medical Sciences, Mashhad 9177948564, Iran
10. International UNESCO Center for Health-Related Basic Sciences and Human Nutrition, Mashhad University of Medical Sciences, Mashhad 9177948564, Iran
* Correspondence: francesco.maione@unina.it (F.M.); askariv@mums.ac.ir (V.R.A.); Tel.: +39-081678429 (F.M.); +98-915-371-9688 (V.R.A.)
† These authors contributed equally to this work.

Abstract: Background: Type-one diabetes (T1D), a chronic autoimmune disease with marked inflammatory responses, is associated with infertility complications and implications. Based on the anti-diabetic, antioxidant, and anti-hyperlipidemic potential of *Portulaca oleracea* (PO), this study aimed to evaluate the protective effect of this plant extract on streptozotocin-induced type-I-diabetes-associated reproductive system dysfunction and inflammation. Methods: Male rats were randomly divided into four experimental groups: control, diabetic, and treatment/s (PO extract at 100 or 300 mg/kg/daily). Then food and water consumption, body, testis and epididymis weights, histopathological evaluation, seminiferous tubules diameter, sperm count and motility, glucose levels, sex hormones, and inflammatory and oxidative stress markers were evaluated. Results: Our results showed that streptozotocin-induced diabetes significantly increased food and water consumption; increased glucose, MDA, TGF-β1, and TNF-α levels; and decreased the seminiferous tubules diameter, sperm count and motility, levels of LH, testosterone, total thiol, VEGF, and SOD activity. Interestingly, PO extract (phytochemically characterized by using liquid chromatography–mass spectrometry to detect bioactive molecules) significantly ameliorated these parameters and histopathological indexes' damage in rats. Conclusion: Even if more preclinical assessments are needed to better characterize the mechanism/s of action, the results of this study will pave the way for the rational use of PO on diabetic-associated clinical complications and implications.

Keywords: diabetes mellitus; infertility; inflammation; oxidative stress; *Portulaca oleracea*

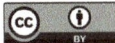

1. Introduction

Diabetes mellitus (DM) is considered one of the most critical and fast-increasing prevalence health concerns worldwide [1]. The prevalence of diabetes, according to the international diabetes federation, was 463 million in 2016, and it is predicted to reach 578 million patients in 2030 and 700 million patients in 2045 [2]. Type-one DM, a chronic autoimmune disease associated with marked inflammatory responses, is characterized by insulin deficiency due to loss of the insulin-producing β cells of the pancreatic Langerhans islets with a consequent disorder in glucose metabolism [3]. In addition, DM is related to the long-term severe damage and failures to various organs that cause complications, including retinopathy, nephropathy, peripheral neuropathy, cardiovascular disorders, and sexual dysfunction [4]. The disturbance of the male reproductive system and infertility is one of the most important and concerning complications of DM. Several animal and human studies have emphasized the detrimental effects of DM on sexual functions and parameters [5,6].

Portulaca oleracea L. (PO), commonly called purslane or hogweed, is an annual grassy plant belonging to *Portulacaceous* that has been widely used as a potherb in Central European, Mediterranean, and Asian countries [7–11]. PO possess numerous active components, including flavonoids such as kaempferol and apigenin; terpenoids such as Portuloside A and B; organic acids such as α-linolenic acid and palmitic acids; and minerals and vitamins [12]. In addition, several pharmacological activities have been reported for PO, including antioxidant, anti-inflammatory, anti-cancer, immune-modulating, and analgesic properties [7–13]. Additionally, it has been demonstrated that PO exerts antidiabetic, glucose-lowering, and insulin-elevating effects in preclinical settings and investigations [14,15]. However, to date, no experimental evidence has been provided for its beneficial effects against diabetes-induced infertility, reproductive dysfunction, and inflammation. On these bases, in this study, we aimed to evaluate the effects of standardized hydroalcoholic extracts from the aerial part of *Portulaca oleracea* on streptozotocin-induced type-I-diabetes-associated reproductive system dysfunction and inflammation.

2. Results

Collectively, 30 chemicals were characterized in the aerial parts of the hydroethanolic extract of PO, substantially including alkaloids (dopa; noradrenalin; and oleraceins A, B, C, and D), flavonoids, terpenoids (portulosides A and portulene), and vitamins (ascorbic acid, α-tocopherol, and riboflavin). Identified compounds are represented in Table 1. The total ion chromatogram of PO extract is also illustrated in Figure 1.

Table 1. The peak of chemicals in the hydroethanol extract of *Portulaca oleracea*, using positive mode LC–MS.

Peak No.	Compound Identification	t_R (min)	M+H (*m/z*)	Reference
1	Portulacanone D	26.9	299.76	[16]
2	Noradrenaline	37.0	170.7	[17]
3	Dopa	15.0	198.12	[18]
4	Oleraceins A	62.5	504.66	[18]
5	Oleraceins B	9.5	533.76	[18]
6	Oleraceins C	64.1	666.06	[18]
7	Oleraceins D	13.1	696.84	[18]
8	Adenosine	19.8	268.8	[18]
9	(3R)-3,5-Bis(3-methoxy-4-hydroxyphenyl)-2,3-dihydro-2(1H)-pyridinone	89.3	342.36	[19]
10	Aurantiamide acetate	36.4	445.8	[20]
11	Cyclo(L-tyrosinyl-L-tyrosinyl)	67.7	327.24	[20]
12	Portuloside A	72.2	332.22	[21]
13	Portulene	66.3	337.02	[22]
14	Lupeol	66.5	427.5	[22]

Table 1. *Cont.*

Peak No.	Compound Identification	t_R (min)	M+H (*m/z*)	Reference
15	(3S)-3-O-(β-D-Glucopyranosyl)-3,7-dimethylocta-1,6-dien-3-ol	67.8	318.12	[23]
16	Friedelane	54.9	413.34	[24]
17	Quercetin	39.4	303.18	[25]
18	Myricetin	55.1	318.24	[25]
19	Genistin	65.4	433.20	[26]
20	Indole-3-carboxylic acid	77.8	162.90	[16]
21	Palmitic acid	62.2	256.14	[27]
22	Stearic acid	37.8	285.18	[27]
23	Caffeic acid	65.8	181.08	[28]
24	Riboflavin	35.0	376.62	[29]
25	Vitamin C	28.5	177.00	[29]
26	α-Tocopherol	67.1	431.22	[27]
27	Hesperidin	76.8	611.58	[30]
28	Portulacerebroside A	64.6	843.18	[24]
29	β-Sitosterol	48.7	415.32	[22]
30	β-Carotene	37.5	538.74	[27]

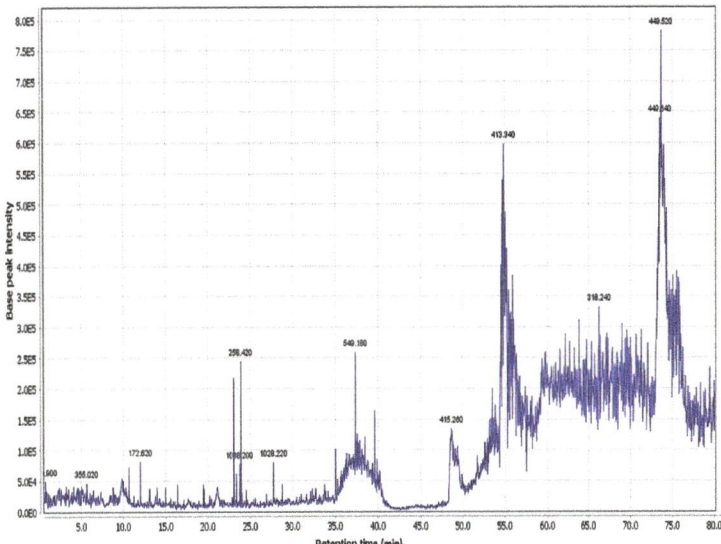

Figure 1. The total ion chromatogram of the aerial part of hydroethanolic extract of *Portulaca oleracea*.

2.1. The Effects of PO Extract on the Water and Food Consumption of Diabetic Rats

The food and water consumption were markedly elevated in the diabetic group compared to the control group at the end of two, four, six, and eight weeks of treatment ($p < 0.05$ and $p < 0.001$; Figure 2A,B). Furthermore, the PO extract (100 and 300 mg/kg) notably decreased the water consumption compared to the diabetic group at all experimental time-points ($p < 0.01$ and $p < 0.001$; Figure 2A). However, the food consumption was only reduced at the end of the eight weeks of treatment with PO extract (100 and 300 mg/kg) compared to the diabetic group ($p < 0.05$ and $p < 0.01$, respectively; Figure 2B).

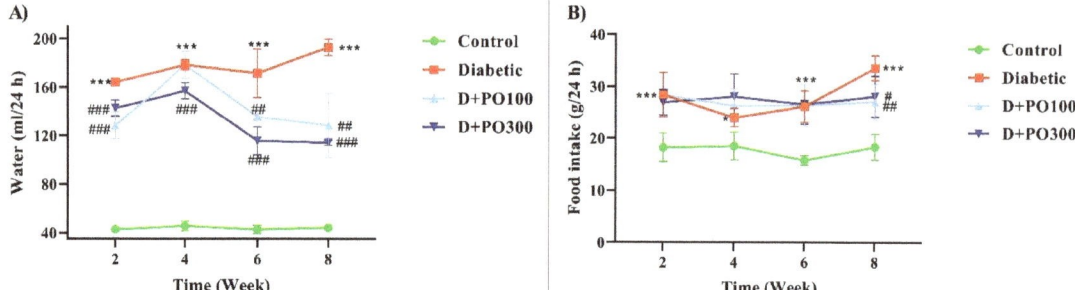

Figure 2. The effects of PO extract on (**A**) water and (**B**) food consumption in diabetic rats. The data are presented as mean ± SD. Repeated measures two-way ANOVA test was carried out with the following Tukey–Kramer's post hoc test; * $p < 0.05$, *** $p < 0.001$ vs. control group; # $p < 0.05$, ## $p < 0.01$, ### $p < 0.001$ vs. diabetic group.

2.2. The Effect of PO Extract on Blood Glucose Level

As reported in Figure 3, the blood glucose level was markedly enhanced in the diabetic group compared to the control group at the end of the zero, four, and eight weeks of treatment ($p < 0.01$ and $p < 0.001$; Figure 3). At the beginning of the study, there were no significant differences in the blood glucose levels of PO extract (100 and 300 mg/kg) and the diabetic group. However, following the four and eight weeks of treatment, PO extract (100 and 300 mg/kg) meaningfully diminished the blood glucose level compared to the diabetic group ($p < 0.001$ for all cases; Figure 3).

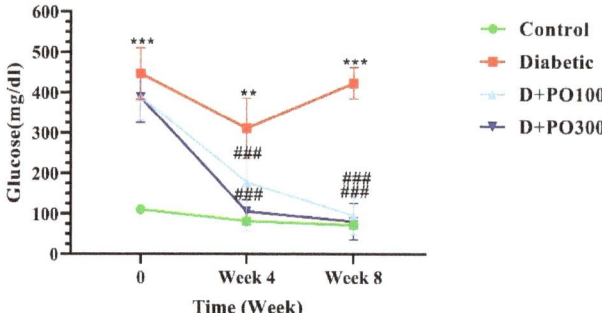

Figure 3. The effects of PO extract on blood glucose levels in diabetic rats. The data are presented as mean ± SD. Repeated measures two-way ANOVA test was carried out with the following Tukey–Kramer's post hoc test; ** $p < 0.01$, *** $p < 0.001$ vs. control group; ### $p < 0.001$ vs. diabetic group.

2.3. The Effect of PO Extract on Body Weight

At the beginning of the study, no significant differences were observed in the body weight between the control, diabetic, and PO extract groups (100 and 300 mg/kg; Figure 4). However, the diabetic group remarkably mitigated the body weight compared to the control group at the end of the two, four, six, and eight weeks of treatment ($p < 0.001$ for all cases, Figure 4). In addition, treatment with PO extract (100 and 300 mg/kg) could not significantly change the body weight compared to the diabetic group at all experimental time-points (Figure 4).

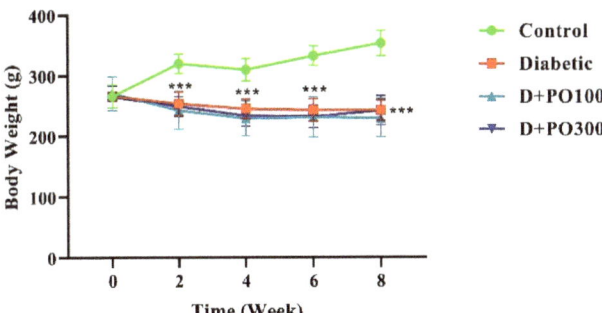

Figure 4. The effects of PO extract on body weight in diabetic rats. The data are presented as mean ± SD. A repeated-measures two-way ANOVA test was carried out with the following Tukey–Kramer's post hoc test; *** $p < 0.001$ vs. control group.

2.4. The Effect of PO Extract on the Testicular Weight and Testicular/Body Weight Index

At the end of the eight-week treatment, no significant differences were observed in the right and left testicular weight between the control, diabetic, and PO extract (100 and 300 mg/kg) groups (Figure 5A,B). Moreover, both the right and left testicular/body weight indexes were considerably augmented in the diabetic group more than the control group following the eight weeks of treatment ($p < 0.001$ for both cases; Figure 5C,D). However, eight weeks of treatment with PO extract (100 and 300 mg/kg) could not prevent the testicular/body weight index compared to the diabetic group (Figure 5C,D).

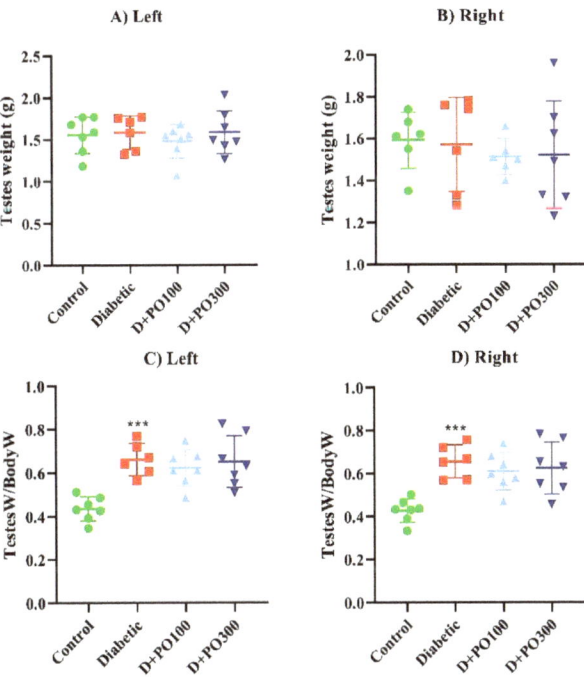

Figure 5. The effects of PO extract on (**A**) left and (**B**) right testicular weight and (**C**) left and (**D**) right testicular/body weight in diabetic rats. The data are presented as mean ± SD. A one-way ANOVA test was carried out with the following Tukey–Kramer's post hoc test; *** $p < 0.001$ vs. control group.

2.5. The Effect of PO Extract on the Epididymis Weight and Epididymis/Body Weight

As shown in Figure 6, the left and right epididymis weight was strikingly attenuated in the diabetic group compared to the control group at the end of the eight weeks ($p < 0.05$ and 0.01, respectively; Figure 6A,B). However, the PO extract (100 and 300 mg/kg) could not significantly change the left and right epididymis weight of the diabetic group following eight weeks of treatment (Figure 6A,B). Additionally, no significant differences were observed in the right and left epididymis/body weight index between the control, diabetic, and PO-extract (100 and 300 mg/kg) groups at the end of the eight weeks (Figure 6A,B).

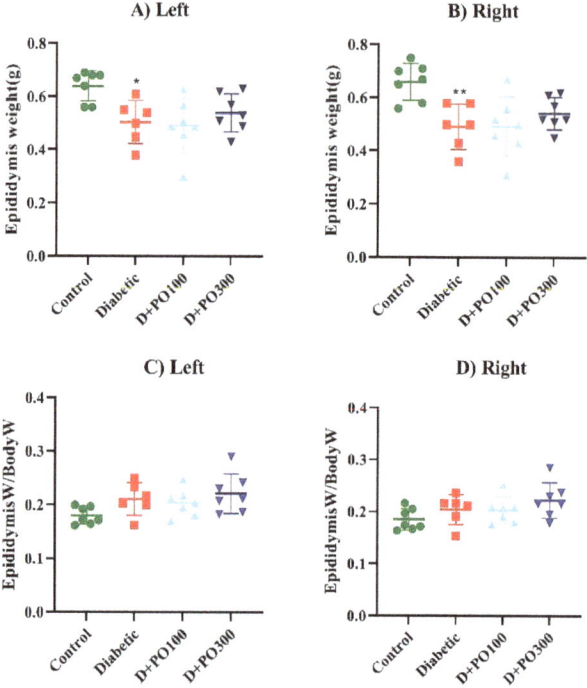

Figure 6. The effects of PO extract on (**A**) left and (**B**) right epididymis weight and (**C**) left and (**D**) right epididymis/body weight in diabetic rats. The data are presented as mean ± SD. A one-way ANOVA test was carried out with the following Tukey–Kramer's post hoc test; * $p < 0.05$, ** $p < 0.01$ vs. control group.

2.6. The Histopathological Evaluations

The results of the H&E staining showed the epithelium disintegration of seminiferous tubules, destruction of Leydig cells, increased space between the seminiferous tubules, and irregularities in the structure of the seminiferous tubules in the diabetic group compared to the control group (Figure 7A–D). However, the PO extract (100 and 300 mg/kg) firmly improved these changes compared to the diabetic group (Figure 7A–D).

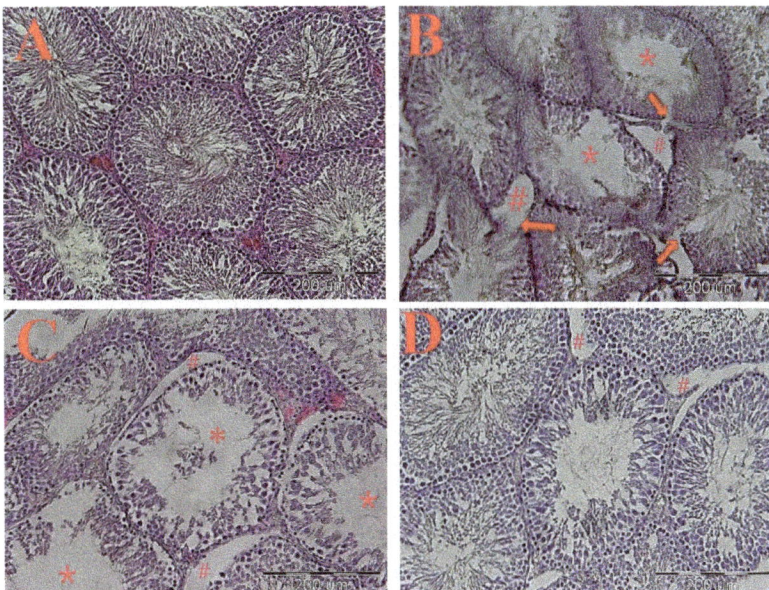

Figure 7. The effects of PO extract on the H&E staining of the transverse section of testicular tissue. (**A**) Control, (**B**) diabetic, (**C**) PO extract (100 mg/kg), and (**D**) PO extract (300 mg/kg). Microscopic view with magnification (20×) of the cross-section of testicular tissue. (**A**) Sham group: spermatogenic tubes with normal structural and cellular order. (**B**) Control group: geometric deformation of tubules, disintegration and rupture of the epithelium of spermatogenic tubules (arrows), reduction of spermatozoid population (*), increase in the distance between tubules, and atrophy and destruction of interstitial cells (Leydig) (#). (**C**) Treatment group with a dose of 100 mg/kg: The decrease in the density of spermatogenic cells is obvious, and there is a decrease in the number of sperm cells (*) and an increase in the distance between tubules (#). (**D**) treatment group with a dose of 300 mg/kg: a slight increase in the distance between tubules.

2.7. The Effect of PO Extract on the Diameter of the Seminiferous Tubules

Our results revealed that the diameter of the seminiferous tubules was meaningfully alleviated in the diabetic group compared to the control group ($p < 0.001$, Figure 8). Moreover, eight weeks of treatment with PO extract (100 and 300 mg/kg) provided a significant increment in the diameter of the seminiferous tubules compared to the diabetic group ($p < 0.01$ and 0.001, respectively, Figure 8).

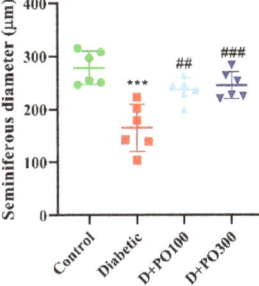

Figure 8. The effects of PO extract on seminiferous diameter in diabetic rats. The data are presented as mean ± SD. A one-way ANOVA test was carried out with the following Tukey–Kramer's post hoc test; *** $p < 0.001$ vs. control group; ## $p < 0.01$, ### $p < 0.001$ vs. diabetic group.

2.8. The Effect of PO Extract on the Count and Motility of Sperm

At the experimental endpoint (eight weeks), the count and motility of sperm were considerably hampered compared to the control group ($p < 0.05$ and 0.01, respectively; Figure 9A,B). However, only the higher dose of PO extract (300 mg/kg) firmly propagated the count and motility of sperm compared to the diabetic group ($p < 0.01$ and 0.05, respectively; Figure 9A,B).

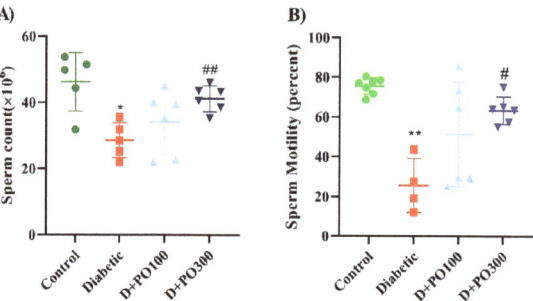

Figure 9. The effects of PO extract on (**A**) numbers and (**B**) motility of sperm in diabetic rats. The data are presented as mean ± SD. A one-way ANOVA test was carried out with the following Tukey–Kramer's post hoc test; * $p < 0.05$, ** $p < 0.01$ vs. control group; # $p < 0.05$, ## $p < 0.01$ vs. diabetic group.

2.9. The Effect of PO Extract on the Levels of LH, FSH, and Testosterone

Our results showed that the diabetic group decreased the LH and testosterone levels significantly compared to the control group ($p < 0.001$ for both cases; Figure 10A,C). Reciprocally, eight weeks of treatment with PO extract (300 mg/kg) strikingly promoted the LH and testosterone levels compared to the diabetic groups ($p < 0.05$ and 0.001, respectively; Figure 10A,C). Furthermore, no significant changes in the FSH level were observed between the four studied groups at the experimental endpoint (eight weeks) (Figure 10C).

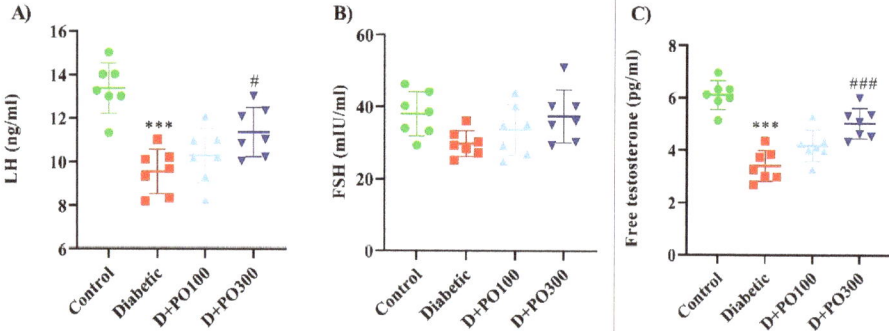

Figure 10. The effects of PO extract on (**A**) LH, (**B**) FSH, and (**C**) testosterone levels in diabetic rats. The data are presented as mean ± SD. A one-way ANOVA test was carried out with the following Tukey–Kramer's post hoc test; *** $p < 0.001$ vs. control group; # $p < 0.05$, ### $p < 0.001$ vs. diabetic group.

2.10. The Effect of PO Extract on the Oxidative and Antioxidative Factors

At the end of the eight weeks, the diabetic group notably elevated the MDA level compared to the control group ($p < 0.001$; Figure 11A), while the PO extract (100 and 300 mg/kg) markedly reduced the MDA level compared to the diabetic group ($p < 0.001$ for both cases, Figure 11A). Our results also revealed that the diabetic group significantly diminished the SOD activity and total thiol content compared to the control group ($p < 0.001$ and 0.05, respectively; Figure 11B,C). However, only the higher dose of PO extract (300 mg/kg) meaningfully enhanced the SOD activity and total thiol content compared to the diabetic group ($p < 0.001$ for both cases; Figure 11B,C).

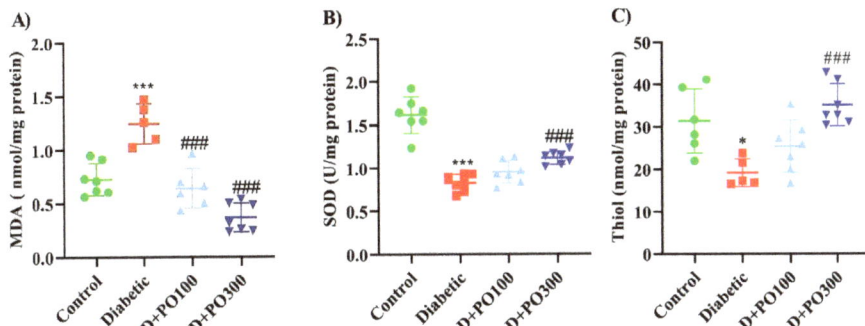

Figure 11. The effects of PO extract on (**A**) MDA, (**B**) SOD, and (**C**) thiol levels in diabetic rats. The data are presented as mean ± SD. A one-way ANOVA test was carried out with the following Tukey–Kramer's post hoc test; * $p < 0.05$, *** $p < 0.001$ vs. control group; ### $p < 0.001$ vs. diabetic group.

2.11. The Effect of PO Extract on TNF-α, VEGF, and TGF-β Levels

As reported in Figure 12A, the TNF-α level was increased in the diabetic group compared to the control group ($p < 0.05$; Figure 12A), while considerably mitigated in the PO extract (300 mg/kg) group compared to the diabetic group ($p < 0.05$; Figure 12A). Our results also demonstrated that the diabetic group considerably attenuated the VEGF level compared to the control group ($p < 0.05$; Figure 12B). However, eight weeks of treatment with PO extract (300 mg/kg) notably propagated the VEGF level compared to the diabetic group ($p < 0.01$, Figure 12B). On the contrary, the TGF-β level was remarkably increased in the diabetic group compared to the control group ($p < 0.001$; Figure 12C), while the PO extracts (100 and 300 mg/kg) considerably mitigated the TGF-β level compared to the diabetic group ($p < 0.01$ and $p < 0.001$, respectively; Figure 12C).

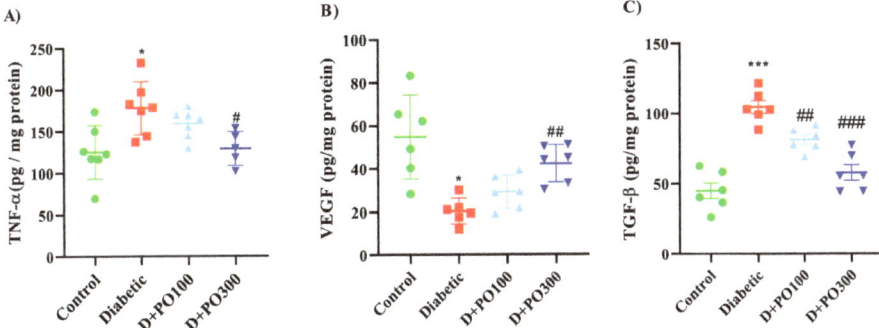

Figure 12. The effects of PO extract on the levels of (**A**) TNF-α, (**B**) VEGF, and (**C**) TGF-β levels in diabetic rats. The data are presented as mean ± SD. A one-way ANOVA test was carried out with the following Tukey–Kramer's post hoc test; * $p < 0.05$, *** $p < 0.001$ vs. control group; # $p < 0.05$, ## $p < 0.01$, ### $p < 0.001$ vs. diabetic group.

3. Discussion

Our study, for the first time, demonstrates the protective effect of *Portulaca oleracea* on streptozotocin-induced type-I-diabetes-associated reproductive system dysfunction and inflammation. Several studies, in both diabetic animal models and on human cavernosal tissue from diabetic patients, have demonstrated that the erectile dysfunction associated with diabetes is a multifactorial condition involving inflammation, oxidative damage and metabolic disorders [31]. Accordingly, our results showed that streptozotocin-induced diabetes leads to increased oxidative stress and inflammatory markers in the testicular tissue and impaired fertility parameters and that PO extract strongly ameliorated these parameters. This seems to be related to the presence of oleraceins (A, B, C, and D), flavonoids, terpenoids (portulosides A and portulene), and vitamins (ascorbic acid, α-tocopherol and riboflavin) chemically characterized for the plant extract.

Pieces of evidence have proved the induction of diabetes and hyperglycemia through a single i.p. injection of streptozotocin in rats [32]. Additionally, Akbarzadeh and co-workers supported that the blood glucose level, food and water consumption, and urine volume were markedly increased, while the body weight and insulin level were reduced, following streptozotocin-induced diabetes in rats [33]. Consistently, streptozotocin-induced diabetes augmented the blood glucose level and food and water consumption, while strikingly decreasing body weight [34]. Our results showed that the streptozotocin-induced diabetes group notably enhanced the blood glucose level and food and water consumption, while significantly reducing the body weight compared to the control group. In addition, PO extract (at both 100 and 300 mg/kg) significantly decreased the blood glucose level and food and water consumption without affecting rat body weight.

According to our results, Lee et al. demonstrated that aqueous extract of PO (300 mg/kg; oral gavage for ten weeks) diminished the blood glucose, triglyceride, low-density lipoprotein (LDL)-cholesterol levels, while elevating the insulin and high-density lipoprotein (HDL)-cholesterol levels in diabetic db/db mice [35] and alloxan-induced diabetic rats [36,37]. Notably, the present study also demonstrates that streptozotocin-induced diabetes leads to the epithelium disintegration of seminiferous tubules, the destruction of Leydig cells, and increased space between the seminiferous tubules, and irregularities in the structure of the seminiferous tubules in the testicular tissue. Moreover, the seminiferous tubules' diameter, sperm count, and sperm motility were diminished in the diabetic group. In line with our results, Ricci and co-workers showed the abnormal histology, seminiferous epithelium cytoarchitecture, occludin distribution pattern, hypertrophy, and abnormally distribution of Leydig cells in the testicular tissue of the streptozotocin-induced diabetes rats. They also reported a decrease in the testosterone and SOD levels in diabetic rats [38]. Consistently, streptozotocin-induced diabetes leads to desquamation of spermatids in the lumen and disorganization of seminiferous tubule germinal epithelium in the testicular tissue.

Furthermore, the LH and testosterone levels and the mean seminiferous tubule diameter were diminished in the diabetic rats [39]. In addition, recent studies reported a decrease in mean seminiferous tubule diameter and sperm count and motility following streptozotocin administration [40–42]. Our results show that PO extract remarkably improved the histopathological changes in the testicular tissue and increased the seminiferous tubule diameter; these results are in accordance with previous reports that demonstrated a protective effect of PO extracts in sperm count and testosterone level in male albino rats [40,43–45].

The male reproductive system is regulated through the hypothalamic–pituitary–testicular axis. The gonadotropin-releasing hormone (GnRH) is secreted by the hypothalamus and stimulates the secretion of LH and FSH from the pituitary gland [46]. As a consequence, LH stimulates the testosterone secretion through Leydig cells, while the FSH regulates spermatogenesis by affecting the Sertoli cells of the testes [47] and testosterone levels [48]. This evidence indicates that there is a relationship between insulin/glucose and LH/FSH levels in serum and that their ratio is affected in diabetes. However, the mechanisms by which insulin, glucose, or both control these hormones are unclear [49].

In our study, we found that the LH and testosterone levels were mitigated, while the FSH level did not change in the streptozotocin-induced diabetes group. Additionally, we found that the higher dose of PO extract (300 mg/kg) firmly propagated the LH and testosterone levels while not changing the FSH level, following streptozotocin-induced diabetes. Similarly, Farag et al. demonstrated that PO seeds' extract (200 and 400 mg/kg) prevented testicular dysfunction, while enhancing testosterone levels following the acrylamide-induced testicular toxicity in rats [50]. In another study, PO seeds and shoot extract (50 mg/kg) significantly increased LH, FSH, and testosterone levels following the doxorubicin-induced testicular toxicity in albino rats [51].

Recent pieces of evidence emphasized the relation between oxidative stress and male infertility. Indeed, DM-1 can affect the spermatogenesis by oxidative damage generating reactive oxygen species (ROS), which either affect the cellular antioxidant defense mechanisms or directly stimulate the inflammatory signaling pathways, ending in testicular apoptosis [52]. Thus, ROS attenuation is crucial for the treatment of reproductive damage in diabetic patients. Additionally, numerous studies emphasized that streptozotocin-induced diabetes elevated lipid peroxidation and ROS levels, while mitigating anti-oxidative markers, including catalase, SOD, glutathione peroxidase, glutathione transferase, and glutathione reductase activities in the testis and epididymal sperm [53,54]. In our preclinical assessment, we showed that streptozotocin-induced diabetes elevated the MDA level, while also attenuating the total thiol content and the SOD activity in the testicular tissue. Moreover, PO extract notably ameliorated the oxidative stress induced by streptozotocin in the testicular tissue of rats. This is in line with previous works that demonstrated the anti-oxidative properties of PO in both male [55,56] and female rodents [57,58].

The last point that we want to discuss is the pivotal role of inflammation in diabetic testicular complications [59] and the stringent involvement of VEGF (an angiotrophic and neurotrophic factor) [60] on spermatogenesis and Sertoli and Leydig cells' physiopathology. The importance of interferon-gamma (IFN-γ), interleukin (IL)-1β, and TNF-α in these physio-pathological mechanisms has been well clarified [61–63]. Furthermore, it has also been revealed that increased TNF-α (in semen) and IL-1β, and IL-6 are associated with decreased sperm count, motility, and morphology [64]. upon the onset and during the progression of diabetes [65,66]. Additionally, it has been reported that VEGF supports germ cell proliferation and survival and regulates endothelial permeability and microcirculation in the testis [67,68]. Moreover, different report highlight that streptozotocin-induced diabetes mitigated the VEGF level, associated with increased apoptosis and testicular damage in rats [69–71]. In our investigation, we found that PO was able to increase the levels of VEGF and to revert the streptozotocin-induced increased of TNF-α and TGF-β levels in testicular tissue. Taken together, these results further corroborate the protective effects of PO on type-I-diabetes-associated reproductive system dysfunction and inflammation.

4. Materials and Methods

4.1. Drugs and Chemicals

Streptozotocin, dimethyl sulfoxide (DMSO), and ethanol were prepared from Sigma-Aldrich Chemical Co. (St. Louis, MO, USA). Ketamine and xylazine were obtained from ChemiDaru Company (Tehran, Iran). Tumor necrosis factor-alpha (TNF-α) and vascular endothelial growth factor (VEGF) and transforming growth factor-beta (TGF-β) ELISA kits were purchased from IBL-International® Company (Hamburg, Germany), and luteinizing hormone (LH), follicle-stimulating hormone (FSH), and testosterone ELISA kits were prepared from CUSABIO Company (Eco-Life Science Ltd., Hong Kong, China). Furthermore, malondialdehyde (MDA), superoxide dismutase (SOD), and total thiol content kits were prepared by Zell Bio Company (Lonsee, Baden-Württemberg, Germany). Other chemicals or reagents were also provided at analytical grades from Santa Cruz Biotechnology (Santa Cruz, Dallas, TX, USA).

4.2. Preparation of Portulaca oleracea Extract and Liquid Chromatography-Mass Spectrometers (LC-MS) Characterisation

Portulaca oleracea (PO) was collected from Sabzevar, Khorasan Razavi province, Iran, in July 2020 and was identified by the pharmacy school at Mashhad University of Medical Sciences (herbarium No. 12-1615-240). First, the extract was prepared by using the maceration method described previously. In brief, 100 g of aerial parts of PO was soaked with one lit 70% ethanol for 48 h at room temperature. Then the extract was concentrated with a rotary evaporator and freeze-dried [7–11]. The yield of the dried extract was 19.5% w/w and stored at $-20\ °C$ until use. Finally, the PO concentrations (100 and 300 mg/kg) were prepared with sterilized distilled water containing 1% v/v DMSO from the raw extract. The liquid chromatography–mass spectrometers (LC–MS) characterization was performed by an AB SCIEX QTRAP (Shimadzu) liquid chromatography coupled with a triple quadrupole Mass Spectrometer and using a Supelco C18 (15 mm × 2.1 mm × 3 μm) column. It was performed according to our previously published methods [12]. The mass spectra were obtained by scanning time of 80 min and in a range of 100 to 1700. The mass spectra were obtained by a scanning time of 80 min and in a range of 100 to 1700. The positive electrospray ionization (ESI) mode was applied for the Mass Spectrometer.

4.3. Animals' Husbandry and Ethics

In this study, 28 healthy male Wistar rats weighing 250–300 g were obtained from the animal care center, Mashhad University of Medical Sciences. The rats were deployed in separated standard cages and ventilated rooms with a 12/12 h natural light–dark cycle, temperature of 24 ± 2 °C, and humidity of 60 ± 3%, with food and water ad libitum. All animals received human care in compliance with Mashhad University of Medical Sciences guidelines (Ethical Approval Code, 980077; Approval Date, 8 August 2019; Approval ID, IR.MUMS.MEDICAL.REC.1398.563). Animal procedures were performed according to ARRIVE guidelines and the Basel declaration, including the 3Rs concept. All methods were carried out to minimize the number of animals used ($n=7$ per group) and their suffering. Experimental study groups were randomized, and their assessments were carried out by researchers blinded to the treatment groups.

4.4. Experimental Diabetes Induction

Diabetes was induced by a single intraperitoneal (i.p.) injection of streptozotocin (50 mg/kg). The streptozotocin solution was freshly prepared in a cold 0.1 M citrate buffer (pH = 4.5). The serum glucose level was measured by using a glucometer after 72 h of streptozotocin injection to confirm the diabetes model. The animals with fasting glucose levels higher than 220 mg/dL and signs of polyuria and polydipsia were considered diabetic [34].

4.5. Study Design

Twenty-eight healthy male Wistar rats (250–300 g) with proven fertility were randomly divided into four experimental groups, as described below:

1. Control group: receiving a single dose of streptozotocin carrier (with a volume equal to 50 mg/kg; i.p.) + PO extract vehicle (oral gavage; for eight weeks).
2. Diabetic group: receiving a single dose of streptozotocin (50 mg/kg; i.p.) + PO extract vehicle (daily oral gavage; for eight weeks).
3. Treatment group-1: receiving a single dose of streptozotocin (50 mg/kg; i.p.) + PO extract (100 mg/kg; daily oral gavage for eight weeks).
4. Treatment group-2: receiving a single dose of streptozotocin (50 mg/kg; i.p.) + PO extract (300 mg/kg; daily oral gavage for eight weeks).

The selected dose was chosen based on preliminary experiments and previous works [8,15,50,72].

4.6. Measurement of Blood Glucose Levels

The 12 h fasting blood glucose level was measured with Accu-Chek Active® glucometer (Roche Diagnostics GmbH, Mannheim, Germany), using the tail vein, at the end of the zero, four, and eight weeks of treatment.

4.7. Sample Preparation

At the experimental endpoint, rats were deeply anesthetized with ketamine (100 mg/kg) and xylazine (10 mg/kg) and acepromazine (3 mg/kg) [12,73]. The blood samples (2 cc) were gathered by intracardiac puncture and then straightly centrifuged at 3000 rpm for 10 min at 4 °C, and the supernatants (sera) were isolated and kept at −20 °C for further investigations. The testicular and epididymis were sequestered and weighed. The testicular tissue homogenate (10% w/v) was provided in 5% potassium chloride and 0.5 mM PMSF, and the protease inhibitor cocktail was then centrifuged at 3000 rpm for 10 min, at 4 °C. The supernatants were collected and stored at −20 °C for further investigations. According to Bradford's method, the total protein concentrations were measured [12,74]. In addition, the epididymis was fixed in 10% v/v buffer formalin for histopathological assessments and was soaked with saline to evaluate the number and motility of sperm.

4.8. Assessment of Hormonal Factors

Enzyme-linked immunosorbent assays (ELISA) for LH, FSH, and testosterone levels were carried out on serum samples according to the manufacturer's instructions [75].

4.9. Assessment of Oxidative and Anti-Oxidative, Inflammatory, Fibrosis and Angiogenesis Biomarkers

The levels of MDA, as an oxidative factor, and the total thiol content and the SOD activity, as anti-oxidative factors, were determined in the testicular tissue by using commercial biochemistry kits according to the manufacturer's instruction [76]. In addition, the levels of TNF-α, as an index of inflammation; VEGF levels, as an angiogenesis marker; and TGF-β, as a fibrotic factor, were measured in testicular tissue by using ELISA assay [7,10–12,77].

4.10. Histological Evaluations and Measurement of the Seminiferous Diameter, Sperm Count and Motility

After sacrifice, the animals' abdomens were opened to weigh and evaluate the fertility parameters, including testicular weight, relative testicular weight, epididymal weight, motility and number of sperm, and protein-level measurement. After the dissection of the lower region, the tail of the epididymis was removed and transferred to a container containing physiological serum. After dissecting the tail and removing the sperm, the remaining tissue fragments were separated from the suspension. The resulting sperm suspension was counted at a ratio of 1:20 to calculate the number of sperm under a light microscope, using a NeoBar slide. The testicular tissue was fixed with 10% v/v buffered formalin, and the histological process, including dehydrating, clearing, and embedding, was carried out. After that, the microscopic sections (5 μm) were prepared and stained with Hematoxylin and Eosin (H&E) and evaluated by optical microscopy. The average seminiferous diameter (μm) was determined for each testis [78].

4.11. Statistical Analysis

All collected data were analyzed by using Graph Pad Prism® 8 (Graph Pad Software, San Diego, CA, USA) software and expressed as mean ± SD. Initially, the normality of the data distribution was evaluated by using the Kolmogorov–Simonov test. In the next step, the biochemical and oxidative result comparison was carried out using a one-way analysis of variance (ANOVA) with Tukey–Kramer's post hoc test. In addition, a comparison of the results of blood glucose levels, weight, and food and water consumption was made by using the repeated measures two-way ANOVA test with Tukey–Kramer's post hoc test. The probability (P) values were considered statistically significant when $p \leq 0.05, 0.01$, and 0.001. By data normalization, animal weight was used for randomization and group allocation to reduce unwanted sources of variations. No animals and related ex vivo samples were excluded from the analysis. An in vivo study was carried out to generate groups of equal size ($n = 7$ of independent values), using a randomization and blinded analysis.

5. Conclusions

The results of this study demonstrate, for the first time, the protective effect of *Portulaca oleracea* (phytochemically characterized by using liquid chromatography–mass spectrometry to detect bioactive molecules) on streptozotocin-induced type I diabetes–associated reproductive system dysfunction and inflammation. These effects are most likely attributable to (i) the decreasing of blood glucose level and testicular tissue damage, (ii) the improvement of inflammatory factors, and (iii) the modulation of sex hormones level and fertility potential. Therefore, these findings indicate the promising beneficial role of PO extract as an efficient therapeutic agent for treating diabetic infertility. However, further preclinical studies aimed to identify the mechanism/s of action, and, potentially, clinical trials are necessary to support and corroborate this evidence.

Author Contributions: V.B.R., H.R., A.S., L.E., A.E.-b., F.M. and V.R.A. wrote the first draft of the manuscript. H.R., A.S., H.R.K., M.R.M., V.B.R., S.E., L.E., A.E.-b., F.M. and V.R.A. carried out the experimental protocols. All authors have read and agreed to the published version of the manuscript.

Funding: This study was financially supported by Mashhad University of Medical Sciences (Grant Number: 980077). A.S. is supported by the Dompé Farmaceutici S.p.A fellowship for PhD program in "Nutraceuticals, functional foods and human health" (University of Naples Federico II).

Institutional Review Board Statement: All animals received human care in compliance with Mashhad University of Medical Sciences guidelines (Ethical approval code: 980077, Approval date: 8 August 2019, Approval ID: IR.MUMS.MEDICAL.REC.1398.563). Animal procedures were performed according ARRIVE guidelines and the Basel declaration including the 3Rs concept.

Informed Consent Statement: Not applicable.

Data Availability Statement: The datasets generated and/or analyzed during the current study are available from the corresponding author upon reasonable request.

Acknowledgments: This study was financially supported by Mashhad University of Medical Sciences (Grant Number: 980077). A.S. is supported by Dompé Farmaceutici S.p.A fellowship for PhD program in "Nutraceuticals, functional foods and human health" (University of Naples Federico II).

Conflicts of Interest: The authors declare no conflict of interest. This study was conducted, and the subsequent paper was written, in the absence of any commercial or financial relationships that could be construed as a potential conflict of interest.

Sample Availability: Samples of the compounds are available from the authors.

References

1. Kaul, K.; Tarr, J.M.; Ahmad, S.I.; Kohner, E.M.; Chibber, R. Introduction to diabetes mellitus. *Adv. Exp. Med. Biol.* **2012**, *771*, 1–11. [CrossRef] [PubMed]
2. Saeedi, P.; Petersohn, I.; Salpea, P.; Malanda, B.; Karuranga, S.; Unwin, N.; Colagiuri, S.; Guariguata, L.; Motala, A.A.; Ogurtsova, K.; et al. Global and regional diabetes prevalence estimates for 2019 and projections for 2030 and 2045: Results from the International Diabetes Federation Diabetes Atlas, 9th edition. *Diabetes Res. Clin. Pract.* **2019**, *157*, 107843. [CrossRef]
3. Eizirik, D.L.; Colli, M.L.; Ortis, F. The role of inflammation in insulitis and beta-cell loss in type 1 diabetes. *Nat. Rev. Endocrinol.* **2009**, *5*, 219–226. [CrossRef]
4. Zheng, Y.; Ley, S.H.; Hu, F.B. Global aetiology and epidemiology of type 2 diabetes mellitus and its complications. *Nat. Rev. Endocrinol.* **2018**, *14*, 88–98. [CrossRef] [PubMed]
5. Ding, G.L.; Liu, Y.; Liu, M.E.; Pan, J.X.; Guo, M.X.; Sheng, J.Z.; Huang, H.F. The effects of diabetes on male fertility and epigenetic regulation during spermatogenesis. *Asian J. Androl.* **2015**, *17*, 948–953. [CrossRef] [PubMed]
6. Corona, G.; Giorda, C.B.; Cucinotta, D.; Guida, P.; Nada, E. Sexual dysfunction at the onset of type 2 diabetes: The interplay of depression, hormonal and cardiovascular factors. *J. Sex. Med.* **2014**, *11*, 2065–2073. [CrossRef]

7. Baradaran Rahimi, V.; Rakhshandeh, H.; Raucci, F.; Buono, B.; Shirazinia, R.; Samzadeh Kermani, A.; Maione, F.; Mascolo, N.; Askari, V.R. Anti-Inflammatory and Anti-Oxidant Activity of Portulaca oleracea Extract on LPS-Induced Rat Lung Injury. *Molecules* **2019**, *24*, 139. [CrossRef]
8. Baradaran Rahimi, V.; Mousavi, S.H.; Haghighi, S.; Soheili-Far, S.; Askari, V.R. Cytotoxicity and apoptogenic properties of the standardized extract of *Portulaca oleracea* on glioblastoma multiforme cancer cell line (U-87): A mechanistic study. *EXCLI J.* **2019**, *18*, 165–186. [CrossRef]
9. Rahimi, V.B.; Ajam, F.; Rakhshandeh, H.; Askari, V.R. A Pharmacological Review on *Portulaca oleracea* L.: Focusing on Anti-Inflammatory, Anti-Oxidant, Immuno-Modulatory and Antitumor Activities. *J. Pharmacopunct.* **2019**, *22*, 7–15. [CrossRef]
10. Rahimi, V.B.; Askari, V.R.; Shirazinia, R.; Soheili-Far, S.; Askari, N.; Rahmanian-Devin, P.; Sanei-Far, Z.; Mousavi, S.H.; Ghodsi, R. Protective effects of hydro-ethanolic extract of *Terminalia chebula* on primary microglia cells and their polarization (M1/M2 balance). *Mult. Scler. Relat. Disord.* **2018**, *25*, 5–13. [CrossRef]
11. Baradaran Rahimi, V.; Askari, V.R. Promising anti-melanogenic impacts of Portulaca oleracea on B16F1 murine melanoma cell line: An in-vitro vision. *S. Afr. J. Bot.* **2021**, *142*, 477–485. [CrossRef]
12. Jaafari, A.; Baradaran Rahimi, V.; Vahdati-Mashhadian, N.; Yahyazadeh, R.; Ebrahimzadeh-Bideskan, A.; Hasanpour, M.; Iranshahi, M.; Ehtiati, S.; Rajabi, H.; Mahdinezhad, M.; et al. Evaluation of the Therapeutic Effects of the Hydroethanolic Extract of Portulaca oleracea on Surgical-Induced Peritoneal Adhesion. *Mediat. Inflamm.* **2021**, *2021*, 8437753. [CrossRef]
13. Zhou, Y.X.; Xin, H.L.; Rahman, K.; Wang, S.J.; Peng, C.; Zhang, H. *Portulaca oleracea* L.: A review of phytochemistry and pharmacological effects. *BioMed Res. Int.* **2015**, *2015*, 925631. [CrossRef] [PubMed]
14. Bai, Y.; Zang, X.; Ma, J.; Xu, G. Anti-Diabetic Effect of *Portulaca oleracea* L. Polysaccharideandits Mechanism in Diabetic Rats. *Int. J. Mol. Sci.* **2016**, *17*, 1201. [CrossRef] [PubMed]
15. Boskabady, M.H.; Hashemzehi, M.; Khazdair, M.R.; Askari, V.R. Hydro-ethanolic Extract of *Portulaca oleracea* Affects Beta-adrenoceptors of Guinea Pig Tracheal Smooth Muscle. *Iran. J. Pharm. Res.* **2016**, *15*, 867–874.
16. Yan, J.; Sun, L.R.; Zhou, Z.Y.; Chen, Y.C.; Zhang, W.M.; Dai, H.F.; Tan, J.W. Homoisoflavonoids from the medicinal plant *Portulaca oleracea*. *Phytochemistry* **2012**, *80*, 37–41. [CrossRef]
17. Chen, J.; Shi, Y.P.; Liu, J.Y. Determination of noradrenaline and dopamine in Chinese herbal extracts from *Portulaca oleracea* L. by high-performance liquid chromatography. *J. Chromatogr. A* **2003**, *1003*, 127–132. [CrossRef]
18. Xiang, L.; Xing, D.; Wang, W.; Wang, R.; Ding, Y.; Du, L. Alkaloids from *Portulaca oleracea* L. *Phytochemistry* **2005**, *66*, 2595–2601. [CrossRef]
19. Tian, J.L.; Liang, X.; Gao, P.Y.; Li, D.Q.; Sun, Q.; Li, L.Z.; Song, S.J. Two new alkaloids from *Portulaca oleracea* and their cytotoxic activities. *J. Asian Nat. Prod. Res.* **2014**, *16*, 259–264. [CrossRef]
20. Liang, X.; Tian, J.; Li, L.; Gao, J.; Zhang, Q.; Gao, P.; Song, S. Rapid determination of eight bioactive alkaloids in *Portulaca oleracea* L. by the optimal microwave extraction combined with positive-negative conversion multiple reaction monitor (+/−MRM) technology. *Talanta* **2014**, *120*, 167–172. [CrossRef]
21. Sakai, N.; Inada, K.; Okamoto, M.; Shizuri, Y.; Fukuyama, Y. Portuloside A, a monoterpene glucoside, from *Portulaca oleracea*. *Phytochemistry* **1996**, *42*, 1625–1628. [CrossRef]
22. Elkhayat, E.S.; Ibrahim, S.R.; Aziz, M.A. Portulene, a new diterpene from *Portulaca oleracea* L. *J. Asian Nat. Prod. Res.* **2008**, *10*, 1039–1043. [CrossRef] [PubMed]
23. Seo, Y.; Shin, J.; Cha, H.J.; Kim, Y.-A.; Ahn, J.-W.; Lee, B.-J.; Lee, D.S. A new monoterpene glucoside from *Portulaca oleracea*. *Bull. Korean Chem. Soc.* **2003**, *24*, 1475–1477. [CrossRef]
24. Xin, H.-L.; Xu, Y.-F.; Hou, Y.-H.; Zhang, Y.-N.; Yue, X.-Q.; Lu, J.-C.; Ling, C.-Q. Two Novel Triterpenoids from *Portulaca oleracea* L. *Helv. Chim. Acta* **2008**, *91*, 2075–2080. [CrossRef]
25. Xu, X.; Yu, L.; Chen, G. Determination of flavonoids in *Portulaca oleracea* L. by capillary electrophoresis with electrochemical detection. *J. Pharm. Biomed. Anal.* **2006**, *41*, 493–499. [CrossRef]
26. Zhu, H.; Wang, Y.; Liu, Y.; Xia, Y.; Tang, T. Analysis of Flavonoids in *Portulaca oleracea* L. by UV-Vis Spectrophotometry with Comparative Study on Different Extraction Technologies. *Food Anal. Methods* **2010**, *3*, 90–97. [CrossRef]
27. Palaniswamy, U.R.; McAvoy, R.J.; Bible, B.B. Stage of harvest and polyunsaturated essential fatty acid concentrations in purslane (*Portulaca oleraceae*) leaves. *J. Agric. Food Chem.* **2001**, *49*, 3490–3493. [CrossRef]
28. Yang, Z.; Liu, C.; Xiang, L.; Zheng, Y. Phenolic alkaloids as a new class of antioxidants in *Portulaca oleracea*. *Phytother. Res.* **2009**, *23*, 1032–1035. [CrossRef]
29. Uddin, M.K.; Juraimi, A.S.; Hossain, M.S.; Nahar, M.A.; Ali, M.E.; Rahman, M.M. Purslane weed (*Portulaca oleracea*): A prospective plant source of nutrition, omega-3 fatty acid, and antioxidant attributes. *Sci. World J.* **2014**, *2014*, 951019. [CrossRef]
30. Cheng, Z.; Wang, D.; Zhang, W.; Du, Y.; Wang, Y.; Zhai, Y.; Ying, X.; Kang, T. LC determination and pharmacokinetic study of the main phenolic components of *Portulaca oleracea* L. extract in rat plasma after oral administration. *Nat. Prod. Res.* **2012**, *26*, 2247–2250. [CrossRef]
31. Elçioğlu, H.K.; Kabasakal, L.; Özkan, N.; Çelikel, Ç.; Ayanoğlu-Dülger, G. A study comparing the effects of rosiglitazone and/or insulin treatments on streptozotocin induced diabetic (type I diabetes) rat aorta and cavernous tissues. *Eur. J. Pharmacol.* **2011**, *660*, 476–484. [CrossRef]
32. Furman, B.L. Streptozotocin-Induced Diabetic Models in Mice and Rats. *Curr. Protoc. Pharmacol.* **2015**, *70*, 5–47. [CrossRef] [PubMed]

33. Akbarzadeh, A.; Norouzian, D.; Mehrabi, M.R.; Jamshidi, S.; Farhangi, A.; Verdi, A.A.; Mofidian, S.M.; Rad, B.L. Induction of diabetes by Streptozotocin in rats. *Indian J. Clin. Biochem.* **2007**, *22*, 60–64. [CrossRef] [PubMed]
34. Vasconcelos, C.F.; Maranhão, H.M.; Batista, T.M.; Carneiro, E.M.; Ferreira, F.; Costa, J.; Soares, L.A.; Sá, M.D.; Souza, T.P.; Wanderley, A.G. Hypoglycaemic activity and molecular mechanisms of *Caesalpinia ferrea* Martius bark extract on streptozotocin-induced diabetes in Wistar rats. *J. Ethnopharmacol.* **2011**, *137*, 1533–1541. [CrossRef] [PubMed]
35. Lee, A.S.; Lee, Y.J.; Lee, S.M.; Yoon, J.J.; Kim, J.S.; Kang, D.G.; Lee, H.S. *Portulaca oleracea* Ameliorates Diabetic Vascular Inflammation and Endothelial Dysfunction in db/db Mice. *Evid. Based Complement. Altern. Med.* **2012**, *2012*, 741824. [CrossRef] [PubMed]
36. Ramadan, B.K.; Schaalan, M.F.; Tolba, A.M. Hypoglycemic and pancreatic protective effects of *Portulaca oleracea* extract in alloxan induced diabetic rats. *BMC Complement. Altern. Med.* **2017**, *17*, 37. [CrossRef] [PubMed]
37. Barakat, L.A.; Mahmoud, R.H. The antiatherogenic, renal protective and immunomodulatory effects of purslane, pumpkin and flax seeds on hypercholesterolemic rats. *N. Am. J. Med. Sci.* **2011**, *3*, 411–417. [CrossRef]
38. Ricci, G.; Catizone, A.; Esposito, R.; Pisanti, F.A.; Vietri, M.T.; Galdieri, M. Diabetic rat testes: Morphological and functional alterations. *Andrologia* **2009**, *41*, 361–368. [CrossRef]
39. Sönmez, M.F.; Karabulut, D.; Kilic, E.; Akalin, H.; Sakalar, C.; Gunduz, Y.; Kara, A.; Dundar, M. The effects of streptozotocin-induced diabetes on ghrelin expression in rat testis: Biochemical and immunohistochemical study. *Folia Histochem. Cytobiol.* **2015**, *53*, 26–34. [CrossRef]
40. Kotian, S.R.; Kumar, A.; Mallik, S.B.; Bhat, N.P.; Souza, A.D.; Pandey, A.K. Effect of Diabetes on the Male Reproductive System—A Histomorphological Study. *J. Morphol. Sci.* **2019**, *36*, 017–023. [CrossRef]
41. Khaki, A.; Fathiazad, F.; Nouri, M.; Khaki, A.; Maleki, N.A.; Khamnei, H.J.; Ahmadi, P. Beneficial effects of quercetin on sperm parameters in streptozotocin-induced diabetic male rats. *Phytother. Res.* **2010**, *24*, 1285–1291. [CrossRef] [PubMed]
42. Afifi, M.; Almaghrabi, O.A.; Kadasa, N.M. Ameliorative Effect of Zinc Oxide Nanoparticles on Antioxidants and Sperm Characteristics in Streptozotocin-Induced Diabetic Rat Testes. *BioMed Res. Int.* **2015**, *2015*, 153573. [CrossRef] [PubMed]
43. Obinna, V.; Kagbo, H.; Agu, G. Effects of Lipophilic and Hydrophilic leaf extracts of *Portulaca oleracea* Linn. (Purslane) on male reproductive parameters in albino rats. *Am. J. Physiol. Biochem. Pharmacol.* **2019**, *9*, 21–32. [CrossRef]
44. Xu, Y.; Lei, H.; Guan, R.; Gao, Z.; Li, H.; Wang, L.; Song, W.; Gao, B.; Xin, Z. Studies on the mechanism of testicular dysfunction in the early stage of a streptozotocin induced diabetic rat model. *Biochem. Biophys. Res. Commun.* **2014**, *450*, 87–92. [CrossRef] [PubMed]
45. Ghaheri, M.; Miraghaee, S.; Babaei, A.; Mohammadi, B.; Kahrizi, D.; Saivosh Haghighi, Z.M.; Bahrami, G. Effect of Stevia rebaudiana Bertoni extract on sexual dysfunction in Streptozotocin-induced diabetic male rats. *Cell. Mol. Biol.* **2018**, *64*, 6–10. [CrossRef]
46. Rastrelli, G.; Maggi, M.; Corona, G. Pharmacological management of late-onset hypogonadism. *Expert Rev. Clin. Pharmacol.* **2018**, *11*, 439–458. [CrossRef] [PubMed]
47. Aladamat, N.; Tadi, P. Histology, Leydig Cells. In *StatPearls*; StatPearls Publishing Copyright © 2022; StatPearls Publishing LLC: Treasure Island, FL, USA, 2021.
48. Acién, P.; Acién, M. Disorders of Sex Development: Classification, Review, and Impact on Fertility. *J. Clin. Med.* **2020**, *9*, 3555. [CrossRef]
49. Ballester, J.; Muñoz, M.C.; Domínguez, J.; Rigau, T.; Guinovart, J.J.; Rodríguez-Gil, J.E. Insulin-dependent diabetes affects testicular function by FSH- and LH-linked mechanisms. *J. Androl.* **2004**, *25*, 706–719. [CrossRef]
50. Farag, O.M.; Abd-Elsalam, R.M.; El Badawy, S.A.; Ogaly, H.A.; Alsherbiny, M.A.; Ahmed, K.A. *Portulaca oleracea* seeds' extract alleviates acrylamide-induced testicular dysfunction by promoting oxidative status and steroidogenic pathway in rats. *BMC Complement. Med. Ther.* **2021**, *21*, 122. [CrossRef]
51. Hozayen, W.G.; Ahmed, O.M.; Abo Sree, H.T.; Ahmed, M.B. Effects of ethanolic purslane shoot and seed extracts on doxorubicin-induced testicular toxicity in albino rats. *Life Sci. J.* **2013**, *10*, 2550–2558.
52. Abdel-Aziz, A.M.; Abozaid, S.M.M.; Yousef, R.K.M.; Mohammed, M.M.; Khalaf, H.M. Fenofibrate ameliorates testicular damage in rats with streptozotocin-induced type 1 diabetes: Role of HO-1 and p38 MAPK. *Pharmacol. Rep.* **2020**, *72*, 1645–1656. [CrossRef] [PubMed]
53. Shrilatha, B.; Muralidhara. Early oxidative stress in testis and epididymal sperm in streptozotocin-induced diabetic mice: Its progression and genotoxic consequences. *Reprod. Toxicol.* **2007**, *23*, 578–587. [CrossRef] [PubMed]
54. Shrilatha, B. Occurrence of oxidative impairments, response of antioxidant defences and associated biochemical perturbations in male reproductive milieu in the Streptozotocin-diabetic rat. *Int. J. Androl.* **2007**, *30*, 508–518. [CrossRef]
55. Samarghandian, S.; Borji, A.; Farkhondeh, T. Attenuation of Oxidative Stress and Inflammation by *Portulaca oleracea* in Streptozotocin-Induced Diabetic Rats. *J. Evid. Based Complement. Altern. Med.* **2017**, *22*, 562–566. [CrossRef] [PubMed]
56. Yang, X.; Yan, Y.; Li, J.; Tang, Z.; Sun, J.; Zhang, H.; Hao, S.; Wen, A.; Liu, L. Protective effects of ethanol extract from *Portulaca oleracea* L on dextran sulphate sodium-induced mice ulcerative colitis involving anti-inflammatory and antioxidant. *Am. J. Transl. Res.* **2016**, *8*, 2138–2148.
57. Ahangarpour, A.; Lamoochi, Z.; Fathi Moghaddam, H.; Mansouri, S.M. Effects of Portulaca oleracea ethanolic extract on reproductive system of aging female mice. *Int. J. Reprod. Biomed.* **2016**, *14*, 205–212. [CrossRef] [PubMed]

58. Yahyazadeh Mashhadi, S.N.; Askari, V.R.; Ghorani, V.; Jelodar, G.A.; Boskabady, M.H. The effect of *Portulaca oleracea* and α-linolenic acid on oxidant/antioxidant biomarkers of human peripheral blood mononuclear cells. *Indian J. Pharmacol.* **2018**, *50*, 177–184. [CrossRef] [PubMed]
59. Coştur, P.; Filiz, S.; Gonca, S.; Çulha, M.; Gülecen, T.; Solakoğlu, S.; Canberk, Y.; Çalışkan, E. Êxpression of inducible nitric oxide synthase (iNOS) in the azoospermic human testis. *Andrologia* **2012**, *44* (Suppl. S1), 654–660. [CrossRef]
60. Calvo, P.M.; Pastor, A.M.; de la Cruz, R.R. Vascular endothelial growth factor: An essential neurotrophic factor for motoneurons? *Neural Regen. Res.* **2018**, *13*, 1181–1182. [CrossRef]
61. Tsalamandris, S.; Antonopoulos, A.S.; Oikonomou, E.; Papamikroulis, G.-A.; Vogiatzi, G.; Papaioannou, S.; Deftereos, S.; Tousoulis, D. The Role of Inflammation in Diabetes: Current Concepts and Future Perspectives. *Eur. Cardiol. Rev.* **2019**, *14*, 50–59. [CrossRef]
62. Azenabor, A.; Ekun, A.O.; Akinloye, O. Impact of Inflammation on Male Reproductive Tract. *J. Reprod. Infertil.* **2015**, *16*, 123–129. [PubMed]
63. Sarkar, O.; Bahrainwala, J.; Chandrasekaran, S.; Kothari, S.; Mathur, P.P.; Agarwal, A. Impact of inflammation on male fertility. *Front. Biosci.* **2011**, *3*, 89–95. [CrossRef]
64. Sanocka, D.; Jedrzejczak, P.; Szumała-Kaekol, A.; Fraczek, M.; Kurpisz, M. Male genital tract inflammation: The role of selected interleukins in regulation of pro-oxidant and antioxidant enzymatic substances in seminal plasma. *J. Androl.* **2003**, *24*, 448–455. [CrossRef] [PubMed]
65. Albasher, G. Modulation of reproductive dysfunctions associated with streptozocin-induced diabetes by *Artemisia judaica* extract in rats fed a high-fat diet. *Mol. Biol. Rep.* **2020**, *47*, 7517–7527. [CrossRef] [PubMed]
66. Yigitturk, G.; Acara, A.C.; Erbas, O.; Oltulu, F.; Yavasoglu, N.U.K.; Uysal, A.; Yavasoglu, A. The antioxidant role of agomelatine and gallic acid on oxidative stress in STZ induced type I diabetic rat testes. *Biomed. Pharmacother.* **2017**, *87*, 240–246. [CrossRef] [PubMed]
67. Tabecka-Lonczynska, A.; Mytych, J.; Solek, P.; Kulpa-Greszta, M.; Sowa-Kucma, M.; Koziorowski, M. Vascular endothelial growth factor (VEGF-A) and fibroblast growth factor (FGF-2) as potential regulators of seasonal reproductive processes in male European bison (*Bison bonasus*, Linnaeus 1758). *Gen. Comp. Endocrinol.* **2018**, *263*, 72–79. [CrossRef]
68. Anand, R.J.; Paust, H.J.; Altenpohl, K.; Mukhopadhyay, A.K. Regulation of vascular endothelial growth factor production by Leydig cells in vitro: The role of protein kinase A and mitogen-activated protein kinase cascade. *Biol. Reprod.* **2003**, *68*, 1663–1673. [CrossRef]
69. Sisman, A.R.; Kiray, M.; Camsari, U.M.; Evren, M.; Ates, M.; Baykara, B.; Aksu, I.; Guvendi, G.; Uysal, N. Potential novel biomarkers for diabetic testicular damage in streptozotocin-induced diabetic rats: Nerve growth factor Beta and vascular endothelial growth factor. *Dis. Markers* **2014**, *2014*, 108106. [CrossRef]
70. Long, L.; Qiu, H.; Cai, B.; Chen, N.; Lu, X.; Zheng, S.; Ye, X.; Li, Y. Hyperglycemia induced testicular damage in type 2 diabetes mellitus rats exhibiting microcirculation impairments associated with vascular endothelial growth factor decreased via PI3K/Akt pathway. *Oncotarget* **2018**, *9*, 5321–5336. [CrossRef]
71. Tunçkiran, A.; Cayan, S.; Bozlu, M.; Yilmaz, N.; Acar, D.; Akbay, E. Protective effect of vascular endothelial growth factor on histologic changes in testicular ischemia-reperfusion injury. *Fertil. Steril.* **2005**, *84*, 468–473. [CrossRef]
72. He, Y.; Long, H.; Zou, C.; Yang, W.; Jiang, L.; Xiao, Z.; Li, Q.; Long, S. Anti-nociceptive effect of *Portulaca oleracea* L. ethanol extracts attenuated zymosan-induced mouse joint inflammation via inhibition of Nrf2 expression. *Innate Immun.* **2021**, *27*, 230–239. [CrossRef]
73. Baradaran Rahimi, V.; Askari, V.R.; Mousavi, S.H. Ellagic acid dose and time-dependently abrogates d-galactose-induced animal model of aging: Investigating the role of PPAR-gamma. *Life Sci.* **2019**, *232*, 116595. [CrossRef] [PubMed]
74. Ernst, O.; Zor, T. Linearization of the bradford protein assay. *JoVE J. Vis. Exp.* **2010**, *38*, e1918. [CrossRef]
75. Saviano, A.; Casillo, G.M.; Raucci, F.; Pernice, A.; Santarcangelo, C.; Piccolo, M.; Ferraro, M.G.; Ciccone, M.; Sgherbini, A.; Pedretti, N.; et al. Supplementation with ribonucleotide-based ingredient (Ribodiet®) lessens oxidative stress, brain inflammation, and amyloid pathology in a murine model of Alzheimer. *Biomed. Pharmacother.* **2021**, *139*, 111579. [CrossRef] [PubMed]
76. Askari, V.R.; Rahimi, V.B.; Zargarani, R.; Ghodsi, R.; Boskabady, M.; Boskabady, M.H. Anti-oxidant and anti-inflammatory effects of auraptene on phytohemagglutinin (PHA)-induced inflammation in human lymphocytes. *Pharmacol. Rep.* **2021**, *73*, 154–162. [CrossRef] [PubMed]
77. Ghadiri, M.; Baradaran Rahimi, V.; Moradi, E.; Hasanpour, M.; Clark, C.C.T.; Iranshahi, M.; Rakhshandeh, H.; Askari, V.R. Standardised pomegranate peel extract lavage prevents postoperative peritoneal adhesion by regulating TGF-β and VEGF levels. *Inflammopharmacology* **2021**, *29*, 855–868. [CrossRef]
78. Roshankhah, S.; Jalili, C.; Salahshoor, M.R. Effects of Crocin on Sperm Parameters and Seminiferous Tubules in Diabetic Rats. *Adv. Biomed. Res.* **2019**, *8*, 4. [CrossRef] [PubMed]

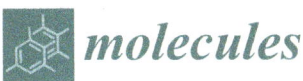

Article

Calceolarioside A, a Phenylpropanoid Glycoside from *Calceolaria* spp., Displays Antinociceptive and Anti-Inflammatory Properties

Stefano Pieretti [1,*], Anella Saviano [2], Adriano Mollica [3], Azzurra Stefanucci [3], Anna Maria Aloisi [4] and Marcello Nicoletti [5]

1. National Centre for Drug Research and Evaluation, Istituto Superiore di Sanità, 00161 Rome, Italy
2. ImmunoPharmaLab, Department of Pharmacy, School of Medicine and Surgery, University of Naples Federico II, 80131 Naples, Italy; anella.saviano@unina.it
3. Department of Pharmacy, University "G. d'Annunzio" of Chieti-Pescara, 66100 Chieti, Italy; a.stefanucci@unich.it (A.S.); adriano.mollica@unich.it (A.M.)
4. Department Medicine, Surgery and Neuroscience, University of Siena, 53100 Siena, Italy; annamaria.aloisi@unisi.it
5. Department of Environmental Biology, Sapienza University of Rome, 00185 Rome, Italy; marcello.nicoletti@uniroma1.it
* Correspondence: stefano.pieretti@iss.it; Tel.: +39-06-4990-2451

Abstract: Phenylpropanoid glycosides are a class of natural substances of plant origin with interesting biological activities and pharmacological properties. This study reports the antinociceptive and anti-inflammatory effects of calceolarioside A, a phenylpropanoid glycoside previously isolated from various Calceolaria species. In models of acute nociception induced by thermal stimuli, such as the hot plate and tail flick test, calceolarioside administered at doses of 1, 5, and 10 µg in the left cerebral ventricles did not modify the behavioral response of mice. In an inflammatory based persistent pain model as the formalin test, calceolarioside A at the high dose tested (100 µg/paw) reduced the licking activity induced by formalin by 35% in the first phase and by 75% in the second phase of the test. In carrageenan-induced thermal hyperalgesia, calceolarioside A (50 and 100 µg/paw) was able to significantly reverse thermal hyperalgesia induced by carrageenan. The anti-inflammatory activity of calceolarioside A was then assessed using the zymosan-induced paw edema model. Calceolarioside A (50 and 100 µg/paw) induced a significant reduction in the edema from 1 to 4 h after zymosan administration. Measuring IL-6, TNFα, and IL-1β pro-inflammatory cytokines released from LPS-stimulated THP-1 cells, calceolarioside A in a concentration-dependent manner reduced the release of these cytokines from THP-1 cells. Taken together, our results highlight, for the first time, the potential and selective anti-inflammatory properties of this natural-derived compound, prompting its rationale use for further investigations.

Keywords: calceolarioside A; nociception; inflammation; phenylpropanoid glycosides; Calceolaria

1. Introduction

Plant-derived molecules are a primary source of drugs, also evaluated as possible drugs for anti-inflammatory effects. Research on new plant-derived compounds is driven by the fact that, although several agents are available to treat various inflammatory diseases, their prolonged use can cause serious adverse effects. Nonsteroidal anti-inflammatory drugs (NSAIDs) inhibit the early stages of prostaglandin biosynthesis through cyclooxygenase (COX) inhibition. NSAIDs are essential drugs used to fight inflammation, but chronic use of NSAIDs is linked to cardiovascular, gastrointestinal, and renal toxicities [1,2]. Similarly, the use of corticosteroids leads to hypertension, hyperglycemia, osteoporosis, and stunting [3], and the development of safer anti-inflammatory agents remains a topic of great interest. Many studies on plant species in folk medicine for inflammation have

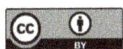

recognized the potential of natural products as possible anti-inflammatory drugs [4]. The anti-inflammatory effects of plant-derived molecules are exerted through their action on critical regulatory molecules, including cyclooxygenase (COX), lipoxygenase (LOX), and cytokines [5,6].

Phenylpropanoid glycosides (PPGs) are acylated glycoconjugates carrying a substituted arylalkyl aglycon, and acylation occurs mainly on the primary hydroxyl group with a residue derived from cinnamoyl. Phenylpropanoid glycosides are secondary metabolites widely distributed in plants with potential therapeutic properties including anti-inflammatory, analgesic, immunomodulatory, and radical scavenging [7,8].

In a previous paper, the common presence of phenylpropanoid glycosides has been reported, i.e., verbascoside (actoside), forsythoside A, isoarenarioside, and calceolarioside A–E from the methanolic extract of several Chilean Calceolaria species [9,10]. The antinociceptive and anti-inflammatory properties of verbascoside and forsythoside A have already been described [7,8], whereas no literature data are available on the effects induced by isoarenarioside or calceolarioside A-E on nociception or inflammation. Therefore, as a starting point in the pharmacological characterization of these compounds, the present study aimed to investigate, for the first time, the antinociceptive potential of calceolarioside A (Figure 1) in thermal and inflammatory models of nociception. We also evaluated calceolarioside A anti-inflammatory effects in an animal model of edema and on LPS-induced cytokine release from human macrophages. The results illustrate the antinociceptive and anti-inflammatory properties of the natural compound calceolarioside A and may help in the development of a new therapeutic strategy for pain and inflammation, particularly in view of its reduction in cytokine release from human macrophages.

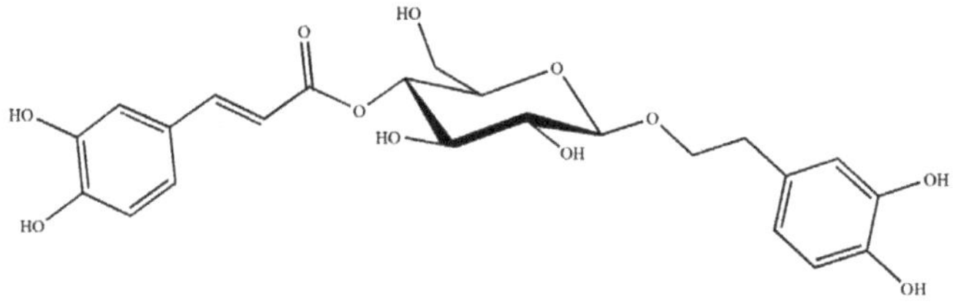

Calceolarioside A

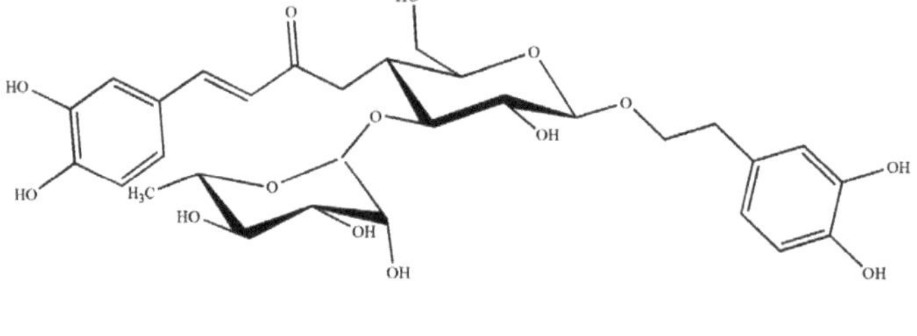

Verbascoside

Figure 1. Structures of calceolarioside A and verbascoside.

2. Results

2.1. Effects of Calceolarioside A in Animal Models of Nociception

Hot plate and tail-flick tests were employed to assess drug effects on nociception [11]. In our experiments, we administered calceolarioside A at doses of 1, 5, and 10 µg in the left cerebral ventricles of mice who underwent the hot plate and the tail-flick tests. The results obtained in these experiments are reported in Figure 2. After central administration, regardless of the dose used, calceolarioside A did not modify the behavioral response to thermal nociceptive stimuli, both in the hot plate and in the tail-flick test (Figure 2).

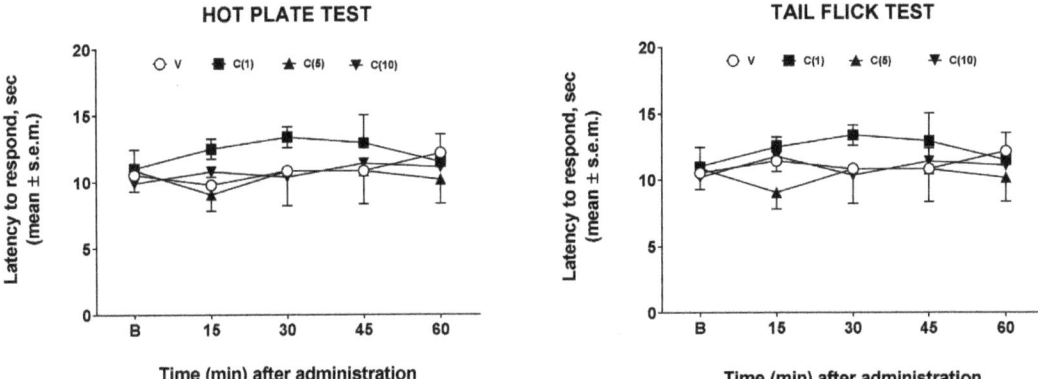

Figure 2. Effects induced by calceolarioside A administered i.c.v. at doses of 1, 5, and 10 µg (C(1–10)) in the hot plate (**left panel**) and tail flick test (**right panel**). Calceolarioside A did not change the response to thermal nociceptive stimuli. Statistical analysis was performed by using two-way ANOVA followed by Dunnett's multiple comparisons test. N = 7.

Then, we investigated the effects of calceolarioside A in another nociception model, e.g., the formalin test [12]. This test can be considered an inflammatory-based persistent pain model. In this case, we administered calceolarioside A at doses of 10, 50, and 100 µg s.c. in the hind paw of the mouse 30 min before formalin. The results of these experiments are shown in Figure 3.

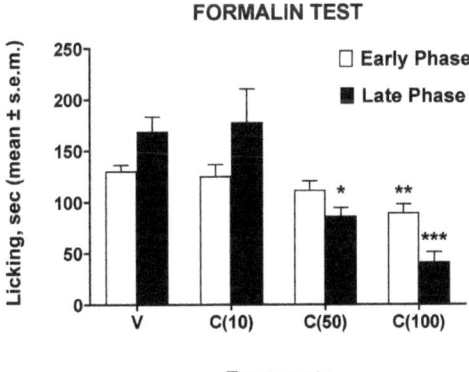

Figure 3. Effects induced by calceolarioside A administered s.c. into the mice hind paw at doses of 10, 50, and 100 µg (C(10–100)), 30 min before the formalin (1%, 20 µL/paw). Statistical analysis of the early and late phase was performed by using one-way ANOVA followed by Dunnett's multiple comparisons test. * $p < 0.05$, ** $p < 0.01$, and *** $p < 0.001$ vs. V (vehicle-treated animals). N = 7.

In the formalin test, administration of calceolarioside A at a dose of 10 µg did not change the animals' behavioral response induced by formalin. Calceolarioside A (50 µg) induced a nonsignificant reduction (by 14%, compared to the control group) in the licking time induced by the aldehyde in the early phase of the test, while it was able to reduce significantly (by 49%, compared to the control group) the noxious response in the late phase. These effects on the early and late phase induced by calceolarioside A were even more evident after the administration of the 100 μg dose, capable of significantly reducing the nociceptive effect of formalin both in the early (by 31%, compared to the control group) and in the late phase (by 75%, compared to the control group) of the test.

From the results obtained in the formalin test, an effect of calceolarioside A in this model of persistent inflammation is highlighted. However, studies on inflammatory pain use compounds with strong antigenic potential such as carrageenans, sulfated polysaccharides extracted from seaweed. Paw injection of this compound induces thermal and mechanical allodynia and hyperalgesia for at least several hours [11]. Therefore, we used carrageenan to reduce the nociceptive threshold to study the possible anti-hyperalgesic effects of calceolarioside A. Carrageenan induced a strong hyperalgesic effect under our experimental condition, 3–4 h after its administration. Thus, we administered s.c. calceolarioside A at doses of 10, 50, and 100 μg s.c. into the mice hind paw, 2.5 h after carrageenan. The anti-hyperalgesic effects of calceolarioside A could be observed in carrageenan-induced hyperalgesia (Figure 4). Treatment with calceolarioside A at 50 and 100 μg was able to significantly reduce thermal hyperalgesia induced by carrageenan, 3 and 4 h after its administration, compared to the control group (Figure 4).

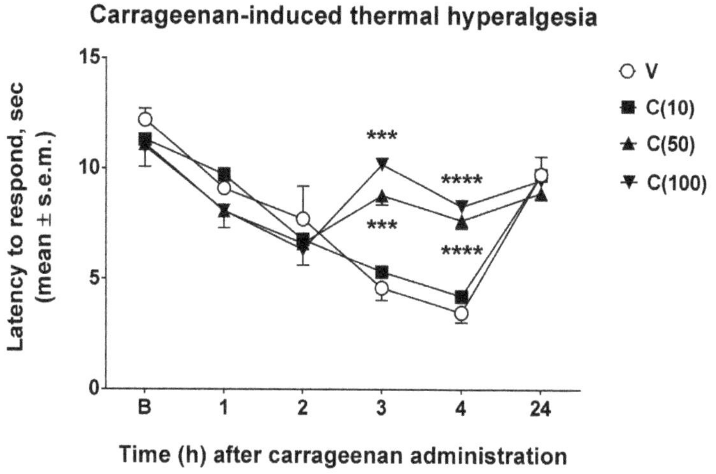

Figure 4. Effects induced by calceolarioside A on carrageenan-induced thermal hyperalgesia. Calceolarioside A was administered s.c. into the mice hind paw at doses of 10, 50, and 100 μg (C(10–100)), 2.5 h after carrageenan (20 μL of 1% carrageenan) administration in the same paw. Statistical analysis was performed by using two-way ANOVA followed by Dunnett's multiple comparisons test. *** $p < 0.001$ and **** $p < 0.0001$ vs. V (vehicle-treated animals). N = 7.

2.2. Effects of Calceolarioside A in Animal Model of Edema

Following the observed antinociceptive effects of calceolarioside A in inflammatory pain models, we aimed to understand if calceolarioside A is able to counteract the formation of edema. Zymosan-induced paw edema is a well-known experimental model to study acute inflammation and the mechanisms of inflammatory pain [13]. Herein, we addressed whether calceolarioside A inhibits zymosan-induced paw edema. Mice were pretreated with different doses of calceolarioside (10, 50, and 100 μg) s.c. into the mice hind paw, 30 min before zymosan s.c. injection in the same manner, and edema were evaluated from 1 to 24 h after the stimulus. As shown in Figure 5, the edema formation was significantly inhibited by calceolarioside A tested at 50 and 100 μg/paw.

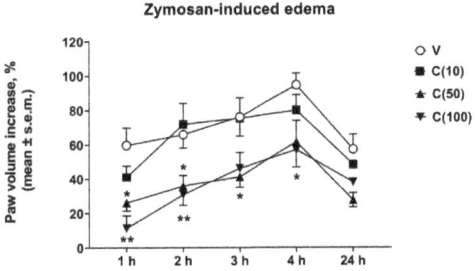

Figure 5. Effects induced by calceolarioside A administered s.c. into the mice hind paw at doses of 10, 50, and 100 μg (C(10–100)), 30 min before zymosan (2.5% w/v in saline, 20 μL/paw) administration in the same paw. Statistical analysis was performed by using two-way ANOVA followed by Dunnett's multiple comparisons test. * $p < 0.05$ and ** $p < 0.01$ vs. V (vehicle-treated animals). N = 7.

2.3. Calceolarioside A Effects on LPS-Induced Cytokine Release from Human Macrophage

LPS is a TLR4-specific agonist described as a potent inducer of inflammatory responses in macrophages [14]. To see whether cytokine production is influenced by calceolarioside A, THP-1 cells were treated with an increasing amount of calceolarioside A in the presence of LPS and cytokine secretion was measured from the medium of the cells using ELISA methods. In addition, the toxicity of calceolarioside A on THP-1 cells was accessed to determine the adequate calceolarioside working concentrations. When the cell viability of THP-1 cells was higher than 90%, samples were considered noncytotoxic and adequate for further analysis. The results obtained in these experiments are reported in Figure 6. In agreement with previous reports [14], we found that LPS treatment significantly induced the production of IL-6, TNFα, and IL-1β pro-inflammatory cytokines (Figure 6). While calceolarioside A, at the tested concentrations, did not affect the production of the aforementioned cytokines in THP 1 cells (data not shown) without any effect on macrophages, it significantly reduced the LPS-induced secretion of these cytokines in THP-1 cells in a concentration-dependent manner (Figure 6).

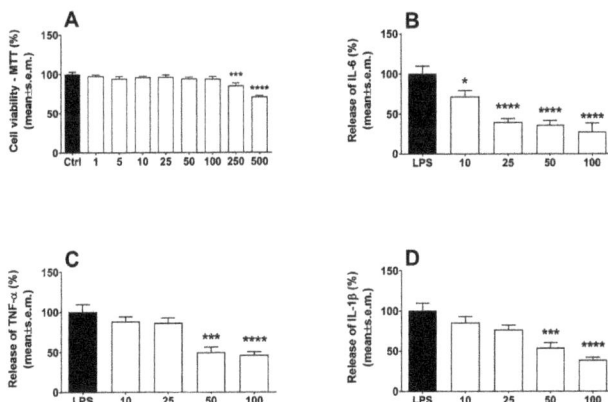

Figure 6. Effects induced by calceolarioside A on cell viability (**A**) and LPS-induced IL-6 (**B**), TNF-α (**C**), and IL-1β (**D**) release in macrophages. Macrophages were exposed for 24 h to 10, 25, 50, and 100 μg mL^{-1} of calceolarioside A. Results were obtained from three separate experiments performed in duplicate and reported as mean ± SEM. Statistical analysis was performed by one-way ANOVA followed by Dunnett's multiple comparisons test. * $p < 0.05$, *** $p < 0.001$, and **** $p < 0.0001$ vs. LPS.

3. Discussion

The results of our study demonstrate, for the first time, the selective and stimulus-dependent antinociceptive and anti-inflammatory effects of calceolarioside A. These effects confirm that PPGs are a class of natural substances capable of inducing interesting analgesic and anti-inflammatory effects, observed for various compounds isolated from different plant species [7,8]. As far as calceolarioside A is concerned, very little data are available in the literature on its biological effects. In a previous study, it was found that calceolarioside A induced a dose-related aggregant effect on rabbit platelets, partly dependent upon a calcium-dependent mechanism [15]. More recently, it was reported that calceolarioside A induced moderate antibacterial activity against *Bacillus cereus NRRLB 3711* [16], antifungal activity against *Malassenzia* spp. [17], and collagenase inhibitory activity [18] and putative anti-viral activity against COVID-19 from docking and molecular dynamics simulation data [19].

Other literature data on calceolarioside A may help us to provide a hypothesis on the mechanism by which this compound induces the antinociceptive and anti-inflammatory effects observed in our experiments. In a study examining the protective effect on adriamycin-induced cardiomyocyte toxicity, calceolarioside A significantly inhibited the adriamycin-induced cell death and caspase-3 activation, decreased the level of intracellular reactive oxygen species, and was more effective than those observed with the other antioxidants, including probucol, ascorbic acid, and alpha-tocopherol [20]. Another study later confirmed the antioxidant properties of calceolarioside A. As a part of research for antioxidative constituents from the genus *Buddleja*, Ahmad et al. [21] investigated the antioxidative activities of calceolarioside A isolated from *Buddleja davidii*. In fresh prepared rat kidney homogenates, calceolarioside A displayed strong scavenging potential for HO$^{\bullet}$, total ROS, and scavenging of ONOO– [21]. Production of ROS and reactive nitrogen species (RNS) is central to the progression of many inflammatory diseases, and ROS act as both a signaling molecule and a mediator of inflammation [22]. ROS produced in oxidative metabolism and some natural or artificial chemicals have been reported to initiate the inflammatory process, resulting in the synthesis and secretion of proinflammatory cytokines [22]. The activation of nuclear factor-kappa B/active protein-1 (NF-κB/AP-1) and production of pro-inflammatory cytokines, mainly IL-1β, IL-12, IL-6, and TNF-α, have been, for instance, documented to play a critical role in the inflammatory and pain process, resulting in several chronic diseases [23]. In a recent study, and in line with what we observed in the experiments conducted on THP-1 cells, calceolarioside A was not cytotoxic to either mouse spleen cells or U266 cells, and strongly inhibited IgE production in U266 cells and IL-2 production in mouse spleen cells, in a dose-dependent manner [24].

Thus, the antioxidant effects of calceolarioside A could explain the antinociceptive and anti-inflammatory effects observed in our in vivo and in vitro experiments. However, other hypotheses can also be formulated. In 1988, Zhou and collaborators [25] reported the isolation of several phenylpropanoid glycosides from *Digitalis purpurea* and *Penstemon linarioides*, including calceolarioside A. These compounds were tested for their inhibitory activity against PKCα, and calceolarioside A was found to be the most active in inhibiting PKCα with IC$_{50}$ values of 0.6 mM. PKCα has been implicated in various cellular functions, including proliferation, apoptosis, differentiation, motility, pain, and inflammation. The roles of central PKC in various pain states have intensively been investigated during the past decade. PKCα is an essential regulator of ion channel and membrane excitability in DRG neurons [26], and it has been reported that phosphorylated PKC increases in DRGs of MIA-induced rat joint pain [27]. Interestingly, the intraplantar injection of chelerythrine chloride, a PKC inhibitor, dose-dependently inhibited bee venom-induced nociception and inflammation in rats [28], and these findings resemble that which occurred in our in vivo experiments after calceolarioside A administration.

4. Materials and Methods

4.1. Drugs

Calceolarioside A (Figure 1) was obtained from *Calceolaria hypericina* Poepp. ex D. C., as previously reported [9]. The aerial parts of *Calceolaria hypericina* Poepp. ex D. C. were collected in Cuesta Zapata, V region, Chile, and identified at the Universidad Federico Santa Maria, Valparaiso, Chile where a specimen was deposited. In the general procedure, the aerial parts were extracted with EtOH at room temperature and, after evaporation, the residue of the extract separated by counter-current distribution with a biphasic solvent system composed of EtOAt:n-BuOH:H_2O in a suitable composition. The presence of calceolarioside A and other phenylpropanoid glycosides was determined by HPLC [9]. Calceolarioside A was stored at $-20\ °C$ until its use for in vivo and in vitro experiments. Carrageenan and zymosan A were purchased from Sigma-Aldrich (Milan, Italy). Dimethyl sulfoxide (DMSO) and formalin were purchased from Merck (Rome, Italy). Unless otherwise stated, all the other reagents were purchased from Carlo Erba (Milan, Italy).

4.2. Animals and Experimental Protocols

Male CD-1 mice (Harlan, Italy) of 3–4 weeks (25 g) were used for all the experiments. Mice were housed in colony cages, under standard conditions of light, temperature, and relative humidity for at least 1 week before starting experimental sessions. All experiments were performed according to Legislative Decree 27/92 and approved by the local ethics committee (Approval number 198/2013-B). Animal studies were performed in accordance to the ARRIVE guidelines [29].

4.3. Hot Plate Test

The hot-plate test was performed as described earlier [30]. A transparent plastic cylinder (14 cm diameter, 31 cm height) was used to confine the mouse on the heated ($55 \pm 0.5\ °C$) surface of the plate. The baseline latency was calculated as a mean of three readings recorded before testing at intervals of 15 min. The animals were placed on the hot plate 15 min after the i.c.v. injection of the vehicle (DMSO 1% solution in saline) or calceolarioside A (1, 5, and 10 µg), and the latencies to paw licking, rearing, or jumping were measured 15, 30, 45, and 60 min after administration. A cut-off time of 60 s was used to avoid tissue injury. The injection volume was 5 µL/mouse.

4.4. Tail Flick Test

The tail flick latency was obtained using a commercial unit (Ugo Basile, Gemonio, Italy), consisting of an infrared radiant light source (100 W, 15 V bulb) focused onto a photocell utilizing an aluminum parabolic mirror [31,32]. During the trials, the mice were gently hand-restrained using leather gloves. Radiant heat was focused 3–4 cm from the tip of the tail, and the latency (s) of the tail withdrawal to the thermal stimulus was recorded. The measurement was interrupted if the latency exceeded the cut-off time (15 s). The baseline latency was calculated as the mean of three readings recorded before testing at intervals of 15 min, and the time course of latency was determined at 15, 30, 45, and 60 min after i.c.v. injection of vehicle (DMSO 1% solution in saline) or calceolarioside A (1, 5, and 10 µg/5 µL). The injection volume was 5 µL/mouse.

4.5. Formalin Test

The procedure used has been previously described [33,34]. Subcutaneous (s.c.) injection of a dilute solution of formalin (1%, 20 µL/paw) into the mice hind paw evokes nociceptive behavioral responses, such as licking or biting the injected paw, which are considered indices of pain. The nociceptive response shows a biphasic trend, consisting of an early phase occurring from 0 to 10 min after the formalin injection, due to the direct stimulation of peripheral nociceptors, followed by a late prolonged phase occurring from 10 to 40 min, which reflects the response to inflammatory pain. During the test, the mouse was placed in a plexiglass observation cage (30 cm × 14 cm × 12 cm), 1 h before the formalin administration to allow it to acclimatize to its surroundings. Immediately after the formalin injection, the mouse was returned to the plexiglass observation cage, and nociceptive behavior was continuously measured using a stopwatch for 5 min intervals for a total testing time of 40 min. The total time(s) that the animal spent licking or biting its paw during the formalin-induced early and late phase of nociception was recorded. Calceolarioside A was dissolved in DMSO:saline (ratio 1:3 v/v) and then administered s.c. into the mice hind paw at a dose of 10, 50, and 100 µg in a volume of 20 µL, 30 min before the formalin (1%, 20 µL/paw).

4.6. Carrageenan-Induced Thermal Hyperalgesia

The plantar test (Ugo Basile, Italy) was used to measure the sensitivity to a noxious heat stimulus to assess thermal hyperalgesia after carrageenan administration [34,35]. A constant radiant heat source was directed on a mouse footpad until its withdrawal, foot drumming, or licking. A timer started automatically when the heat source was activated and a photocell stopped the timer when the mouse withdrew its hind paw. Animals were acclimatized to their environment for 1 h before the measurements of paw withdrawal latency (PWL), when exploratory behavior had ceased. The heat intensity was adjusted to obtain a baseline between 10 and 15 s, and a 30 s cut-off was used to avoid tissue damage. A total of 3 readings were taken from each paw and averaged. Animals were first tested to determine their baseline PWL to respond; 2 h later, each animal received an s.c. injection of 20 µL of 1% carrageenan into the dorsal surface of the right hind paw. The PWL (s) of each animal to the plantar test was determined again at 1, 2, 3, 4, and 24 h after the carrageenan injection. Mice received an s.c. injection of calceolarioside A (10, 50, or 100 µg/20 µL paw) into the dorsal surface of the right hind paw, 2.5 h after carrageenan. Calceolarioside A was dissolved in DMSO:saline (ratio 1:3 v/v).

4.7. Zymosan-Induced Paw Edema

Mice received an s.c. administration (20 µL/paw) of zymosan A (2.5% w/v in saline) into the dorsal surface of the right hind paw [36]. Paw volume was measured 3 times before the injections and at 1, 2, 3, 4, and 24 h thereafter using a hydroplethysmometer apparatus (Ugo Basile, Italy). The increase in paw volume was then evaluated as the percentage difference between the paw volume at each time point and the basal paw volume. Calceolarioside A dissolved in DMSO:saline (ratio 1:3 v/v) at increasing doses (1, 10, or 100 µg/20 µL paw) was administered s.c. into the dorsal surface of the right hind paw 30 min before zymosan.

4.8. Assay of Calceolarioside Anti-Inflammatory Activity on LPS-Stimulated Macrophage

Human peripheral blood monocytic cell line THP-1 was purchased from the American Type Culture Collection (Bethesda, MD, USA). Cells were maintained in RPMI-1640 medium supplemented with 2 mM L-glutamine and 100 U mL^{-1} of streptomycin-penicillin and 10% heat-inactivated fetal bovine serum (Sigma Aldrich, St. Louis, MO, USA) at 37 °C with 5% CO_2. THP-1 cells were plated in 6-well culture plates at 1×10^6 cells/well and were differentiated to macrophages using 100 ng mL^{-1} of phorbol-12-myristate-13-acetate (PMA, St. Louis, MO, USA) for 24 h with serum-free RPMI-1640 at 37 °C. After 72 h, the cells were treated with LPS at a final concentration of 0.1 µg mL^{-1} to stimulate cytokine production and with calceolarioside A at 10, 25, 50, and 100 µg mL^{-1}. After 24 h of incubation, the supernatant was removed and centrifuged to remove any cell residues. The IL-6, IL-1β, and TNFα release was quantified using an ELISA, according to the manufacturer's protocol (R&D Systems, Minneapolis, MN, USA).

In parallel, the effects of calceolarioside A on the viability of the LPS-stimulated macrophages were assessed using the 3-(4,5-dimethylthiazol-2-yl)-2,5-diphenyltetrazolium bromide (MTT) assay. After 24 h of exposure to calceolarioside A 1, 5, 10, 25, 50, 100, 250, and 500 µg mL^{-1}, 20 µL of MTT (1 mg mL^{-1} in PBS) was added to each well and incubated continuously for 4 h under normal culture conditions. The cells were then treated with 100 µL of DMSO. The absorbance was measured at 570 nm using a microplate reader (Thermo MK3, Winosky, VT, USA). Data were expressed as a percentage of the value obtained for the solvent control (0.1% DMSO), which was set to 100%.

To reduce any variation from differences in cell density, the ELISA results were normalized to the MTT values. The concentration of cytokines of the positive control (cells only treated with LPS) was defined as 100%. All results from the tested calceolarioside A were then calculated as a percentage of the positive control [37].

5. Conclusions

In this study, we demonstrated for the first time the antinociceptive and anti-inflammatory effects of calceolarioside A. Calceolarioside A induced stimulus-dependent antinociceptive effects, as it reduced nociception induced by inflammatory stimuli but not by thermal nociceptive stimuli. This effect could be secondary to its anti-inflammatory properties, demonstrated in vivo in an edema model and in vitro in human macrophages. These data confirm the analgesic and anti-inflammatory properties of PPGs and indicate that this class of natural compound might represent a new therapeutic strategy for fighting pain-associated inflammatory diseases.

Author Contributions: Conceptualization, S.P., A.M.A. and M.N.; methodology, S.P., A.M. and A.M.A.; validation, A.M.A. and A.M.; formal analysis, S.P.; investigation, A.S. (Anella Saviano), A.S. (Azzurra Stefanucci) and S.P.; resources, A.S. (Anella Saviano) and A.S. (Azzurra Stefanucci); data curation, A.S. (Anella Saviano), S.P. and A.S. (Azzurra Stefanucci); writing—original draft preparation, S.P. and A.M.; writing—review and editing, A.M.A. and M.N.; visualization, A.S. (Anella Saviano) and A.S. (Azzurra Stefanucci); supervision, S.P., A.M.A. and M.N.; project administration, S.P. and A.M.A.; funding acquisition, S.P. All authors have read and agreed to the published version of the manuscript.

Funding: This research was funded by Istituto Superiore di Sanità, Rome, Italy, via the intramural research supporting fund.

Institutional Review Board Statement: The animal study protocol was approved by the Institutional Review Board of Istituto Superiore di Sanità (Approval number 198/2013-B) for studies involving animals.

Informed Consent Statement: Not applicable.

Data Availability Statement: Data relating to this research are available upon request.

Conflicts of Interest: The authors declare no conflict of interest.

Sample Availability: Samples of calceolarioside A are available from the authors.

References

1. Furman, D.; Campisi, J.; Verdin, E.; Carrera-Bastos, P.; Targ, S.; Franceschi, C.; Ferrucci, L.; Gilroy, D.W.; Fasano, A.; Miller, G.W.; et al. Chronic inflammation in the etiology of disease across the life span. *Nat. Med.* **2019**, *25*, 1822–1832. [CrossRef] [PubMed]
2. Bindu, S.; Mazumder, S.; Bandyopadhyay, U. Non-steroidal anti-inflammatory drugs (NSAIDs) and organ damage: A current perspective. *Biochem. Pharmacol.* **2020**, *180*, 114147. [CrossRef] [PubMed]
3. Rice, J.B.; White, A.G.; Scarpati, L.M.; Wan, G.; Nelson, W.W. Long-term Systemic Corticosteroid Exposure: A Systematic Literature Review. *Clin. Ther.* **2017**, *39*, 2216–2229. [CrossRef]
4. Yatoo, M.I.; Gopalakrishnan, A.; Saxena, A.; Parray, O.R.; Tufani, N.A.; Chakraborty, S.; Tiwari, R.; Dhama, K.; Iqbal, H.M.N. Anti-Inflammatory Drugs and Herbs with Special Emphasis on Herbal Medicines for Countering Inflammatory Diseases and Disorders-A Review. *Recent Pat. Inflamm. Allergy Drug Discov.* **2018**, *12*, 39–58. [CrossRef]
5. Yahfoufi, N.; Alsadi, N.; Jambi, M.; Matar, C. The Immunomodulatory and Anti-Inflammatory Role of Polyphenols. *Nutrients* **2018**, *10*, 1618. [CrossRef] [PubMed]
6. Milia, E.; Bullitta, S.M.; Mastandrea, G.; Szotáková, B.; Schoubben, A.; Langhansová, L.; Quartu, M.; Bortone, A.; Eick, S. Leaves and Fruits Preparations of *Pistacia lentiscus* L.: A Review on the Ethnopharmacological Uses and Implications in Inflammation and Infection. *Antibiotics* **2021**, *10*, 425. [CrossRef] [PubMed]
7. Pan, J.; Yuan, C.; Lin, C.; Jia, Z.; Zheng, R. Pharmacological activities and mechanisms of natural phenylpropanoid glycosides. *Pharmazie* **2003**, *58*, 767–775. [CrossRef]
8. Kurkin, V.A. Phenylpropanoids from medicinal plants: Distribution, classification, structural analysis, and biological activity. *Chem. Nat. Compd.* **2003**, *39*, 123–153. [CrossRef]

9. Nicoletti, M.; Galeffi, C.; Messana, I.; Marini-Bettolo, G.B.; Garbarino, J.A.; Gambaro, V. Phenylpropanoid glycosides from *Calceolaria hypericina*. *Phytochemistry* **1988**, *27*, 639–641. [CrossRef]
10. Di Fabio, A.; Bruni, A.; Poli, F.; Garbarino, J.A.; Chamy, M.C.; Piovano, M.; Nicoletti, M. The Distribution of Phenylpropanoid Glycosides in Chilean *Calceolaria* spp. *Biochem. Syst. Ecol.* **1995**, *23*, 179–182. [CrossRef]
11. Barrot, M. Test and models of nociception and pain in rodents. *Neuroscience* **2012**, *211*, 39–50. [CrossRef]
12. Capone, F.; Aloisi, A.M. Refinement of pain evaluation techniques. The formalin test. *Ann. Ist. Super. Sanita* **2004**, *40*, 223–229. [PubMed]
13. Suo, J.; Linke, B.; Meyer dos Santos, S.; Pierre, S.; Stegner, D.; Zhang, D.D.; Denis, C.V.; Geisslinger, G.; Nieswandt, B.; Scholich, K. Neutrophils mediate edema formation but not mechanical allodynia during zymosan-induced inflammation. *J. Leukoc. Biol.* **2014**, *96*, 133–142. [CrossRef]
14. Rossol, M.; Heine, H.; Meusch, U.; Quandt, D.; Klein, C.; Sweet, M.J.; Hauschildt, S. LPS-Induced Cytokine Production in Human Monocytes and Macrophages. *Crit. Rev. Immunol.* **2011**, *31*, 379–446. [CrossRef] [PubMed]
15. Capasso, A.; Di Giannuario, A.; Pieretti, S.; Nicoletti, M. Platelet Aggregation Induced by Calceolarioside A in vitro: Role of platelet Intracellular Calcium. *Planta Med.* **1993**, *59*, 337–339. [CrossRef] [PubMed]
16. Kirmizibekmez, H.; Kúsz, N.; Karaca, N.; Demirci, F.; Hohmann, J. Secondary Metabolites from the Leaves of *Digitalis viridiflora*. *Nat. Prod. Commun.* **2017**, *12*, 59–61. [CrossRef] [PubMed]
17. Mishra, R.K.; Mishra, V.; Pandey, A.; Tiwari, A.K.; Pandey, H.; Sharma, S.; Pandey, A.C.; Dikshit, A. Exploration of anti-*Malassezia* potential of *Nyctanthes arbor-tristis* L. and their application to combat the infection caused by Mala s1 a novel allergen. *BMC Complement. Altern. Med.* **2016**, *16*, 114. [CrossRef] [PubMed]
18. Morikawa, T.; Inoue, N.; Nakanishi, Y.; Manse, Y.; Matsuura, H.; Okino, K.; Hamasaki, S.; Yoshikawa, M.; Muraoka, O.; Ninomiya, K. Collagen synthesis-promoting and collagenase inhibitory activities of constituents isolated from the rhizomes of *Picrorhiza kurroa* Royle ex Benth. *Fitoterapia* **2020**, *143*, 104584. [CrossRef] [PubMed]
19. Adem, Ş.; Eyupoglu, V.; Sarfraz, I.; Rasul, A.; Zahoor, A.F.; Ali, M.; Abdalla, M.; Ibrahim, I.M.; Elfiky, A.A. Caffeic acid derivatives (CAFDs) as inhibitors of SARS-CoV-2: CAFDs-based functional foods as a potential alternative approach to combat COVID-19. *Phytomedicine* **2021**, *85*, 153310. [CrossRef]
20. Kim, D.S.; Kim, H.R.; Woo, E.R.; Kwon, D.Y.; Kim, M.S.; Chae, S.W.; Chae, H.J. Protective effect of calceolarioside on adriamycin-induced cardiomyocyte toxicity. *Eur. J. Pharmacol.* **2006**, *541*, 24–32. [CrossRef] [PubMed]
21. Ahmad, I.; Ahmad, N.; Wang, F.J. Antioxidant phenylpropanoid glycosides from Buddleja davidii. *Enzyme Inhib. Med. Chem.* **2009**, *24*, 993–997. [CrossRef] [PubMed]
22. Mittal, M.; Siddiqui, M.R.; Tran, K.; Reddy, S.P.; Malik, A.B. Reactive oxygen species in inflammation and tissue injury. *Antioxid. Redox Signal.* **2014**, *20*, 1126–1167. [CrossRef] [PubMed]
23. Zhang, J.M.; An, J. Cytokines, inflammation, and pain. *Int. Anesthesiol. Clin.* **2007**, *45*, 27–37. [CrossRef] [PubMed]
24. Chen, Y.; Xue, G.; Liu, F.; Gong, X. Immunosuppressive effect of extracts from leaves of *Fraxinus Mandshurica* Rupr. *Bioengineered* **2017**, *8*, 212–216. [CrossRef] [PubMed]
25. Zhou, B.N.; Bahler, B.D.; Hofmann, G.A.; Mattern, M.R.; Johnson, R.K.; Kingston, D.G. Phenylethanoid glycosides from *Digitalis purpurea* and *Penstemon linarioides* with PKCalpha-inhibitory activity. *J. Nat. Prod.* **1998**, *61*, 1410–1412. [CrossRef] [PubMed]
26. He, Y.; Wang, Z.J. Nociceptor beta II, delta, and epsilon isoforms of PKC differentially mediate paclitaxel-induced spontaneous and evoked pain. *J. Neurosci.* **2015**, *35*, 4614–4625. [CrossRef]
27. Koda, K.; Hyakkoku, K.; Ogawa, K.; Takasu, K.; Imai, S.; Sakurai, Y.; Fujita, M.; Ono, H.; Yamamoto, M.; Fukuda, I.; et al. Sensitization of TRPV1 by protein kinase C in rats with monoiodoacetate-induced joint pain. *Osteoarthr. Cartil.* **2016**, *24*, 1254–1262. [CrossRef]
28. Chen, H.S.; Lei, J.; He, X.; Qu, F.; Wang, Y.; Wen, W.W.; You, H.; Arendt-Nielsen, L. Peripheral involvement of PKA and PKC in subcutaneous bee venom-induced persistent nociception, mechanical hyperalgesia, and inflammation in rats. *Pain* **2008**, *135*, 31–36. [CrossRef] [PubMed]
29. Kilkenny, C.; Browne, W.J.; Cuthill, I.C.; Emerson, M.; Altman, D.G. Improving bioscience research reporting: The ARRIVE guidelines for reporting animal research. *PLoS Biol.* **2010**, *8*, e1000412. [CrossRef]
30. Biancalani, C.; Giovannoni, M.P.; Pieretti, S.; Cesari, N.; Graziano, A.; Vergelli, C.; Cilibrizzi, A.; Di Giannuario, A.; Colucci, M.; Mangano, G.; et al. Further studies on arylpiperazinyl alkyl pyridazinones: Discovery of an exceptionally potent, orally active, antinociceptive agent in thermally induced pain. *J. Med. Chem.* **2009**, *52*, 7397–7409. [CrossRef]
31. DellaValle, A.; Stefanucci, A.; Scioli, G.; Szűcs, E.; Benyhe, S.; Pieretti, S.; Minosi, P.; Sturaro, C.; Calò, G.; Zengin, G.; et al. Selective MOR activity of DAPEA and Endomorphin-2 analogues containing a (R)-γ-Freidinger lactam in position two. *Bioorg. Chem.* **2021**, *115*, 105219. [CrossRef] [PubMed]
32. Mollica, A.; Costante, R.; Novellino, E.; Stefanucci, A.; Pieretti, S.; Zador, F.; Samavati, R.; Borsodi, A.; Benyhe, S.; Vetter, I.; et al. Design, Synthesis and Biological Evaluation of Two Opioid Agonist and Cav 2.2 Blocker Multitarget Ligands. *Chem. Biol. Drug Des.* **2015**, *86*, 156–162. [CrossRef] [PubMed]
33. Maione, F.; Colucci, M.; Raucci, F.; Mangano, G.; Marzoli, F.; Mascolo, N.; Crocetti, L.; Giovannoni, M.P.; Di Giannuario, A.; Pieretti, S. New insights on the arylpiperazinylalkyl pyridazinone ET1 as potent antinociceptive and anti-inflammatory agent. *Eur. J. Pharmacol.* **2020**, *888*, 173572. [CrossRef] [PubMed]

34. Mollica, A.; Costante, R.; Stefanucci, A.; Pinnen, F.; Lucente, G.; Fidanza, S.; Pieretti, S. Antinociceptive profile of potent opioid peptide AM94, a fluorinated analogue of biphalin with non-hydrazine linker. *J. Pept. Sci.* **2013**, *19*, 233–239. [CrossRef] [PubMed]
35. Hargreaves, K.; Dubner, R.; Brown, F.; Flores, C.; Joris, J. A new and sensitive method for measuring thermal nociception in cutaneous hyperalgesia. *Pain* **1988**, *32*, 77–88. [CrossRef]
36. Rinaldi, F.; Del Favero, E.; Rondelli, V.; Pieretti, S.; Bogni, A.; Ponti, J.; Rossi, F.; Di Marzio, L.; Paolino, D.; Marianecci, C.; et al. ph-sensitive niosomes: Effects on cytotoxicity and on inflammation and pain in murine models. *J. Enzyme Inhib. Med. Chem.* **2017**, *32*, 538–546. [CrossRef] [PubMed]
37. Mollica, A.; Scioli, G.; Della Valle, A.; Cichelli, A.; Novellino, E.; Bauer, M.; Kamysz, W.; Llorent-Martínez, E.J.; Fernández-de Córdova, M.L.; Castillo-López, R.; et al. Phenolic Analysis and In Vitro Biological Activity of Red Wine, Pomace and Grape Seeds Oil Derived from *Vitis vinifera* L. cv. Montepulciano d'Abruzzo. *Antioxidants* **2021**, *10*, 1704. [CrossRef] [PubMed]

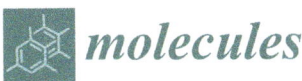

Article

In Vitro Bioaccessibility and Anti-Inflammatory Activity of a Chemically Characterized *Allium cepa* L. Extract Rich in Quercetin Derivatives Optimized by the Design of Experiments

Hammad Ullah [1,†], Alessandro Di Minno [1,2,†], Cristina Santarcangelo [1,†], Ariyawan Tantipongpiradet [1], Marco Dacrema [1], Rita di Matteo [1], Hesham R. El-Seedi [3,4], Shaden A. M. Khalifa [5], Alessandra Baldi [1], Antonietta Rossi [1] and Maria Daglia [1,4,*]

1 Department of Pharmacy, University of Napoli Federico II, Via D. Montesano 49, 80131 Naples, Italy
2 CEINGE-Biotecnologie Avanzate, Via Gaetano Salvatore 486, 80145 Naples, Italy
3 Pharmacognosy Group, Department of Pharmaceutical Biosciences, Uppsala University, Biomedical Centre, Box 591, SE 751 24 Uppsala, Sweden
4 International Research Center for Food Nutrition and Safety, Jiangsu University, Zhenjiang 212013, China
5 Department of Molecular Biosciences, The Wenner-Gren Institute, Stockholm University, SE 106 91 Stockholm, Sweden
* Correspondence: maria.daglia@unina.it
† These authors contributed equally to this work.

Abstract: *Allium cepa* L. is a highly consumed garden crop rich in biologically active phenolic and organosulfur compounds. This study aimed to assess the *in vitro* bioaccessibility and anti-inflammatory effect of a chemically characterized *A. cepa* extract rich in quercetin and its derivatives. Different varieties of *A. cepa* were studied; based on the highest total phenolic content, the "Golden" variety was selected. Its extracts, obtained from the tunicate bulb, tunic, and bulb, were subjected to determination of quercetin and its derivatives with LC-MS analysis and based on the highest total quercetin content, the tunic extract was utilized for further experiments. The extraction method was optimized through a design of experiment (DoE) method via full factorial design, which showed that 40% ethanol and 1 g tunic/20 mL solvent are the best extraction conditions. HPLC analysis of the optimized tunic extract identified 14 flavonols, including 10 quercetin derivatives. As far as *in vitro* bioaccessibility was concerned, the increases in some quercetin derivatives following the gastro-duodenal digestion process support the bioaccessibility of these bioactive compounds. Moreover, the extract significantly inhibited the production of PGE2 in stimulated J774 cell lines, while no effects of the tunic extract were observed against the release of IL-1β, TNF-α, and nitrites. The study provided insights into the optimized extraction conditions to obtain an *A. cepa* tunic extract rich in bioavailable quercetin derivatives with significant anti-inflammatory effects against PGE2.

Keywords: *Allium cepa* L.; quercetin; bioaccessibility; design of experiments; anti-inflammatory activity

1. Introduction

Allium cepa L. (Amaryllidaceae), also known as onion, is the second most important garden crop after the tomato, with production of approximately 101 million tons worldwide in 2019 [1]. The increased production and consumption of this crop owing to increased consumer demand is mainly due to its well-known nutritional and functional properties [2]. In fact, onion is one of the most popular ingredients in foods worldwide, is used in many traditional medicines, and is considered safe for humans, being consumed as a vegetable and herbal medicine since ancient times [3]. Hippocrates, the Greek physician, prescribed *A. cepa* as a diuretic, to battle pneumonia, and as a wound healer. In Indian, Turkish, and Pakistani traditional medicine, *A. cepa* has been used as a decotion as a blood purifier, for scurvy prevention, as an antimicrobial substance, for digestive, metabolic, and skin problems, and for insect bites [4]. Modern use of *A. cepa* includes *inter alia*, antioxidant, antithrombotic, antiplatelet, anticoagulant, and anti-inflammatory activities [5,6], anti-diabetic, hypoglycemic, anti-hyperlipidemic, and anti-hypertensive effects [7], and antimicrobial and immunoprotective properties [8].

Chemically, *A. cepa* contains a variety of bioactive compounds such as carbohydrate prebiotics (fructooligosaccharides), ascorbic acids, organosulfur compounds (diallyl monosulfide, diallyl disulfide, diallyl trisulfide, and diallyl tetrasulfide), and flavonoids (quercetin, luteolin, kaempferol, and anthocyanin). The flavonols most represented in onion are quercetin and its derivatives (i.e., quercetin aglycone, quercetin-3-monoglucoside, quercetin-4′-monoglucoside, quercetin-3,4′diglucoside, quercetin 7,4′-diglucoside, quercetin 3,7,4′-triglucoside, dihydroquercetin-3-monoglucoside, isorhamnetin 3-monoglucoside, isorhamnetin 4′-monoglucoside, and isorhamnetin 3,4′-diglucoside). Although quercetin is a flavonol ubiquitously present in vegetables and fruits, it is particularly concentrated in onions. In fact, *A. cepa* has 3 to 10 times higher content of quercetin (300 mg/kg), occurring mainly in the outer dry and semi-dry layers (tunics) as a result of sunlight exposure [9], than other vegetables commonly considered good sources of quercetin such as *Brassica oleracea* L. (100 mg/kg), *Malus domestica* Borkh. (50 mg/kg), and *Vaccinium caesariense* Mack. (40 mg/kg) [2,10].

Recent studies showed that the estimated intake of quercetin (expressed as quercetin aglycone equivalents) ranges from 3 to 40 mg/day in Western diets and can reach the intake of 250 mg/day in high fruit and vegetable consumers. Differently, the recommended doses of quercetin in food supplements range from 200 to 1000 mg/day. After the intake of quercetin and its derivatives, the human quercetin plasma concentrations are in the nanomolar range after the consumption of quercetin-rich foods, while human quercetin plasma concentrations increase to micromolar range upon quercetin-based food supplement intake. The different human quercetin plasma concentrations can be justified by the different intake of quercetin with diet and food supplements and the rather high half-lives of quercetin metabolites, ranging from 11 to 28 h, which help to achieve considerable plasma levels following food supplement consumption [11–13]. Only after adequate intake is quercetin reported to exert many physiological activities, including antioxidant, anti-inflammatory, analgesic, immunomodulatory, neuroprotective, anti-obesity, hepatoprotective, anti-diabetic, and anti-apoptotic activities, through the modulation of metabolism, regulation of DNA transcription, and activation of apoptosis [14].

Today the main source of quercetin used as an ingredient in dietary supplements is *Sophora japonica* L. but given the high demand of the market for quercetin-based food supplements, the possibility of producing extracts with a high content of quercetin from low-cost vegetables or by-products of the agri-food industry can be an excellent strategy to diversify the sources of quercetin. Therefore, considering onion's high production and low cost, this crop can be considered a good source to obtain quercetin-rich extracts, to be used as food supplements and functional food ingredients [15].

In this context, the aim of this study was to develop an *A. cepa* extract rich in quercetin and its derivatives to be used as a food supplement and functional food ingredient. Thus, since the chemical composition of *A. cepa* changes based on different varieties and agronomic conditions of the region in which onion is grown, extracts obtained from different *A. cepa* varieties were tested to evaluate the total polyphenol content (TPC). The variety that provided the extract with the highest TPC was selected. Then, to select the onion part containing the highest concentrations of quercetin and its derivatives, the most represented quercetin derivatives (quercetin 3,4′-diglucoside; quercetin 3-monoglucoside; quercetin 4′-monoglucoside, quercetin 4′-methyl-3′- glucoside, and quercetin aglycone) were identified and quantified in extracts obtained from different parts of the selected onion variety (i.e., tunicate bulb, bulb, and tunic). Based on the highest quercetin content, onion tunics obtained from the selected variety were extracted with an extraction method optimized through design of experiment (DoE). Finally, in view of possible applications as a food supplement and functional food ingredient, this onion tunic extract was submitted to determine its metabolic profiling, *in vitro* bioaccessibility, and anti-inflammatory activity.

2. Results

2.1. Content of Total Polyphenols in Tunicate Bulb Extracts Obtained from Different A. cepa Varieties

Total polyphenols content (TPC) in the extracts obtained from four different *A. cepa* varieties is reported in Table 1. Golden variety extract resulted in having the highest TPC in comparison with the other varieties and was selected for further experiments.

Table 1. Total polyphenol content (TPC) in four different *A. cepa* variety extracts.

Variety	Total Polyphenol Content (mg GAE/100 g)
Golden	44.03 ± 1.19 [a]
Yellow Elenka	35.77 ± 0.45 [b]
White Cenol	13.80 ± 0.81 [c]
White Orizaba	17.36 ± 0.74 [d]

Results are means ± standard deviations ($n = 3$). Different superscript letters (a, b, c, and d) indicate a statistically significant difference in TPC between four A. cepa extracts ($p < 0.05$). Statistical analysis results are reported in Table S2.

2.2. Determination of the Main Quercetin and Its Derivatives in Tunicate Bulb, Tunic, and Bulb Extracts Obtained from A. cepa Golden Variety

The extracts obtained from the tunicate bulb, tunic, and bulb of the *A. cepa* Golden variety were analyzed using RP-HPLC-PDA-ESI-MSn (Figure 1). The main peaks were identified as reported in Table 2.

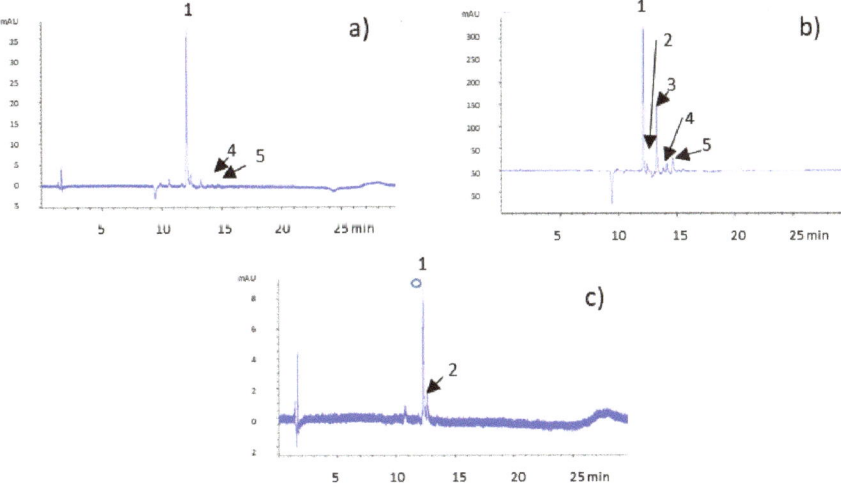

Figure 1. Chromatogram of *A. cepa* Golden variety extracts recorded at 370 nm. (**a**) Tunicate bulb extract, (**b**) tunic extract, and (**c**) bulb extract. Peaks shown are: (1) quercetin 3,4′-diglucoside, (2) quercetin 3-monoglucoside, (3) quercetin 4′-monoglucoside, (4) quercetin 4′-methyl-3′- glucoside, and (5) quercetin aglycone.

Peak 1 was identified as quercetin 3 4′-diglucoside with a parent ion at m/z 625, whose fragmentation pattern consisted of fragment ions at m/z 463 and 301, indicating the loss of two hexose residues (−162 amu) and formation of a fragment ion [M-H-301]⁻ which represents quercetin aglycone [16]. Peaks 2 and 3, presenting the same parent ion at m/z 463 but with different retention times, were assigned to quercetin 3-monoglucoside and quercetin 4′-monoglucoside, respectively. Fragmentation pattern analysis was carried out on the ions at m/z 301, 151, and 135 in line with literature data proposed for quercetin-associated flavonols [17]. Peak 4 showed [M-H]⁻ at m/z 477 and fragments with m/z 315 and 151, which correspond to quercetin 4′-methyl-3′- glucoside. Peak 5 was identified as quercetin aglycone based on the [M-H]$^-$ ion at m/z 301 and fragment ions 179 and 151, a typical fragmentation pattern for quercetin [18]. The tunicate bulb extract chromatogram presented peaks 1, 4, and 5. The tunic extract chromatogram presents all five of the identified compounds, while in the bulb extract chromatogram, peaks 3, 4, and 5 are missing.

Table 2. Identified compounds in *A. cepa* extracts according to (RT), UV-vis (λ max), and MS and MSn data (m/z and fragments MS/MS).

Peak	RT (min)	Compound	λ Max (nm)	m/z [M-H]$^-$	Fragments [M-H]$^-$
1	11.96	quercetin 3 4′-diglucoside	208, 265, 346	625	463, 301
2	13.18	quercetin 3-glucoside	206, 246, 357	463	301, 151, 135
3	13.59	quercetin 4′-glucoside	210, 253, 366	463	301, 151, 135
4	13.97	quercetin 4′-methyl-3′-glucoside	204, 253, 360	477	315, 151
5	14.82	quercetin aglycone	209, 255, 371	301	151

Thus, the five quercetin derivatives identified were quantified in three different batches of *A. cepa* Golden variety extracts, obtained from the tunicate bulb, tunic, and bulb extracts, respectively. Their concentrations were expressed as equivalents of quercetin aglycone since the aim of their quantification was the evaluation of the overall concentration of quercetin derivatives to select the onion part with the highest concentration of quercetin. The concentration of quercetin and its derivatives was calculated using a calibration curve obtained using five solutions at known concentrations (ranging from 5 and 200 µg/mL) of standard quercetin (the equation of the calibration curve was: y = 17.692x − 71.407 and R^2 = 0.9957). The results, reported in Table 3, demonstrate that tunic extract showed the highest concentration of quercetin derivatives (3.35 ± 0.53 mg/g) in comparison with the concentrations recorded for bulb and tunicate bulb extracts.

Table 3. Concentrations of quercetin derivatives (expressed as mg of quercetin aglycone/g of extract) in three different batches (batch 1, 2, and 3) of *A. cepa* Golden variety bulb, tunicate bulb, and tunic extracts and mean of the total content of quercetin derivatives expressed as quercetin equivalent.

Compound	Tunicate Bulb Extract			Tunic Extract			Bulb Extract		
	Batch 1	Batch 2	Batch 3	Batch 1	Batch 2	Batch 3	Batch 1	Batch 2	Batch 3
Quercetin 3 4′-O-diglucoside	0.22 ± 0.07	0.31 ± 0.02	0.22 ± 0.03	1.28 ± 0.11	2.09 ± 0.32	1.33 ± 0.46	0.17 ± 0.05	0.13 ± 0.07	0.18 ± 0.05
quercetin 3-O-glucoside	-	-	-	0.23 ± 0.03	0.23 ± 0.03	0.23 ± 0.03	0.09 ± 0.01	0.09 ± 0.01	0.09 ± 0.01
quercetin 4-O-glucoside	-	-	-	1.33 ± 0.63	1.00 ± 0.28	0.98 ± 0.27	-	-	-
isorhamnetin 4′-glucoside	0.09 ± 0.02	0.09 ± 0.01	0.09 ± 0.03	0.21 ± 0.05	0.17 ± 0.02	0.17 ± 0.09	-	-	-
quercetin aglycone	0.09 ± 0.03	0.09 ± 0.01	0.14 ± 0.03	0.49 ± 0.03	0.41 ± 0.02	0.35 ± 0.03	-	-	-
Total content of quercetin derivatives expressed as quercetin equivalent (mg/g)		0.49 ± 0.05 [a]			3.50 ± 0.41 [b]			0.25 ± 0.03 [a]	

Data regarding the concentration of quercetin derivatives are expressed as mean ± standard deviation of quercetin equivalent of three replicates (n = 3), while total content of quercetin derivatives is expressed as mean ± standard deviation of the sum of quercetin derivatives of the three batches. Different superscript letters (a and b) indicate a statistically significant difference between three *A. cepa* extracts ($p < 0.05$). Statistical analysis results are reported in Table S3.

2.3. Optimization of the Extraction Method of the Tunic Extract Obtained from A. cepa Golden Variety by Means of Design of Experiments (DoE)

As the *A. cepa* Golden variety tunic extract had the highest concentration of quercetin and its derivatives, it was selected for the subsequent optimization of the extraction method. A full factorial design technique was applied to investigate three independent variables: (1) the percentage of ethanol in the extraction mixture, (2) the S/L ratio, and (3) the time of extraction, acting on the dependent variable, the total content of quercetin, and its derivatives expressed as equivalent of quercetin aglycone occurring in tunic *A. cepa* extract. The effects of each independent variable were evaluated at two different levels, while three repeats were carried out at the center point to evaluate the experimental error. Regression analysis of the model showed that it is characterized by a good fit, strength, and predictive power (Figure 2a). Only two variables (% of ethanol in the extraction mixture and S/L ratio) had a positive influence on the dependent variable, while the time of extraction variable did not influence the dependent variable itself (Figure 2b). The response surface plot (Figure 2c) showed a linear model, which reveals that within the experimental domain studied, the best conditions to obtain a tunic *A. cepa* extract with the highest quercetin concentration (26.6 ± 2.484 mg/g of quercetin aglycone equivalents) are the greater amount of ethanol in the extraction mixture (40%) and the higher S/L ratio (1 g in 20 mL).

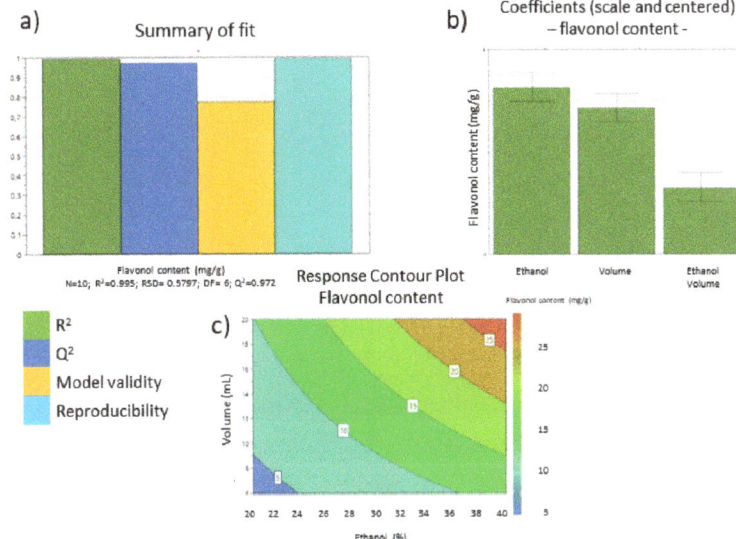

Figure 2. Optimization of tunic A. cepa extraction method using DoE. Summary of fit plots (**a**), regression coefficients of the developed model (**b**), and surface response plot (**c**).

2.4. Tunic A. cepa Extract Metabolic Profiling through RP-HPLC-PDA-ESI-MSn Analysis

Tunic *A. cepa* extracts metabolic profiling was determined by RP-HPLC-PDA-ESI-MSn analysis (Figure 3).

In the optimization of the chromatographic method to be used to determine the metabolic profile of the extract, a different reverse-phase stationary phase, which provides better selectivity and retention to improve the separation of the different flavonols, was used as an alternative to the C18 stationary phase used in the first part of this study. In total, 14 compounds were identified, all flavonols, as reported in Table 4. Peaks 1 and 2 with a parent ion at m/z 317 were assigned to dihydroisorhamnetin or 3'-O-Methyltaxifolin, which provided the fragment ions at m/z 299 [M-H-18] and 191 [M-H-126] deriving from the loss of a water molecule and trihydroxybenzoic group, respectively [19]. Peaks 3, 4, 5, and 6 were identified as quercetin dihexoside with a parent ion with m/z 625. This breaks down into fragments at m/z 463 and 301 due to the subsequential loss of two hexoside moieties (−162 amu) to obtain quercetin aglycone [20]. Peak 7 shows a [M-H]$^-$ ion at m/z 463 assigned to quercetin hexoside, which produced a quercetin aglycone fragment with an m/z 301 derived from losing a hexosyl sugar moiety [18]. Peaks 8 and 9 represent quercetin hexoside dimer with a parent ion at m/z 927 and a fragmentation pattern including the ions with m/z 463 and 301 that correspond to quercetin dihexoside and quercetin aglycone, respectively [18]. Peak 10 presents a fragment at m/z 301, which indicates that these compounds originate from quercetin. The characteristic product ions at m/z 271, 255, 179, and 151 lead to the aglycones' identification as quercetin [18]. Peak 11 presents [M-H]$^-$ at m/z 753 with characteristic product ions at m/z 299 and 271, identified as rhamnocitrin 3-rhamninoside. Peak 12 was tentatively identified as rhamnocitrin by the molecular ion [M−H]$^-$ at m/z 299 and fragment ion at m/z 271, which reflect decarbonylation, i.e., [M-H-CO]$^-$. Kaempferide (13) and chrysoeriol (14) were tentatively identified by their molecular ion [M−H]$^-$ at m/z 299 and fragmentation ions at m/z 284, 255, and 227, or m/z 226 and 211, respectively [21].

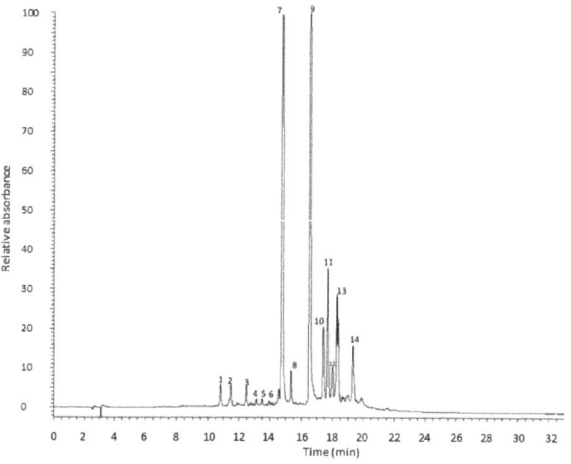

Figure 3. HPLC chromatogram of tunic *A. cepa* extract recorded at 370 nm.

Table 4. Identified compounds in tunic *A. cepa* extract of Golden variety according to their retention time (RT), UV–vis (λ Max), MS, and MSn data (m/z and fragments MS/MS).

Peak	RT (min)	Compound	λ Max (nm)	m/z [M-H]$^-$	Fragments [M-H]$^-$
1	10.82	Dihydroisorhamnetin or 3′-O-Methyltaxifolin	225, 294	317	299, 191
2	11.48	Dihydroisorhamnetin or 3′-O-Methyltaxifolin	206, 246, 357	317	299, 191
3	12.50	quercetin dihexoside derivative	267, 294, 327	625	463, 301
4	13.05	quercetin dihexoside derivative	204, 253, 360	625	463, 301
5	13.47	quercetin dihexoside derivative	287, 377, 472	625	463, 301
6	13.95	quercetin dihexoside derivative	290, 378	625	463, 301
7	14.73	quercetin hexoside derivative	231, 252, 307	463	301
8	15.33	quercetin hexoside dimer	293, 356, 377	927	463, 301
9	16.50	quercetin hexoside dimer	255, 303, 368	927	463, 301
10	17.33	Quercetin	204, 301, 367	301	271, 255, 179, 151
11	17.67	Rhamnocitrin 3-rhamninoside	205, 301, 364	754	299, 271
12	17.98	Rhamnocitrin	252, 300, 364	299	271
13	18.27	Kaempferide	204, 301, 362	299	284, 255, 227
14	19.32	Chrysoeriol	204, 301, 360	299	226, 211

2.5. In Vitro Bioaccessibility of Quercetin and Its Derivatives Identified in the Tunic A. cepa Golden Variety Extract

The extract was submitted to *in vitro* simulated gastro-duodenal digestion and was then analyzed through RP-HPLC-PDA-ESI-MSn analysis. The peak area corresponding to quercetin and its derivatives was recorded before and after gastro-duodenal digestion, and an increase in the peak area of quercetin and its derivatives was found, with the exception of peaks 4, 5, and 6, which, after the digestion process, are no longer present in the chromatogram. The results are reported in Table 5.

Table 5. Mean relative peak area and percentage increase of quercetin and its derivatives identified in *A. cepa* Golden variety tunic extract before and after gastro-duodenal digestion process.

Compound	Peak Area before Digestion	Peak Area after Digestion	Increase % Peak Area
quercetin dihexoside derivative	30,850 ± 1451	47,936 ± 932	155.4%
quercetin hexoside derivative	337,332 ± 2290	937,801 ± 3829	278.0%
quercetin hexoside dimer	42,237 ± 987	59,954 ± 1267	141.9%
quercetin hexoside dimer	539,102 ± 3128	218,649 ± 3721	−40.6%
Quercetin	106,915 ± 3121	384,291 ± 4563	359.4%

Peak area expressed as mean ± standard deviation ($n = 3$).

2.6. In Vitro Anti-Inflammatory Effects of A. cepa Extract

To assess the anti-inflammatory properties of A. cepa extract, a murine macrophage cell line J774, stimulated with LPS (10 µg/mL, 24 h) as a well-known proinflammatory stimulus, was used. Anti-inflammatory activities were assessed by measuring the levels of proinflammatory mediators such as PGE_2, IL-1β, nitrites, and TNF-α. Pre-incubation of J774 macrophages with A. cepa extract (2 h before LPS) inhibited the production of PGE_2 induced by LPS significantly and in a concentration-dependent manner (0.1, 0.5, 0.75, and 1 mg/mL) (Figure 4A), while it reduced IL-1β release, but not in a significant manner (Figure 4B). Conversely, treatment with A. cepa extract did not display an inhibitory effect on the production of nitrites and TNF-α induced by LPS. In order to rule out any alteration in cell viability, an MTT assay was performed and did not show any statistical reduction of cell viability after treatment with the extract (data not shown).

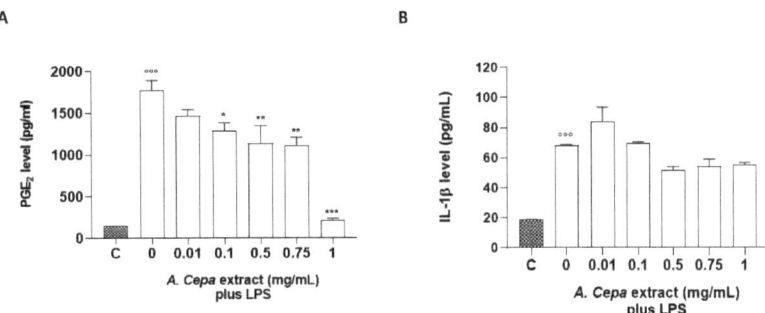

Figure 4. Cont.

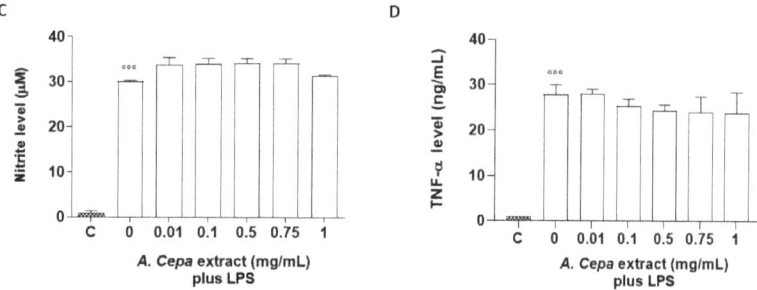

Figure 4. Effect of the *A. cepa* extract on LPS-induced PGE$_2$, IL-1β, nitrite, and TNF-α production. J774 cells were pre-treated for 2 h with increasing concentrations of the extract (0.01, 0.05, 0.1, 0.5, 0.75, and 1.0 mg/mL) prior to LPS stimulation (10 μg/mL) for 24 h. Unstimulated J774 cells acted as a negative control. Nitrites (**C**), stable end-products of NO, were measured in the supernatants by the Griess reaction, whereas PGE$_2$ (**A**), IL-1β (**B**), and TNF-α (**D**) were measured by ELISA. °°° $p < 0.001$ vs. unstimulated cells C, *** $p < 0.001$, ** $p < 0.01$, and * $p < 0.05$ vs. LPS alone.

3. Discussion

In this work, a chemically characterized *A. cepa* extract rich in quercetin and its derivatives was obtained from an onion tunic with a conventional extraction method optimized by DoE. Then, in view of possible applications as a food supplement ingredient, the extract was subjected to preliminary *in vitro* studies, such as the determination of its bioaccessibility and anti-inflammatory activity. First, four extracts obtained from different *A. cepa* varieties were tested to evaluate the TPC and select the variety that provided the extract with the highest content of polyphenols. Then, five different quercetin derivatives (quercetin 3,4′-diglucoside, quercetin 3-monoglucoside, quercetin 4′-monoglucoside, quercetin 4′-methyl-3′- glucoside, and quercetin aglycone) were identified and quantified in extracts obtained from the tunicate bulb, tunic, and bulb, to select the onion part containing the highest concentrations of quercetin and its derivatives, with tunic providing the richest part compared to tunicate bulb and bulb. Then, profiling of the flavonoids present in the tunic *A. cepa* Golden variety extract was performed. Fourteen compounds were identified. Furthermore, the increases in some quercetin derivatives following the gastro-duodenal digestion process support the bioaccessibility of these bioactive compounds. In particular, the chromatographic peak areas of quercetin and its monoglucoside derivatives were found to increase after the *in vitro* simulated gastro-duodenal digestion process, while those corresponding to dihexoside derivatives were not recorded in the chromatogram of the digested extract. These results can be explained by both the degradation of dihexoside derivatives to quercetin and its monoglucoside derivatives and the possible release of quercetin derivatives from the onion matrix. These results are unsurprising, as it is known that onion tunics contain plant cell wall (PCW) components, mainly pectic polysaccharides as inferred from the levels of uronic acid, galactose, arabinose and rhamnose, and glucose with minor quantities of xylose and mannose described by Ng et al. [22], and these PCW components can have a protective role towards polyphenols by affecting their release in the human digestive system [23]. Voragen et al. [24] reported that pectins play an important role in creating PCW and affect properties such as porosity, surface charge, ionic balance, and pH, which in turn can affect the interactions between polyphenols and PCW. Although the mechanisms that ultimately drive such interactions are still not fully understood, they appear to be shaped by a variety of factors, the most important of which are the physicochemical properties of their partners, such as their morphology (surface area and porosity/pore shape), chemical composition (sugar ratio, solubility, and non-sugar components), and molecular architecture (molecular weight, degree of esterification, functional groups, and conformation). Although knowledge regarding the interactions between intracellular flavonols and onion tunic PCW is unknown, these results lead to the hypothesis that the noncovalent interactions (i.e., electrostatic interactions, hydrogen bonds, and hydrophobic effect) between onion flavonols and PCW components break during digestion, releasing the polyphenols and increasing their bioavailability. Thus, in view of possible applications for this extract as a food supplement ingredient, no coating agents are required to preserve the bioactive components, as often suggested to preserve polyphenols occurring in vegetable extracts. Furthermore, the increased concentrations of bioactive compounds observed following the digestion process further support the use of *A. cepa* extract as an ingredient for dietary supplements. In the European Union, 200 mg/day of quercetin is the maximum accepted dose as an ingredient for food supplements, with 60% gastrointestinal absorption. Only 5 to 10% of quercetin is absorbed in the small intestine, whereas 90 to 95% is absorbed in the colon. Once ingested, it passively diffuses from the intestinal lumen to enterocytes, where it is metabolized and distributed to tissues through systemic circulation. Taking into account the absolute bioavailability, which was estimated at ~45% (through the oral administration of 14C-labeled quercetin), the possibility of increasing the intake of quercetin through this *A. cepa* extract, naturally rich in this component which does not degrade as a result of digestion, but instead increases in bioaccessibility, can lead to advantages that other extracts obtained from different food matrices do not have.

Regarding the anti-inflammatory properties, our data suggest prevalent activity on PGE_2 with concentration-dependent inhibition. As a member of the family of prostaglandins, PGE_2 is synthetized from Arachidonic Acid (AA) by the phospholipase A_2 and cyclooxygenase enzymes (COX). Previously published studies have focused on the activity of flavonols, especially quercetin and its derivates, with particular attention to AA. In a study by Lesjak et al. [25], both the activity of quercetin (and its derivatives) on the COX-2 pathway and its ability to inhibit COX-1 and 12-LOX pathways were studied. Quercetin and its derivatives also demonstrated a concentration-dependent inhibitor potential on 12-HHT, TXB_2, and PGE_2 inflammatory mediators. However, the maximal anti-inflammatory effect was achieved by the monomethylated metabolite of quercetin, tamaraxetin. The effect of this metabolite was entirely comparable to that observed with aspirin. This metabolite is synthetized within enterocytes, with quercetin acting as a substrate for catechol-O-methyltransferases (COMT) that convert quercetin into its monomethylated derivative. Thus, the good bioaccessibility of quercetin and its derivatives present in this onion tunic extract, which favors the absorption of such bioactive compounds and their passage into the systemic circulation, allows us to hypothesize that this extract may have anti-inflammatory effects *in vivo*, which must be confirmed by human studies.

In contrast with the presented data, two studies have reported that quercetin and its metabolites act as *in vivo* and *in vitro* COX-1 activators and, thus, can promote the synthesis of eicosanoids. However, (1) compelling evidence argues for the information provided by our group as being in line with current knowledge in the area (reviewed in ref. [26]), and (2) the concentrations employed in these studies to identify the mechanistic and structural basis for bioflavonoids functioning as high affinity reducing co-substrates/activators of COXs, are lower than the ones reported here.

We believe that the results of this research have some practical implications. Every year in the European Union, more than 0.5 million tons of onion waste are produced [15]. Following proper treatments, onion waste can be used for fodder preparation or as fertilizer. However, most onion waste products remain underutilized despite being rich in bioactive compounds that could be used in the health product industry as food supplements and herbal medicine ingredients. Therefore, the development of a quercetin-rich extract obtained with a conventional extraction method that is easily used industrially and which does not conflict with existing European legislation on novel food [27] could be a good strategy to produce economically and environmentally sustainable products increasingly demanded by the market.

Moreover, currently, marketed food supplements contain quercetin in the aglycone form, although quercetin glucoside derivatives show higher absorption efficiency in the small intestine (absorption by approximately 52%) compared to the aglycone form (absorption by approximately 24%) [28]. Therefore, the availability of a quercetin-based extract containing, in addition to the aglycone form, its glycoside derivatives with good bioaccessibility can represent added value as it allows better absorption of quercetin and, therefore, higher efficacy.

Finally, although the data presented here derive from pre-clinical *in vitro* studies that must be confirmed with *in vivo* studies and clinical studies, the results relating to the anti-inflammatory activity of the extract that has an inhibitory activity on the release of PGE_2 dose-dependent are promising as PGE_2 is involved in acute inflammation and inflammatory immune diseases via different mechanisms.

The main limitation of our study is the lack of studies and clinical trials investigating the clinical significance of the *in vitro* results reported here and identifying subjects who could maximally benefit from an *A. cepa* extract (subjects affected by low-grade inflammation, e.g., sarcopenic, depressed, and insulin resistance). To this end, further investigations are being carried out on tunic *A. cepa* extract, and the results of these studies might support the use of this extract in low-grade inflammatory stages.

4. Materials and Methods

4.1. Chemicals and Reagents

All the compounds used for *in vitro* gastric and duodenal digestion processes are reported below: potassium chloride (KCl), dihydrogen potassium phosphate (KH_2PO_4), sodium carbonate ($NaHCO_3$), magnesium chloride ($MgCl_2$), ammonium carbonate (NH_4)CO_3, calcium chloride ($CaCl_2$), sodium chloride (NaCl), hydrochloric acid (HCl), and sodium hydroxide (NaOH). All were provided by Carlo Erba (Milan, Italy). Pancreatin from porcine pancreas (extract of pig bile), pepsin from porcine gastric mucosa, porcine bile extract, formic acid solution (1M), water, methanol, LC-MS grade acetonitrile, and sodium monobasic dehydrated phosphate (NaH_2PO_4 $2H_2O$), were sourced from Sigma-Aldrich, Merck KGaA (Milan, Italy). PVDF filters (0.22 and 0.45 µm) were purchased from Euroclone S.p.A (Milan, Italy).

4.2. Sampling

Four local varieties of *A. cepa*, namely Golden, Yellow Elenka, White Cenol, and White Orizaba, grown in the Oltrepò Pavese area (Lombardia Region, Italy), were obtained from the producers in the summer of 2021. The onions were stored at a cold-room temperature of 4 °C until the extraction process.

4.3. Identification of Local A. cepa Varieties Rich in Polyphenols

4.3.1. *A. cepa* Extraction Procedure

For each variety, three *A. cepa* tunicate bulbs were selected and cut with a knife to obtain a representative sample. The following extraction protocol was applied: a 5g sample was mixed with 100 mL of hydroalcoholic solution $CH_3OH/H_2O/CH_3COOH$ (95:4:1 $v/v/v$) and blended for 10 min in an ice bath with a mixer (Bluesky BBL-500-13) to obtain a homogeneous suspension. Finally, 1 mL of solution was filtrated with 0.45 µm and 0.22 µm PTFE filters.

4.3.2. Folin–Ciocalteu Assay

The total polyphenol content analysis of the onion extracts obtained from four varieties was performed using Folin–Ciocalteu reagent according to Singleton et al. 1965 [29], with modifications [30] as follows: the reaction was initiated by the addition of 10 µL of the sample with 50 µL Folin–Ciocalteu reagent, 200 µL of 15% (w/v) sodium carbonate, and 740 µL of water in a microtube of 1.5 mL. The reaction medium was stored in the dark for 2 h at 25 °C. Absorbance was measured at 750 nm (FLUOstar Omega microplate reader, BMG Labtech GmbH, Ortenberg, Germany) against a blank sample. A gallic acid calibration curve was prepared with 5–500 µg/mL ($r^2 = 0.999$). The resulting total polyphenol amounts were expressed as mg gallic acid equivalents in comparison to a gram of *A. cepa* extract (mg GAE/g). All samples were analyzed in triplicate.

4.4. Extraction, Identification, and Quantification of Quercetin and Its Derivatives in Different Parts of A. cepa (Tunicate Bulb, Tunic, and Bulb)

4.4.1. RP-HPLC-PDA-ESI-MSn Analysis

Three different extracts were obtained from the tunicate bulb, tunic, and bulb of *A. cepa*, the Golden variety, using the protocol described in Section 4.3.1. Chromatographic analyses were performed using a Thermo Finnigan Surveyor Plus HPLC apparatus equipped with a quaternary pump, a Surveyor UV–Vis photodiode array detector (PDA), and an LCQ Advantage max ion trap mass spectrometer (Thermo Fisher Scientific, Waltham, MA, USA), coupled through an ESI source. RP-HPLC-PDA-ESI-MS/MS data were acquired under negative ionization modes using Xcalibur software. The ion trap operated in full scan (100–2000 m/z), data-dependent scan, and MSn modes; when greater discrimination was required, additional targeted MS^2 and MSn experiments were performed on selected molecular ions. To optimize the MS operating conditions, a preliminary experiment was performed: 10 μg/mL quercetin-3-glucoside (H_2O/MeOH: 50/50 with 0.1% formic acid) solution were directly infused in the ESI interface at a flow rate of 25 μL/min into the mass spectrometer. Optimized conditions were as follows: sheath gas 60, capillary temperature 220 °C, auxiliary gas 25, spray voltage 5 kV, and capillary voltage −26.13 V. Separation was assessed using a Luna Omega PS C18 100 A° (150 × 2.1 mm; particle size 3 μm), connected with an adequate precolumn, both sourced from Phenomenex (Torrance, CA, USA). The mobile phase was water, with 0.1% formic acid (eluent A) and methanol (eluent B), eluted in a gradient as follows: from 10% to 80% B in 10 min, 80% in an isocratic mode for 10 min, from 80% to 10% B in 5 min, ending with a 5 min isocratic run at 10% B. The run time was 35 min in total, which included reconditioning the column. The flow rate was kept to 0.3 mL/min, the autosampler was set to 4 °C, and the column was set to 25 °C. A 5 μL injection volume was used. Chromatogram measurements were taken at 214, 254, and 370 nm; spectral data were taken between 200 and 800 nm for every peak. Compounds were characterized based on their UV–Vis and mass spectra, checking the molecular ion and fragment ions against fragmentation patterns of standard molecules, where possible, and with molecules described in the literature.

4.4.2. RP-HPLC-PDA Quantitative Analysis

The content of quercetin and derivatives was assessed with the same methods described in Section 4.4.1 using Agilent 1100 HPLC apparatus (Agilent, Waldbronn, Germany), equipped with a quaternary pump, autosampler, and photodiode array detector (PDA). Data were acquired using Chemstation software. All analyses were performed in triplicate. Quercetin aglycone was selected as an external standard. A calibration curve was prepared using a stock solution of quercetin aglycone (1 mg/L) in ethanol and diluted to obtain five concentrations in a range of 5–200 μg/mL ($r^2 = 0.996$). The content of different quercetin derivatives was expressed as the quercetin equivalent (μg/mL quercetin/g extract). The validation of the method was performed following ICH procedures [31] (Table S1).

4.5. Optimization and Characterization of Tunic A. cepa Extract Golden Variety Composition

4.5.1. Optimization of Tunic *A. cepa* Extraction by Design of Experiments (DoE)

Extraction of the tunic *A. cepa Golden variety* extract was performed in triplicate at room temperature using a hydroalcoholic solution at pH 2.5 under constant stirring. The solution was protected from light to prevent potential degradation of the flavonoids. Some factors affecting the extraction yield were investigated by means of DoE methodology, using MODDE Pro 11 Software (Umetrics, Umeå, Sweden). A three-factor, two-level, full factorial design study was utilized to study the impact of the sample amount/hydroalcoholic solution volume (S/L) ratio (1:6, 1:20 g/mL), time of extraction (120–140 min), and percentage of ethanol in the extraction mixture (20–40%), on the yield of quercetin and its derivative concentration from tunic *A. cepa* extract, expressed as quercetin equivalent content through HPLC-PDA analysis. A total of 11 experiments were carried out, including a triplicate measurement at the center point used to estimate experimental error. The obtained extracts were analyzed through the HPLC-PDA method to achieve the content of quercetin and its derivatives expressed as a quercetin aglycone equivalent (mg/g extract).

4.5.2. Metabolic Profile of Optimized Tunic *A. cepa* Golden Variety Extract

Analysis of the metabolic profile of optimized tunic *A. cepa* Golden variety extract was performed using the same method and conditions reported in Section 4.4.1 with some modifications. The separation of the compound was performed with a Kinetex XB-C18 100 A column (150 × 4.6 mm; particle size 5 µm), protected by its corresponding guard column, both from Phenomenex, California, USA. Gradient elution was executed with acidified water (0.1% formic acid) as mobile phase A and methanol as mobile phase B at a flow rate of 0.6 mL/min. The elution gradient started from 10% B to 80% B in 15 min, followed by a 16 min isocratic run of 80% B, 80% B to 10% B in 1 min, and finally, an isocratic run of 10% B for 1 min. Compounds were characterized based on their UV–Vis and mass spectra, checking the molecular ion and fragment ions against fragmentation patterns of standard molecules, where possible, and with molecules described in the literature.

4.6. In Vitro Bioaccessibility by Simulated Gastro-Duodenal Digestion

In vitro simulated digestion was performed following the protocol of Minekus et al. 2014 [32] with some modifications. The *A. cepa* Golden variety tunic extract was added to 10 mL of bidistilled water and mixed with 7.5 mL of simulated gastric fluid (SGF) with pepsin (25,000 U/mL) and HCL 1M until reaching a pH of 3.00 ± 0.02. Finally, distilled water was used to make up a volume of 20 mL, and the solution was incubated at 37 °C for 2 h in a shaking water bath. At the end of the gastric phase, 20 mL of the digested extract were mixed with 11 mL (Simulated Intestinal Fluid, SIF). Pancreatin was added (800 U/mL) with porcine bile (160 mM), and the solutions were adjusted with NaOH 1 M to obtain a final pH of 7. Finally, the sample was made up to a 40 mL final volume and incubated at 37 °C for 2 h. The gastro-duodenal digested sample was freeze-dried and stored at 4 °C prior to HPLC-MS analysis.

4.7. Cell Culture

The murine monocyte/macrophage J774 cell line (Sigma-Aldrich, Merck KGaA (Milan, Italy) was grown in Dulbecco's modified Eagles medium (DMEM) supplemented with 2 mM glutamine, 25 mM Hepes, penicillin (100 U/mL), streptomycin (100 µg/mL), 10% foetal bovine serum (FBS), and 1.2% Na pyruvate. Cells were plated to a seeding density of 5.0×10^5 in 24 multiwell or 1.0×10^5 in 96 multiwell plates. Cells were pre-treated (for 2 h) with increasing concentrations of *A. cepa* extract (0.01–1 mg/mL) and stimulated with LPS from Escherichia coli, Serotype 0111:B4, (10 µg/mL) for 24 h [30].

4.7.1. Nitrite, PGE2, IL-1β, and TNF-α Assay

After 24 h of incubation, the supernatants were collected for nitrite, PGE2, IL-1β, and TNF-α measurements. The nitrite concentrations in the samples were measured by the Griess reaction by adding 100 µL of Griess reagent (0.1% naphthylethylenediamide dihydrochloride in H_2O and 1% sulphanilamide in 5% concentrated H_3PO_4; vol. 1:1) to 100 µL samples. The optical density at 540 nm (OD540) was measured using an ELISA microplate reader (Thermo Scientific, Multiskan GO, Waltham, MA, USA). Nitrite concentrations were calculated by comparison with the OD540 of standard solutions of sodium nitrite prepared in a culture medium. PGE2, IL-1β, and TNF-α levels were measured with commercially available ELISA kits according to the manufacturer's instructions (R&D system and Cayman Chemical, Bertin Pharma, Montigny Le Bretonneux, France).

4.7.2. Cell Viability

Cell respiration, an indicator of cell viability, was assessed by the mitochondrial-dependent reduction of 3-(4,5-dimethylthiazol-2-yl)-2,5-diphenyltetrazolium bromide (MTT) to formazan. After stimulation with LPS in the absence or presence of test compounds for 24 h, cells were incubated in 96-well plates with MTT (0.2 mg/mL) for 1 h. The culture medium was removed by aspiration, and the cells were dissolved in DMSO (0.1 mL). The extent of reduction of MTT to formazan within cells was quantified by the measurement of OD650.

4.8. Statistical Analysis

The experiments were performed in triplicate. All results were reported as mean ± standard deviation, and the mean values were compared using one-way ANOVA followed by Tukey's multiple comparison test. For the *in vitro* anti-inflammatory studies, the results are expressed as mean ± standard error (SEM) of the mean of n observations, where n represents the number of experiments performed on different days. Triplicate wells were used for various treatment conditions. The results were analyzed by one-way ANOVA followed by a Bonferroni post hoc test for multiple comparisons. A p-value less than 0.05 was considered significant. All graphs were generated using GraphPad Prism (version 5).

5. Conclusions

In conclusion, considering the growing interest in the development of new economically and environmentally sustainable food products using secondary raw materials, our data support the *in vitro* bioaccessibility of quercetin and its derivatives and the anti-inflammatory effects, particularly on PG metabolites, of an *A. cepa* extract obtained from onion tunic. Our data also demonstrate variation in the distribution of the identified quercetin and its derivatives across the tunicate bulb, bulb, and tunic extracts of the *A. cepa* Golden variety and suggest the importance of a DoE approach in order to obtain an extract rich in bioactive compounds. We believe that the approach followed in the development of this possible ingredient of food supplements and functional foods, in the study of bioaccessibility of its bioactive compounds and biological properties, could be an example for the preparation of other ingredients for the design of healthier foods.

Supplementary Materials: The following supporting information can be downloaded at: https://www.mdpi.com/article/10.3390/molecules27249065/s1, Table S1: Accuracy (Recovery %), Precision (Repeatability and Intermediate precision) and Limits of Detection (LOD) and Quantification LOQ) of the Analytical Procedure for the determination of quercetin in A. cepa Golden variety tunicate bulb, bulb, and tunic extracts; Table S2: Statistical analysis of quantification of total content of polyphenols (expressed as equivalent mg of gallic acid); Table S3: Statistical analysis of quantification of total content of quercetin derivatives expressed as quercetin equivalent (mg/g)

Author Contributions: Conceptualization, M.D. (Marco Dacrema), A.D.M. and A.R.; methodology, A.B., C.S., H.U., M.D. (Maria Daglia) and R.d.M.; software-validation, C.S. and M.D. (Maria Daglia); writing—original draft preparation, A.D.M., A.R., H.U., C.S., M.D. (Marco Dacrema) and M.D. (Maria Daglia); writing—review and editing, A.T., H.R.E.-S. and S.A.M.K. All authors have read and agreed to the published version of the manuscript.

Funding: This research received no external funding.

Institutional Review Board Statement: Not applicable.

Informed Consent Statement: Not applicable.

Conflicts of Interest: The authors declare no conflict of interest.

References

1. FAO. World Food and Agriculture - Statistical Yearbook 2021. 2021. Available online: https://www.ams.usda.gov/mnreports/fvwretail.pdf (accessed on 3 November 2022).
2. Marefati, N.; Ghorani, V.; Shakeri, F.; Boskabady, M.; Kianian, F.; Rezaee, R.; Boskabady, M.H. A Review of Anti-Inflammatory, Antioxidant, and Immunomodulatory Effects of Allium cepa and Its Main Constituents. *Pharm. Biol.* **2021**, *59*, 285–300. [CrossRef]
3. Zhao, X.X.; Lin, F.J.; Li, H.; Li, H.B.; Wu, D.T.; Geng, F.; Ma, W.; Wang, Y.; Miao, B.H.; Gan, R.Y. Recent Advances in Bioactive Compounds, Health Functions, and Safety Concerns of Onion (Allium cepa L.). *Front. Nutr.* **2021**, *8*, 669805. [CrossRef]
4. Teshika, J.D.; Zakariyyah, A.M.; Zaynab, T.; Zengin, G.; Rengasamy, K.R.; Pandian, S.K.; Fawzi, M.M. Traditional and Modern Uses of Onion Bulb (Allium cepa L.): A Systematic Review. *Crit. Rev. Food Sci. Nutr.* **2019**, *59*, S39–S70. [CrossRef]
5. Kim, J.H.; Kim, J.S.; Kim, S.H.; Jeong, S.H.; Jeong, U.Y.; Jung, J.E.; Lee, S.K.; Lee, S.H. Antioxidant and Anti-Inflammatory Effects of Ethanol Extract from Whole Onion (Allium cepa L.) with Leaves. *Agriculture* **2022**, *12*, 963. [CrossRef]
6. Wang, C.K. Health Benefits of Onion Bioactives on Hypercholesterolemia, Cardiovascular Diseases, and Bone Mineral Density. *Food Front.* **2020**, *1*, 107–108. [CrossRef]
7. Galavi, A.; Hosseinzadeh, H.; Razavi, B.M. The Effects of Allium cepa L.(Onion) and Its Active Constituents on Metabolic Syndrome: A Review. *Iran J. Basic Med. Sci.* **2021**, *24*, 3–16.
8. Lebdah, M.; Tantawy, L.; Elgamal, A.M.; Abdelaziz, A.M.; Yehia, N.; Alyamani, A.A.; ALmoshadak, A.S.; Mohamed, M.E. The Natural Antiviral and Immune Stimulant Effects of Allium cepa Essential Oil Onion Extract against Virulent Newcastle Disease Virus. *Saudi J. Biol. Sci.* **2022**, *29*, 1239–1245. [CrossRef]
9. Kumar, M.; Barbhai, M.D.; Hasan, M.; Punia, S.; Dhumal, S.; Rais, N.; Chandran, D.; Pandiselvam, R.; Kothakota, A.; Tomar, M.; et al. Onion (Allium cepa L.) Peels: A Review on Bioactive Compounds and Biomedical Activities. *Biomed. Pharmacother.* **2022**, *146*, 112498. [CrossRef]
10. Hollman, P.C.H.; Arts, I.C.W. Flavonols, Flavones and Flavanols–Nature, Occurrence and Dietary Burden. *J. Sci. Food Agric.* **2000**, *80*, 1081–1093. [CrossRef]
11. Hollman, P.C.; Gaag, M.V.; Mengelers, M.J.; van Trijp, J.M.; de Vries, J.H.; Katan, M.B. Absorption and Disposition Kinetics of the Dietary Antioxidant Quercetin in Man. *Free Radic. Biol. Med.* **1996**, *21*, 703–707. [CrossRef]
12. Manach, C.; Williamson, G.; Morand, C.; Scalbert, A.; Rémésy, C. Bioavailability and Bioefficacy of Polyphenols in Humans. I. Review of 97 Bioavailability Studies. *Am. J. Clin. Nutr.* **2005**, *81*, 230S–242S. [CrossRef]
13. Hai, Y.; Zhang, Y.; Liang, Y.; Ma, X.; Qi, X.; Xiao, W.; Xue, W.; Luo, Y.; Yue, T. Advance on the Absorption, Metabolism, and Efficacy Exertion of Quercetin and Its Important Derivatives: Absorption, Metabolism and Function of Quercetin. *Food Front.* **2020**, *1*, 420–434. [CrossRef]
14. Boots, A.W.; Haenen, G.R.; Bast, A. Health Effects of Quercetin: From Antioxidant to Nutraceutical. *Eur. J. Pharmacol.* **2008**, *585*, 325–337. [CrossRef]
15. FIBRACEP; H2020; CORDIS; European Commission "Valorization of European Onion Waste by-Products into Dietary Fibre-Based Formula with Hypocholesterolemic, Hypoglycemic, and Antioxidant Effects". Report Summary. Available online: https://cordis.europa.eu/project/id/782061/it (accessed on 4 November 2022).
16. Francescato, L.N.; Debenedetti, S.L.; Schwanz, T.G.; Bassani, V.L.; Henriques, A.T. Identification of Phenolic Compounds in Equisetum Giganteum by LC–ESI-MS/MS and a New Approach to Total Flavonoid Quantification. *Talanta* **2013**, *105*, 192–203. [CrossRef]
17. Bonaccorsi, P.; Caristi, C.; Gargiulli, C.; Leuzzi, U. Flavonol Glucoside Profile of Southern Italian Red Onion (Allium cepa L.). *J. Agric. Food Chem.* **2005**, *53*, 2733–2740. [CrossRef]
18. Chen, G.; Li, X.; Saleri, F.; Guo, M. Analysis of Flavonoids in Rhamnus Davurica and Its Antiproliferative Activities. *Molecules* **2016**, *21*, 1275. [CrossRef]
19. Jaganath, I.B.; Mullen, W.; Lean, M.E.; Edwards, C.A.; Crozier, A. In Vitro Catabolism of Rutin by Human Fecal Bacteria and the Antioxidant Capacity of Its Catabolites. *Free Radic. Biol. Med.* **2009**, *47*, 1180–1189. [CrossRef]
20. Ibrahim, R.M.; El-Halawany, A.M.; Saleh, D.O.; el Naggar, E.M.B.; El-Shabrawy, A.E.R.O.; El-Hawary, S.S. HPLC-DAD-MS/MS Profiling of Phenolics from Securigera Securidaca Flowers and Its Anti-Hyperglycemic and Anti-Hyperlipidemic Activities. *Rev. Bras. Farmacogn.* **2015**, *25*, 134–141. [CrossRef]
21. Chernonosov, A.A.; Karpova, E.A.; Lyakh, E.M. Identification of Phenolic Compounds in Myricaria bracteata Leaves by High-Performance Liquid Chromatography with a Diode Array Detector and Liquid Chromatography with Tandem Mass Spectrometry. *Rev. Bras. Farmacogn.* **2017**, *27*, 576–579. [CrossRef]
22. Ng, A.; Smith, A.C.; Waldron, K.W. Effect of Tissue Type and Variety on Cell Wall Chemistry of Onion (Allium cepa L.). *Food Chem.* **1998**, *63*, 17–24. [CrossRef]
23. Siemińska-Kuczer, A.; Szymańska-Chargot, M.; Zdunek, A. Recent Advances in Interactions between Polyphenols and Plant Cell Wall Polysaccharides as Studied Using an Adsorption Technique. *Food Chem.* **2022**, *373*, 131487. [CrossRef]
24. Voragen, A.G.; Coenen, G.J.; Verhoef, R.P.; Schols, H.A. Pectin, a Versatile Polysaccharide Present in Plant Cell Walls. *Struct. Chem.* **2009**, *20*, 263–275. [CrossRef]
25. Lesjak, M.; Beara, I.; Simin, N.; Pintać, D.; Majkić, T.; Bekvalac, K.; Orčić, D.; Mimica-Dukić, N. Antioxidant and Anti-Inflammatory Activities of Quercetin and Its Derivatives. *J. Funct. Foods* **2018**, *40*, 68–75. [CrossRef]

26. Ali, M.; Thomson, M.; Afzal, M. Garlic and Onions: Their Effect on Eicosanoid Metabolism and Its Clinical Relevance. *Prostaglandins Leukot. Essent. Fatty Acids* **2000**, *62*, 55–73. [CrossRef]
27. Regulation (EU) 2015/2283 of the European Parliament and of the Council of 25 November 2015 on Novel Foods, Amending Regulation (EU) No 1169/2011 of the European Parliament and of the Council and Repealing Regulation (EC) No 258/97 of the European Parliament. *Off. J. Eur. Union* **2015**, 1–22.
28. Hollman, P.C.; de Vries, J.H.; van Leeuwen, S.D.; Mengelers, M.J.; Katan, M.B. Absorption of Dietary Quercetin Glycosides and Quercetin in Healthy Ileostomy Volunteers. *Am. J. Clin. Nutr.* **1995**, *62*, 1276–1282. [CrossRef]
29. Singleton, V.L.; Rossi, J.A. Colorimetry of Total Phenolics with Phosphomolybdic-Phosphotungstic Acid Reagents. *Am. J. Enol. Vitic.* **1965**, *16*, 144–158.
30. Ullah, H.; Sommella, E.; Santarcangelo, C.; D'Avino, D.; Rossi, A.; Dacrema, M.; di Minno, A.; di Matteo, G.; Mannina, L.; Campiglia, P.; et al. Hydroethanolic Extract of Prunus Domestica L.: Metabolite Profiling and in Vitro Modulation of Molecular Mechanisms Associated to Cardiometabolic Diseases. *Nutrients* **2022**, *14*, 340. [CrossRef]
31. ICH Harmonised Guideline Validation of Analytical Procedures Q2(R2). Available online: https://database.ich.org/sites/default/files/ICH_Q2-R2_Document_Step2_Guideline_2022_0324.pdf (accessed on 20 November 2022).
32. Minekus, M.; Alminger, M.; Alvito, P.; Ballance, S.; Bohn, T.O.R.S.T.E.N.; Bourlieu, C.; Carrière, F.; Boutrou, R.; Corredig, M.; Dupont, D.; et al. A Standardised Static in Vitro Digestion Method Suitable for Food–an International Consensus. *Food Funct.* **2014**, *5*, 1113–1124. [CrossRef]

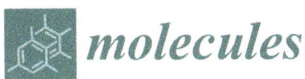

Review

A Selective Review and Virtual Screening Analysis of Natural Product Inhibitors of the NLRP3 Inflammasome

Sherihan El-Sayed [1,2], Sally Freeman [1,*] and Richard A. Bryce [1]

1 Division of Pharmacy and Optometry, School of Health Sciences, Manchester Academic Health Sciences Centre, University of Manchester, Oxford Road, Manchester M13 9PT, UK
2 Department of Medicinal Chemistry, Faculty of Pharmacy, Zagazig University, Zagazig 44519, Egypt
* Correspondence: sally.freeman@manchester.ac.uk; Tel.: +44-7950403456

Abstract: The NLRP3 inflammasome is currently an exciting target for drug discovery due to its role in various inflammatory diseases; however, to date, no NLRP3 inhibitors have reached the clinic. Several studies have used natural products as hit compounds to facilitate the design of novel selective NLRP3 inhibitors. Here, we review selected natural products reported in the literature as NLRP3 inhibitors, with a particular focus on those targeting gout. To complement this survey, we also report a virtual screen of the ZINC20 natural product database, predicting favored chemical features that can aid in the design of novel small molecule NLRP3 inhibitors.

Keywords: NLRP3; IL-1β; inflammation; natural products; docking; design

Citation: El-Sayed, S.; Freeman, S.; Bryce, R.A. A Selective Review and Virtual Screening Analysis of Natural Product Inhibitors of the NLRP3 Inflammasome. *Molecules* 2022, 27, 6213. https://doi.org/10.3390/molecules27196213

Academic Editor: Francesco Maione

Received: 25 August 2022
Accepted: 15 September 2022
Published: 21 September 2022

Publisher's Note: MDPI stays neutral with regard to jurisdictional claims in published maps and institutional affiliations.

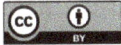

Copyright: © 2022 by the authors. Licensee MDPI, Basel, Switzerland. This article is an open access article distributed under the terms and conditions of the Creative Commons Attribution (CC BY) license (https://creativecommons.org/licenses/by/4.0/).

1. Introduction

The NLRP3 (NOD-, LRR-, and pyrin domain containing 3) inflammasome is one of the most interesting targets implicated in various inflammatory diseases (e.g., Alzheimer's disease, atherosclerosis, and gout). The inflammasome consists of three parts: a sensor molecule, adaptor protein, and effector (Figure 1a). The sensor part of the inflammasome is the PRR (pattern recognition receptor) that triggers inflammasome assembly in response to DAMPs (damage-associated molecular patterns) or PAMPs (pathogen-associated molecular patterns). PRRs can be classified into two main classes: the NOD (nucleotide-binding and oligomerization domain-like receptor (NLR)) family, including, for example, the protein NLRP3; and the non-NLR family, which has members such as the protein AIM2 (absent in melanoma 2). AIM2 can bind directly to the stimulus via the HIN (hemopoietic expression-interferon inducibility-nuclear localization) domain; however, NLRP3 is activated indirectly in response to various stimuli [1]. The adaptor protein is referred to as ASC (apoptosis-associated Speck-like protein containing a CARD) and it consists of a pyrin domain, which binds to the sensor protein via pyrin–pyrin interactions; and a CARD (caspase recruitment and activation) domain, which binds to procaspase-1 via CARD–CARD interactions. The effector is a protease caspase-1 that is responsible for cytokine activation and pyroptosis [1,2].

The NLRP3 inflammasome is a cytoplasmic macromolecule often present in macrophages that regulate the activation of potent inflammatory mediators and is implicated in the pathogenesis of numerous non-infectious diseases. NLRP3 consists of three domains: an N-terminal pyrin (PYD) domain, which binds to ASC; a central adenosine triphosphatase NACHT domain; and a C-terminal leucine-rich repeat (LRR) domain [3]. Although NLRP3 can respond to a wide range of stimuli other than pathogenic molecules, the mechanism of NLRP3 activation has not been fully characterized; there are several theories describing this activation [4]. In many cells, NLRP3 activation passes through two stages: priming and activation. In normal cells, the amount of NLRP3 is insufficient to activate inflammasome assembly, so a priming stage is required, which involves overexpression of the NLRP3 inflammasome components through the activation of the transcription factor NF-κB. The activation of NF-κB can be achieved through various stimuli, for example, the binding of PAMPs such as lipopolysaccharide (LPS) to the membrane-bound receptor TLR4 (toll-like receptor 4). Then, NLRP3 activation occurs through either ion-dependent or ion-independent pathways [5–7].

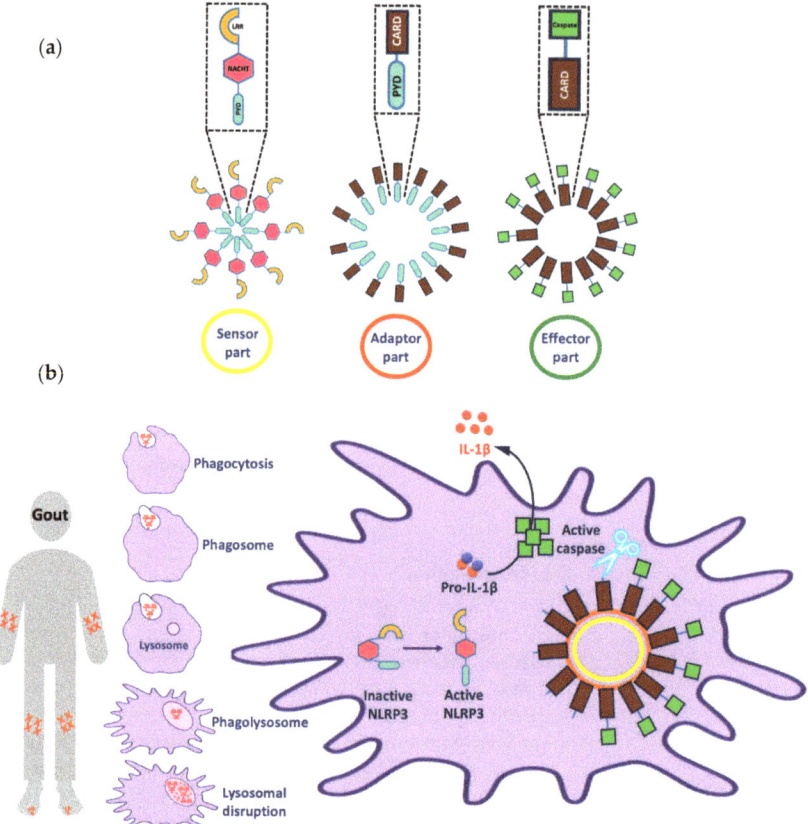

Figure 1. Representation of (**a**) different parts of the NLRP3 inflammasome and (**b**) the activation of the NLRP3 inflammasome by uric acid and implications in gout. Note that this figure was modified from Figure 1 in our recent publication [4].

1.1. Ion-Dependent Activation Pathways

High levels of extracellular ATP, which bind to the P2X purinoceptor 7 (P2X7) channel, increase cell membrane permeability to potassium, which can activate NLRP3 in primed cells. As an example of stimulated inflammation, crystal accumulation due to pathological conditions (e.g., cholesterol, uric acid), foreign inhaled crystals (e.g., silica, asbestos), and proteinaceous aggregates (e.g., amyloid-β) are phagocytosed by lysosome and lead to lysosomal disruption. Cathepsins released after lysosomal damage increase K^+ efflux via an ATP-dependent mechanism [5,8]. Some studies have shown that chloride efflux via volume-regulated anion channels (VRACs) can also trigger NLRP3 activation [9,10]. In addition, mitochondrial stress and increased calcium influx contribute to increased intracellular reactive oxygen species (ROS), which activate NLRP3 [11].

1.2. Ion-Independent Activation Pathways

Inhibition of glycolysis, inhibition of mitochondrial NADH oxidase, and displacement of hexokinase 2 from mitochondria have been linked to NLRP3 activation via an ion-independent mechanism [5]. Once activated, NLRP3 and ASC move from the endoplasmic reticulum and mitochondria, respectively, to form the inflammasome complex in the cytoplasm. The NLRP3 NACHT domain promotes oligomerization of the NLRP3 pyrin domain to bind ASC via pyrin–pyrin interactions. ASC is then converted to a prion-like form and long ASC specks or pyroptosome are produced, which play an important role in NLRP3 activation. Pro-caspase-1 then binds to ASC via CARD–CARD interactions and forms its own prion-like filaments that branch off the ASC filaments. Procaspase-1 consists of two fragments: a p35 fragment, which contains both a CARD domain and p20 subunit, and a p10 fragment. Active caspase-1 is formed after heterodimerization of two molecules of p20 with two molecules of p10. Active caspase-1 then activates pro-IL-1β by its conversion to IL-1β, which is released from the cell and causes tissue damage and/or repair [12,13].

Recently, studies reported that NEK7 (NIMA-related kinase 7), a member of the NIMA ('never in mitosis gene A')-related serine-threonine kinase family, plays a key role in NLRP3 activation. Its binding to the C-terminal LRR domain of NLRP3 during interphase is pivotal for NLRP3-ASC-caspase 1 assembly. NEK7 is a mitotic kinase, which also serves in mitotic spindle formation and centrosome separation in the cell cycle. The amount of NEK7 in macrophages is insufficient to enable its dual action simultaneously; thus, NEK7 activates NLRP3 only in interphase. Interestingly, NLRP3-NEK7 binding is linked to potassium efflux, although the exact mechanism is unknown [3,13,14].

Despite its role in the defense against invading pathogens and in tissue repair, NLRP3 inflammasome activation is implicated in the pathogenesis of a range of serious conditions. Inflammasome-dependent diseases include cancer, metabolic disorders (e.g., type 2 diabetes), diseases caused by the accumulation of crystals (e.g., gout or atherosclerosis), and diseases caused by the formation of protein aggregates (e.g., Alzheimer's disease) [15–18]. Considering in more detail the problem of gout as an example (Figure 1b), we observe that this disease is characterized by the deposition of monosodium urate (MSU) crystals in the joints when its plasma concentration is >420 µM, leading to joint swelling and inflammation. Crystal accumulation activates the immune system, activating the macrophage to remove the accumulated crystals by phagocytosis to form a phagosome. The phagosome fuses with the lysosome in the cytoplasm of the macrophage to form a phagolysosome. Further crystal accumulation in the phagosome leads to lysosomal disruption that activates the sensor part of the NLRP3 inflammasome from its inactive closed form to an active open form. After, the active NLRP3 sensor oligomerizes and binds to the adaptor and effector parts of the inflammasome as mentioned earlier. Finally, this process leads to the release of active IL-1β from the cell, which causes an inflammatory effect and joint pain in gout patients [18–24].

1.3. MCC950 and Analogues as Inhibitors of NLRP3

MCC950 (Figure 2a) is a diaryl sulfonyl urea derivative known as cytokine release inhibitory drug 3 (CRID3). MCC950 is considered as the most potent and selective NLRP3 inhibitor to date, with an IC_{50} of 7.5 nM in mouse bone marrow-derived macrophages (BMDMs) and an IC_{50} of 8.1 nM in human monocyte-derived macrophages (HMDMs) [25,26]. Mechanistic studies revealed that MCC950 binds to the NLRP3^{NACHT} subdomains, hindering the ATPase activity, driving NLRP3 into the inactive closed conformer [27–29]. Moreover, MCC950 can bind to both active (open) and inactive (closed) conformers of NLRP3 [30,31]. Although MCC950 is one of the most potent direct selective inhibitors of NLRP3, the reported renal and hepatic toxicity restricts its therapeutic development, which may be attributed to the furan moiety of MCC950 [32,33]. Therefore, it is essential to develop potent NLRP3 inhibitors with a new chemical scaffold.

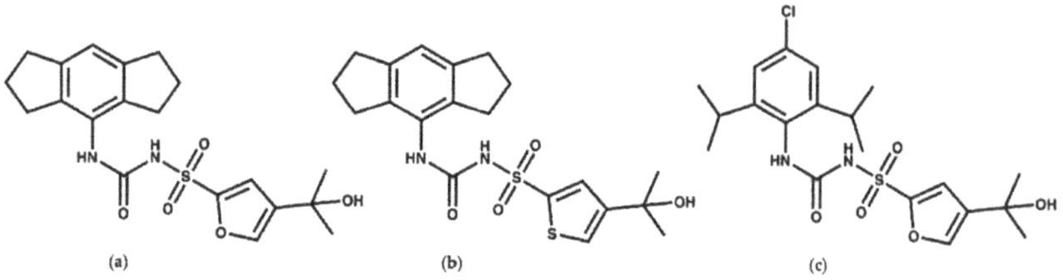

Figure 2. Chemical structures of (**a**) MCC950, (**b**) the thiophene isostere of MCC950 [24], and (**c**) NP3-146.

Keuler and coworkers [34] studied the chemical stability of a series of 12 sulfonyl urea analogues of MCC950 using HPLC, and the affinity of the compounds with NLRP3 was also determined using surface plasmon resonance spectroscopy. Their study revealed that the anionic form of MCC950 and its analogues are more stable than the neutral form. Additionally, Keuler and coworkers reported that the thiophene isostere (Figure 2b) had the same potency and stability as MCC950, which could be of use for the future design of novel inhibitors. Interestingly, their study suggested that the tertiary alcohol group is important both for the chemical stability and activity of the MCC950 analogues [34]. In 2021, a crystal structure of the NACHT domain in complex with NP3-146 (Figure 2c) was solved by Dekker and coworkers [35] (PDB code 7ALV, resolution 2.8 Å). The fluorescent probe NP3-146 inhibits the NLRP3 activity and the release of IL-1β at a concentration of 20 nM [35].

In this piece of work, we started with a short introduction to the NLRP3 inflammasome activation process and its implication in inflammatory diseases. Then, selected natural products reported in the literature as NLRP3 inhibitors will be discussed, with a particular focus in some which target gout. Finally, a virtual screen (VS) of the ZINC20 natural product database was performed to provide insight into the future design of selective NLRP3 inhibitors.

2. Reported NLRP3 Natural Product Inhibitors

Inflammasomes play an important role in the pathogenesis and progression of diseases so they are considered as important therapeutic targets. Inflammasome inhibitors have the potential to treat a number of life-threatening diseases. There are different suggested mechanisms for the inhibition of inflammasome activity. Here, we provide selected examples of natural products (NPs) that have been reported in the literature as NLRP3 inhibitors, with a focus on those relating to gout. For NPs targeting other diseases, we direct the reader elsewhere [36–45].

2.1. Glycyrrhizin and Isoliquirtigenin

ASC oligomerization is a key step in inflammasome activation. Glycyrrhizin (GL) and isoliquirtigenin (ILG) (Figure 3)are flavonoid derivatives from Glycyrrhiza uralensis that exert their inflammasome inhibitory activity either by inhibiting ASC pyroptosome formation or LPS- NF-κB activation [46]. GL can inhibit both NLRP3 and AIM2 inflammasome activation while ILG is a selective inhibitor for NLRP3 inflammasome with an IC_{50} value of 10.1 μM [46,47]. In the study conducted by Hiroe and coworkers [46], the IL-1β release was 3 ng/mL in the ATP-induced NLRP3 inflammasome activation when the cells were treated with 1000 and 1 μM of GL and ILG, respectively. This indicates that ILG is more potent than GL. Moreover, ILG can inhibit IL-1β release in response to MSU-induced NLRP3 activation at a concentration of 10 μM.

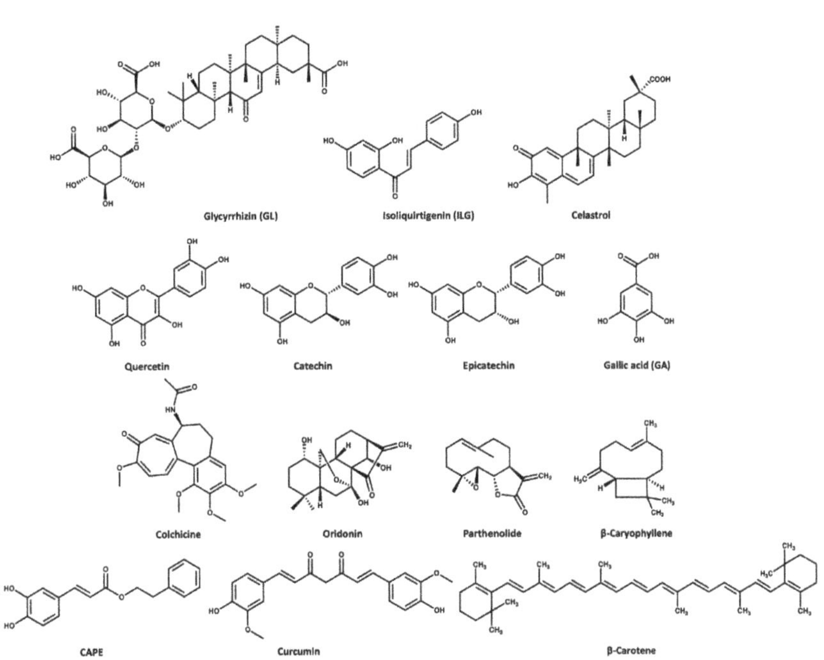

Figure 3. Chemical structures of the selected NPs that are known inhibitors of the NLRP3 inflammasome.

2.2. Celastrol

Celastrol (Figure 3) triterpenoid isolated from the roots of *Tripterygium wilfordii*, shows a promising anti-inflammatory effect. The Chinese National Medical Products Administration has approved the use of *Tripterygium wilfordii* tablets for the treatment of rheumatoid arthritis: a concentration of 25–50 nM of celastrol inhibits the IL-1β release in ATP- and LPS-induced NLRP3 activation [48]. Yu and coworkers [49] reported that a dose of 125 nM of celastrol could inhibit the IL-1β release in vivo and in vitro through preventing the oligomerization of ASC and subsequently NLRP3 activity [49].

2.3. Quercetin and Procyanidins

Quercetin is a dietary flavonoid (Figure 3) present in many fruits and vegetables as glycosides, ethers, or sulfates. Quercetin is known to have beneficial effects on human health [50–52]. Quercetin has been reported to show an anti-inflammatory effect in gouty arthritis caused by MSU, showing inhibition of IL-1β release at a concentration of 30 μM, with reports suggesting that this effect is related to inhibition of the NLRP3 inflammasome [53,54]. Procyanidins are a group of flavonoids that exist as secondary metabolites in fruits (e.g., cherries, grapes). Procyanidins exist in two forms: monomer (catechin and epicatechin (Figure 3), and homopolymer [55,56]. Several studies suggest that the intake of procyanidins (or consuming cherries) helps to decrease joint swelling and pain associated with gout. It has also been reported that procyanidins at a concentration of 10 μM can inhibit NLRP3 activation induced by MSU in vitro [57].

To provide insight into the potential interaction of quercetin and the procyanidins monomers (catechin and epicatechin) with NLRP3, here, we docked each compound in turn into the cofactor site and the known (MCC950) inhibitor binding site in the NACHT domain of NLRP3 [35] using the software OEdocking [58]. Quercetin and the procyanidins did not dock well into the cofactor site; however, quercetin and epicatechin were both a good fit for the inhibitor binding site, with chemgauss4 docking scores of −10.8 and −10.5, respectively (Figure 4). The oxygen atom of the chromen-4-one ring in quercetin and the chroman ring in epicatechin form hydrogen bonds with Arg578, which is one of the key residues for MCC950 binding observed in the crystal and cryo-EM structures (Figure 4a). Moreover, two hydrogen bonds formed between the hydroxyl groups of the ligands and the carboxylate side chain of Glu629 and Asp662 (Figure 4b). This suggests that these polyphenols may be used as lead compounds to design novel selective inhibitors of the NLRP3 inflammasome.

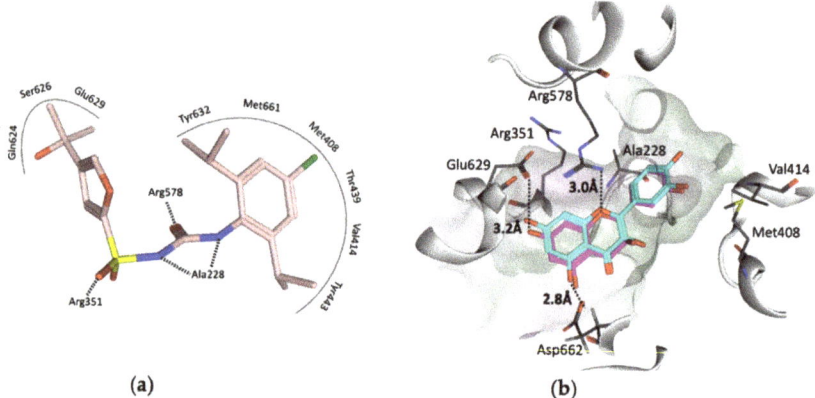

Figure 4. (**a**) Representation of the MCC950–analogue (NP3-146) interactions from the NACHT domain X-ray structure (PDB code 7ALV) [25]. (**b**) Docked poses of quercetin (cyan) and epicatechin (magenta) in the ligand binding site of the NACHT domain. Black dotted lines represent the hydrogen bonds, and the pocket is colored based on the lipophilicity; polar surface (purple) and nonpolar surface (green).

2.4. Gallic Acid

Gallic acid (GA, Figure 3) belongs to the polyphenol class of phytochemicals and is widely distributed in plants such as pomegranates, guava, mulberry, and tea leaves. GA is known for its antioxidant and anti-inflammatory activity [59,60]. A study revealed that GA has anti-inflammatory activity in gouty arthritis due to NLRP3 inhibition. Their study suggested that GA at a concentration of 80 µM can inhibit MSU-mediated NLRP3 activation and inflammasome oligomerization via inhibition of NEK7 binding to NLRP3 in vitro [61]. Moreover, a dose of 100 mg/kg GA was effective in treating knee joint swelling in a mice model by inhibiting the IL-1β release compared to a dose of 1 mg/kg for colchicine [61].

2.5. Colchicine

The *Colchicum autumnale* plant, also known as the autumn crocus, is the natural source of colchicine (Figure 3) Colchicine is a microtubule inhibitor [62], which has been used for the treatment of gout since ancient Egyptian times, receiving approval by the FDA in 2009 [62–64]. Bonaventura and coworkers [65] recently reported that the anti-inflammatory effect of colchicine is related to its ability to inhibit NLRP3 inflammasome oligomerization, which subsequently causes inhibition of the release of cytokines. However, the exact mechanism is unclear, with a suggestion that the microtubule depolymerization by colchicine in immune cells may negatively affect inflammasome oligomerization [65,66].

2.6. Oridonin

Oridonin (Figure 3) is a herbal medicine used for the treatment of inflammatory diseases, for example, gout, peritonitis, and type-2 diabetes. Oridonin's anti-inflammatory activity is due to its covalent binding to cysteine 279 of NACHT through a Michael addition, which prevents the NEK7–NLRP3 interaction (Figure 5). Oridonin inhibits NLRP3 activity with an IC_{50} value of 0.75 µM [67,68].

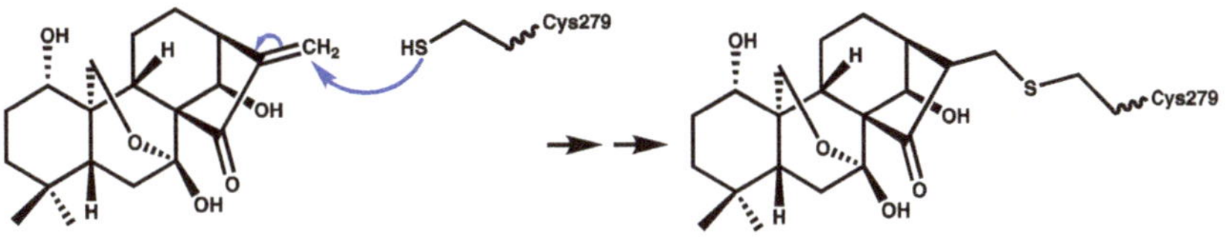

Figure 5. Schematic representation of covalent bond formation between oridonin and cysteine 279 of the NACHT domain.

2.7. Parthenolide

Parthenolide (Figure 3) belongs to the sesquiterpene lactone phytochemical class, which is widely used for the treatment of inflammatory disorders. It has been reported that the anti-inflammatory effect of parthenolide is due to its binding to cysteine residues of caspase-1 so it can inhibit inflammasomes and subsequently cytokine release [69,70]. Juliana and coworkers [70] reported that parthenolide at a concentration of 10 µM can selectively inhibit the ATPase activity of NLRP3 through binding to cysteine in the p20 subunit of caspase-1. In addition, we propose that the mechanism of parthenolide binding to cysteine of caspase-1 may be similar to the oridonin binding to the cysteine residue of NACHT (Figure 5) due to the structural similarity between parthenolide and oridonin.

2.8. β-Caryophyllene

β-Caryophyllene (Figure 3) is a bicyclic sesquiterpene that is most abundant in the essential oils extracted from oregano, cinnamon, rosemary, thyme, basil, mint, cloves, and ginger. β-Caryophyllene shows various biological activities through its binding to cannabinoid receptors [71,72]. Recently, Li and coworkers [73] reported that β-caryophyllene can block the MSU-induced activation of NLRP3 in vivo using a dose of 100 mg/kg. Moreover, their study suggests that the mechanism of action of β-caryophyllene may be through direct binding to NLRP3 or indirect inhibition of NF-κB, caspase-1, ASC, and/or TLR4 [73].

2.9. CAPE

Caffeic acid phenethyl ester (CAPE) (Figure 3) naturally extracted from propolis (a resin made by bees), is proposed to be effective for the treatment of acute gout [74]. CAPE is a small molecule that shows NLRP3 inhibitory activity at a concentration of 10 µM. CAPE exerts its inhibitory activity via direct binding to ASC^{PYD} but not $NLRP3^{PYD}$, thus preventing ASC-NLRP3 oligomerization [74].

2.10. Curcumin

Curcumin (Figure 3) extracted from turmeric (*Curcuma longa*), is used widely as a herbal supplement due to its antioxidant and anti-inflammatory activities [75,76]. Studies have shown that the role of curcumin in inflammatory diseases may be attributed to its inhibitory effect on the NF-κB signaling pathway, which is involved in inflammasome activation [77,78]. Poor water solubility, fast metabolism at physiological pH, and poor bioavailability of curcumin are the main challenges in studying its therapeutic effect; however, it is noted that piperine increases its bioavailability [79]. To overcome these limitations, studies have used metals or polypeptides as a delivery system to improve the solubility and bioavailability of curcumin [78,80]. Zhang and coworkers [78] used tetrahedral framework nucleic acids (TFNAs) as a carrier for curcumin to improve its bioavailability. Then, in vivo testing of the curcumin–TFNAs complex using a mouse model of gout induced by MSU revealed that the complex can manage joint swelling at a concentration of 40 µM.

2.11. β-Carotene

β-Carotene (Figure 3) is a prodrug of retinol (vitamin A) that exists in most fruit and vegetables. In 2020, Yang and coworkers [81] studied the NLRP3 inhibitory activity of β-carotene using gout as a disease model. This study revealed that β-carotene (30 mg/kg in vivo and 20 µM in vitro) can selectively inhibit NLRP3 through its direct binding to the pyrin domain. Of note, oral administration of β-carotene was of benefit in the treatment of gouty arthritis in mice [69,81].

3. Virtual Screening to Identify Possible Natural Product Scaffolds Targeting NLRP3

The study of NPs as treatments for various diseases is of substantial interest to the scientific community; however, there are limitations as many NPs are present at low concentrations in the natural source and have complex structures, making their synthesis challenging [82,83]. Moreover, most NPs are non-selective for certain protein targets and need a high dose to have a therapeutic effect [84]. However, compounds from natural sources could be used as inspiring lead compounds to rationally design novel selective small molecules [85–87]. Chen and coworkers [87] used pterostilbene (IC_{50} > 10 mM), which was extracted from blueberries as a lead compound to develop a more potent NLRP3 inhibitor with an IC_{50} value of 0.56 µM (Figure 6).

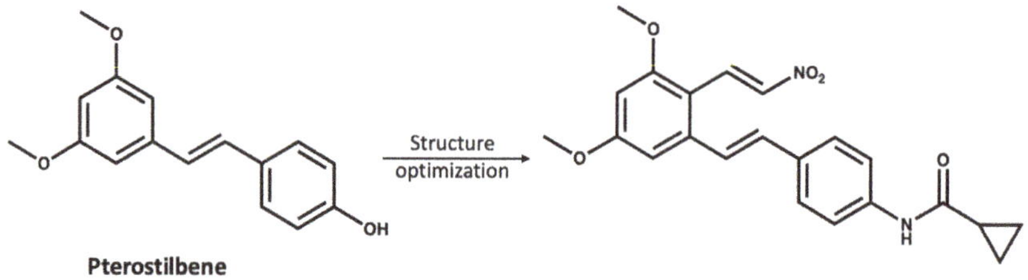

Figure 6. The reported [87] structure optimization of pterostilbene, leading to the discovery of a more potent NLRP3 inhibitor.

In order to identify NP scaffolds that could provide potent specific interactions with NLRP3, in this current work, we performed VS of 100,000 compounds from the ZINC20 natural products database (https://zinc20.docking.org (accessed on 15 August 2022)) using the OpenEye [58] software suite. This subset of ZINC20 was selected according to physical properties (Table S1), then docked into the MCC950 inhibitor binding site and the ADP cofactor site from the crystal structure of the NLRP3-NACHT domain (Figure 7, PDB code 7ALV) [35]. A final selection of compounds for the cofactor site and the inhibitor site are discussed.

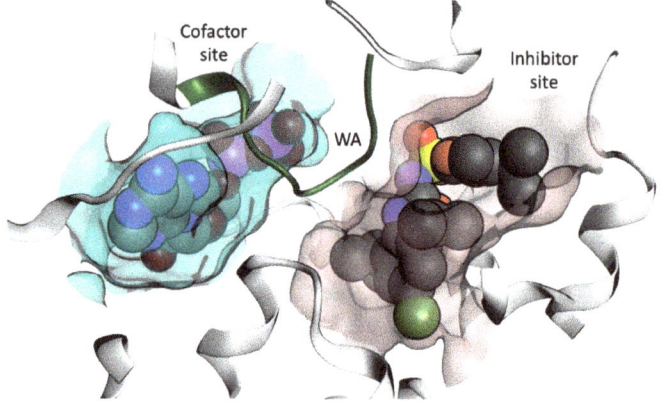

Figure 7. Representation of the cofactor (ADP) site and the inhibitor binding site from the X-ray structure of the NACHT domain of NLRP3 (PDB code 7ALV) [25]. Walker A (WA) site is colored green.

Docking of the subset from the ZINC20 natural products database in both the cofactor and inhibitor sites resulted in the identification of two sets of compounds. The first group of compounds **1–6** showed good binding to the ADP cofactor binding site (Figure 8a and Table S2), which have structural features in common with celastrol. In addition, compounds **1–6** all contain a charged carboxylate group, which is predicted to facilitate binding to the Walker A site, similar to the known NLRP3 inhibitor, CY09 (Figure 8b) [88]. The docking scores for compounds **1–6** ranged from −16.0 to −17.5, similar to the redocked score of −16.3 for ADP in its X-ray pose and better than the docking score of −14.3 for CY09 (Table S2).

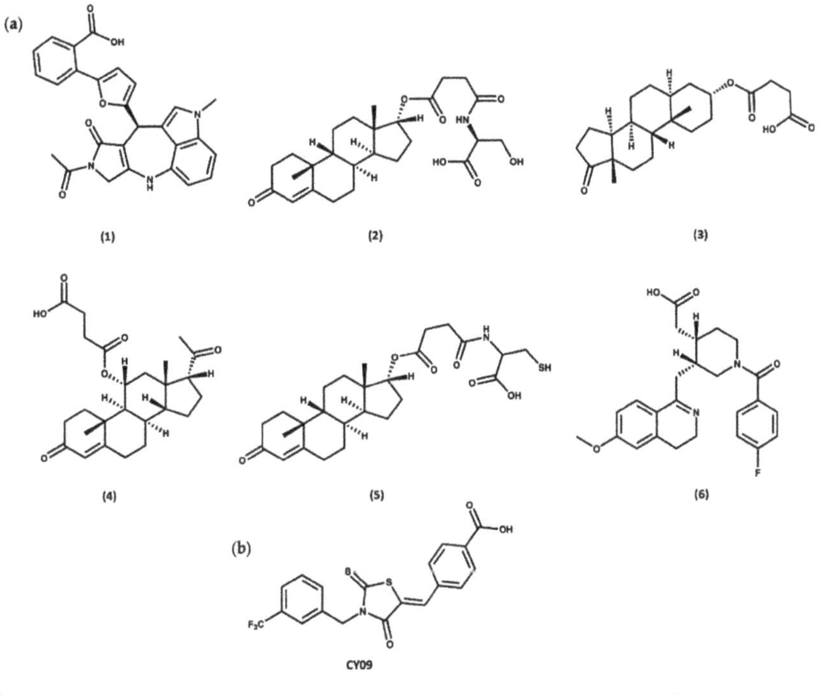

Figure 8. (a) Top-ranked compounds predicted from virtual screening of the ZINC20 NP database to bind to the ADP cofactor site of the NLRP3-NACHT structure. (b) Chemical structure of CY09.

The second group of compounds, ranking top from virtual screening into the known MCC950 ligand binding site, all have a general structure containing an indole ring connected to an aromatic ring through an amide linker; this pharmacophore is denoted in Figure 9a. The indole moiety is a common scaffold in drug discovery, both in synthetic compounds and natural indole alkaloids, with various pharmacological activities [89,90]. The docking scores of this group in the inhibitor site were approximately −14, compared to values of −11.2 and −12.7 for the known inhibitors NP3-146 and MCC950, respectively. Interestingly, these indole compounds, such as **7** and **8** (Figure 9b), have some structural similarity to the recently published compound **J114** (Figure 9c). The latter compound was reported to show both NLRP3 and AIM2 inhibition via inhibition of the interaction between ASC protein and the inflammasome [91]. Yan and coworkers [91] designed compound **J114** (IC_{50} = 0.07 µM) by structure optimization of the hit compound **1** (IC_{50} = 3.1 µM) obtained from high-throughput screening (Figure 9c).

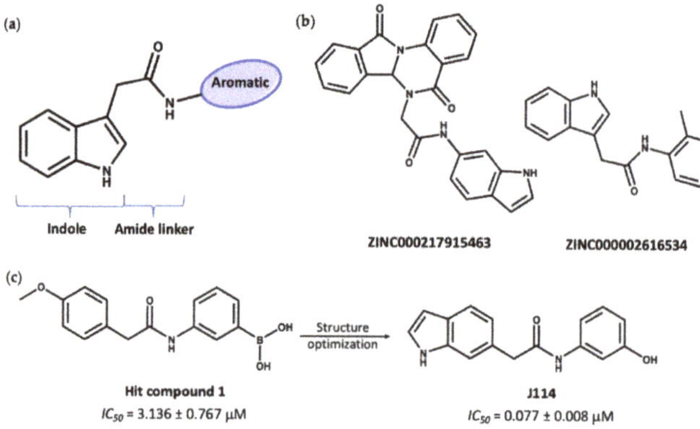

Figure 9. (a) General structure of top-ranked compounds predicted from virtual screening to bind to the MCC950 inhibitor site of the NLRP3-NACHT structure. (b) Structures of compounds **7** (ZINC ID: ZINC000217915463) and **8** (ZINC ID: ZINC000002616534). (c) The reported [91] hit compound **1** and the synthetic active NLRP3 inhibitor, **J114**.

4. Conclusions

Non-steroidal anti-inflammatory drugs (NSAIDs), colchicine, and corticosteroids are the most common approaches to the treatment of acute attacks of gout (British National Formulary (BNF) [92]. Xanthine oxidase inhibitors, for example, allopurinol, are used for the long-term control of gout, which decreases the concentration of uric acid, preventing urate deposition (BNF). According to the American College of Rheumatology guidelines and the BNF, IL-1β inhibitors (e.g., canakinumab) could be used for certain cases of gouty arthritis that cannot be treated with NSAIDs [93]. The biologic canakinumab and other IL-1β inhibitors are orally inactive, so it is urgent to design small orally active leads that inhibit proteins involved in IL-1β release. The NLRP3 inflammasome is a cytoplasmic protein complex that is implicated in IL-1β release and inflammation in various inflammatory diseases, including gout. Many studies have revealed that NPs can directly inhibit NLRP3 activity by binding to the NLRP3^{NACHT} domain (e.g., oridonin) or to NLRP3^{PYD} (e.g., β-carotene). Additionally, NPs can inhibit NLRP3 indirectly through blocking of NLRP3-ASC binding (e.g., ILG, CAPE), inhibition of ASC oligomerization (e.g., celastrol), or inhibition of the NF-κB signaling pathway (β-caryophyllene, curcumin).

To obtain further insights into the preferred scaffolds, we used virtual screening with the ZINC20 database of NPs, resulting in two sets of predicted inhibitors targeting NLRP3. The first group is similar in structure to a known NLRP3 inhibitor either from a natural source (e.g., celastrol), which have a common steroid structure similar to most of the compounds in the first group, or synthetically derived (e.g., CY09) in which the carboxylate group is key to its binding to the Walker A site; these potential inhibitors are predicted to interact with NLRP3 through direct binding to the ADP/ATP site. The second group of compounds, all containing indole rings, have very promising binding energies to the inhibitor site of the NACHT domain. This survey of existing natural product inhibitors of the inflammasome, combined with virtual screening for preferred NP scaffolds targeting NLRP3, highlights the possibilities for the design of novel selective NLRP3 inhibitors inspired by natural products.

Supplementary Materials: The following supporting information can be downloaded at: https://www.mdpi.com/article/10.3390/molecules27196213/s1, Table S1: Filter parameters used to filter ZINC20 natural products subset; Table S2: Docking score and similarity score of the best compounds that bind to the cofactor site (compounds **1–6**) using the structure of the NACHT domain of NLRP3 (PDB code 7ALV) [35].

Author Contributions: Conceptualization, S.F., S.E.-S. and R.A.B.; methodology, S.F., S.E.-S. and R.A.B.; formal analysis, S.E.-S. and R.A.B.; writing—original draft preparation, S.E.-S.; writing—review and editing, S.F. and R.A.B.; supervision, S.F. and R.A.B. All authors have read and agreed to the published version of the manuscript.

Funding: This research was funded by the Egyptian Ministry of Higher Education-Mission Sector through a full PhD scholarship (ADDED MM 14/19) to Sherihan El-Sayed at the University of Manchester. This work also made use of the facilities of the N8 Centre of Excellence in Computationally Intensive Research (N8 CIR) provided and funded by the N8 research partnership and EPSRC (Grant No. EP/T022167/1). The Centre is coordinated by the Universities of Durham, Manchester, and York.

Institutional Review Board Statement: Not applicable.

Informed Consent Statement: Not applicable.

Data Availability Statement: The datasets generated and analyzed in the current study are available from the corresponding author upon reasonable request.

Acknowledgments: The authors would like to acknowledge the assistance given by Research IT and the use of the Computational Shared Facility at The University of Manchester.

Conflicts of Interest: The authors declare no conflict of interest.

References

1. Rathinam, V.A.; Chan, F.K.M. Inflammasome, inflammation, and tissue homeostasis. *Trends Mol. Med.* **2018**, *24*, 304–318. [CrossRef] [PubMed]
2. Guo, H.; Callaway, J.B.; Ting, J.P. Inflammasomes: Mechanism of action, role in disease, and therapeutics. *Nat. Med.* **2015**, *21*, 677–687. [CrossRef] [PubMed]
3. Sharif, H.; Wang, L.; Wang, W.L.; Magupalli, V.G.; Andreeva, L.; Qiao, Q.; Hauenstein, A.V.; Wu, Z.; Núñez, G.; Mao, Y.; et al. Structural mechanism for NEK7-licensed activation of NLRP3 inflammasome. *Nature* **2019**, *570*, 338–343. [CrossRef] [PubMed]
4. El-Sayed, S.; Freeman, S.; Bryce, R.A. Probing the effect of NEK7 and cofactor interactions on dynamics of NLRP3 monomer using molecular simulation. *Prot. Sci.* **2022**. *In press.*
5. Mangan, M.S.; Olhava, E.J.; Roush, W.R.; Seidel, H.M.; Glick, G.D.; Latz, E. Targeting the NLRP3 inflammasome in inflammatory diseases. *Nat. Rev. Drug Discov.* **2018**, *17*, 588–606. [CrossRef]
6. Swanson, K.V.; Deng, M.; Ting, J.P.Y. The NLRP3 inflammasome: Molecular activation and regulation to therapeutics. *Nat. Rev. Immunol.* **2019**, *19*, 477–489. [CrossRef]
7. Tschopp, J.; Schroder, K. NLRP3 inflammasome activation: The convergence of multiple signalling pathways on ROS production? *Nat. Rev. Immunol.* **2010**, *10*, 210–215. [CrossRef]
8. Ribeiro, D.E.; Roncalho, A.L.; Glaser, T.; Ulrich, H.; Wegener, G.; Joca, S. P2X7 receptor signaling in stress and depression. *Int. J. Mol. Sci.* **2019**, *20*, 2778. [CrossRef]
9. Daniels, M.J.; Rivers-Auty, J.; Schilling, T.; Spencer, N.G.; Watremez, W.; Fasolino, V.; Booth, S.J.; White, C.S.; Baldwin, A.G.; Freeman, S.; et al. Fenamate NSAIDs inhibit the NLRP3 inflammasome and protect against Alzheimer's disease in rodent models. *Nat. Commun.* **2016**, *7*, 1–10. [CrossRef]
10. Yang, Y.; Wang, H.; Kouadir, M.; Song, H.; Shi, F. Recent advances in the mechanisms of NLRP3 inflammasome activation and its inhibitors. *Cell Death Dis.* **2019**, *10*, 1–11. [CrossRef]
11. Abais, J.M.; Xia, M.; Zhang, Y.; Boini, K.M.; Li, P.L. Redox regulation of NLRP3 inflammasomes: ROS as trigger or effector? *Antioxid. Redox Signal.* **2015**, *22*, 1111–1129. [CrossRef] [PubMed]
12. Rathinam, V.A.; Vanaja, S.K.; Fitzgerald, K.A. Regulation of inflammasome signaling. *Nat. Immunol.* **2012**, *13*, 333–342. [CrossRef] [PubMed]
13. Shi, H.; Wang, Y.; Li, X.; Zhan, X.; Tang, M.; Fina, M.; Su, L.; Pratt, D.; Bu, C.H.; Hildebrand, S.; et al. NLRP3 activation and mitosis are mutually exclusive events coordinated by NEK7, a new inflammasome component. *Nat. Immunol.* **2016**, *17*, 250–258. [CrossRef] [PubMed]
14. He, Y.; Zeng, M.Y.; Yang, D.; Motro, B.; Núñez, G. NEK7 is an essential mediator of NLRP3 activation downstream of potassium efflux. *Nature* **2016**, *530*, 354–357. [CrossRef]
15. Legrand-Poels, S.; Esser, N.; L'homme, L.; Scheen, A.; Paquot, N.; Piette, J. Free fatty acids as modulators of the NLRP3 inflammasome in obesity/type 2 diabetes. *Biochem. Pharmacol.* **2014**, *92*, 131–141. [CrossRef]
16. Liu, D.; Zeng, X.; Li, X.; Mehta, J.L.; Wang, X. Role of NLRP3 inflammasome in the pathogenesis of cardiovascular diseases. *Basic Res. Cardiol.* **2018**, *113*, 1–14. [CrossRef]
17. Heneka, M.T.; Kummer, M.P.; Stutz, A.; Delekate, A.; Schwartz, S.; Vieira-Saecker, A.; Griep, A.; Axt, D.; Remus, A.; Tzeng, T.C.; et al. NLRP3 is activated in Alzheimer's disease and contributes to pathology in APP/PS1 mice. *Nature* **2013**, *493*, 674–678. [CrossRef]

18. Szekanecz, Z.; Szamosi, S.; Kovács, G.E.; Kocsis, E.; Benkő, S. The NLRP3 inflammasome-interleukin 1 pathway as a therapeutic target in gout. *Arch. Biochem. Biophys.* **2019**, *670*, 82–93. [CrossRef]
19. Martinon, F.; Pétrilli, V.; Mayor, A.; Tardivel, A.; Tschopp, J. Gout-associated uric acid crystals activate the NALP3 inflammasome. *Nature* **2006**, *440*, 237–241. [CrossRef]
20. Busso, N.; So, A. Gout. Mechanisms of inflammation in gout. *Arthritis Res. Ther.* **2010**, *12*, 1–8. [CrossRef]
21. Kingsbury, S.R.; Conaghan, P.G.; McDermott, M.F. The role of the NLRP3 inflammasome in gout. *J. Inflamm. Res.* **2011**, *4*, 39. [PubMed]
22. Liu, L.; Wang, D.; Liu, M.; Yu, H.; Chen, Q.; Wu, Y.; Bao, R.; Zhang, Y.; Wang, T. The development from hyperuricemia to gout: Key mechanisms and natural products for treatment. *Acupunct. Herb. Med.* **2022**, *2*, 25–32. [CrossRef]
23. So, A.K.; Martinon, F. Inflammation in gout: Mechanisms and therapeutic targets. *Nat. Rev. Rheumatol.* **2017**, *13*, 639–647. [CrossRef]
24. Cabău, G.; Crișan, T.O.; Klück, V.; Popp, R.A.; Joosten, L.A. Urate-induced immune programming: Consequences for gouty arthritis and hyperuricemia. *Immunol. Rev.* **2020**, *294*, 92–105. [CrossRef] [PubMed]
25. Zhang, X.; Xu, A.; Lv, J.; Zhang, Q.; Ran, Y.; Wei, C.; Wu, J. Development of small molecule inhibitors targeting NLRP3 inflammasome pathway for inflammatory diseases. *Eur. J. Med. Chem.* **2019**, *185*, 111822. [CrossRef] [PubMed]
26. Coll, R.C.; Robertson, A.A.; Chae, J.J.; Higgins, S.C.; Muñoz-Planillo, R.; Inserra, M.C.; Vetter, I.; Dungan, L.S.; Monks, B.G.; Stutz, A.; et al. A small-molecule inhibitor of the NLRP3 inflammasome for the treatment of inflammatory diseases. *Nature Med.* **2015**, *21*, 248. [CrossRef]
27. Ohto, U.; Kamitsukasa, Y.; Ishida, H.; Zhang, Z.; Murakami, K.; Hirama, C.; Maekawa, S.; Shimizu, T. Structural basis for the oligomerization-mediated regulation of NLRP3 inflammasome activation. *Proc. Natl. Acad. Sci. USA* **2022**, *119*, e2121353119. [CrossRef]
28. Andreeva, L.; David, L.; Rawson, S.; Shen, C.; Pasricha, T.; Pelegrin, P.; Wu, H. NLRP3 cages revealed by full-length mouse NLRP3 structure control pathway activation. *Cell* **2021**, *184*, 6299–6312. [CrossRef]
29. Hochheiser, I.V.; Pilsl, M.; Hagelueken, G.; Moecking, J.; Marleaux, M.; Brinkschulte, R.; Latz, E.; Engel, C.; Geyer, M. Structure of the NLRP3 decamer bound to the cytokine release inhibitor CRID3. *Nature* **2022**, *604*, 184–189. [CrossRef]
30. Tapia-Abellán, A.; Angosto-Bazarra, D.; Martínez-Banaclocha, H.; de Torre-Minguela, C.; Cerón-Carrasco, J.P.; Pérez-Sánchez, H.; Arostegui, J.I.; Pelegrin, P. MCC950 closes the active conformation of NLRP3 to an inactive state. *Nat. Chem. Biol.* **2019**, *15*, 560. [CrossRef]
31. Coll, R.C.; Hill, J.R.; Day, C.J.; Zamoshnikova, A.; Boucher, D.; Massey, N.L.; Chitty, J.L.; Fraser, J.A.; Jennings, M.P.; Robertson, A.A.; et al. MCC950 directly targets the NLRP3 ATP-hydrolysis motif for inflammasome inhibition. *Nat. Chem. Biol.* **2019**, *15*, 556–559. [CrossRef] [PubMed]
32. Østergaard, J.A.; Jha, J.C.; Sharma, A.; Dai, A.; Choi, J.S.; de Haan, J.B.; Cooper, M.E.; Jandeleit-Dahm, K. Adverse renal effects of NLRP3 inflammasome inhibition by MCC950 in an interventional model of diabetic kidney disease. *Clin. Sci.* **2022**, *136*, 167–180. [CrossRef] [PubMed]
33. Li, H.; Guan, Y.; Liang, B.; Ding, P.; Hou, X.; Wei, W.; Ma, Y. Therapeutic potential of MCC950, a specific inhibitor of NLRP3 inflammasome. *Eur. J. Pharmacol.* **2022**, *928*, 175091. [CrossRef] [PubMed]
34. Keuler, T.; Ferber, D.; Marleaux, M.; Geyer, M.; Guütschow, M. Structure–Stability Relationship of NLRP3 Inflammasome-Inhibiting Sulfonylureas. *ACS Omega* **2022**, *7*, 8158–8162. [CrossRef]
35. Dekker, C.; Mattes, H.; Wright, M.; Boettcher, A.; Hinniger, A.; Hughes, N.; Kapps-Fouthier, S.; Eder, J.; Erbel, P.; Stiefl, N.; et al. Crystal Structure of NLRP3 NACHT Domain With an Inhibitor Defines Mechanism of Inflammasome Inhibition. *J. Mol. Biol.* **2021**, *433*, 167309. [CrossRef]
36. Bai, Y.; Mu, Q.; Bao, X.; Zuo, J.; Fang, X.; Hua, J.; Zhang, D.; Jiang, G.; Li, P.; Gao, S.; et al. Targeting NLRP3 Inflammasome in the Treatment Of Diabetes and Diabetic Complications: Role of Natural Compounds from Herbal Medicine. *Aging Dis.* **2021**, *12*, 1587. [CrossRef]
37. Bagherniya, M.; Khedmatgozar, H.; Fakheran, O.; Xu, S.; Johnston, T.P.; Sahebkar, A. Medicinal plants and bioactive natural products as inhibitors of NLRP3 inflammasome. *Phytother. Res.* **2021**, *35*, 4804–4833. [CrossRef]
38. Lee, J.H.; Kim, H.J.; Kim, J.U.; Yook, T.H.; Kim, K.H.; Lee, J.Y.; Yang, G. A Novel Treatment Strategy by Natural Products in NLRP3 Inflammasome-Mediated Neuroinflammation in Alzheimer's and Parkinson's Disease. *Int. J. Mol. Sci.* **2021**, *22*, 1324. [CrossRef]
39. Hua, F.; Shi, L.; Zhou, P. Phenols and terpenoids: Natural products as inhibitors of NLRP3 inflammasome in cardiovascular diseases. *Inflammopharmacology* **2022**, *30*, 137–147. [CrossRef]
40. Ding, N.; Wei, B.; Fu, X.; Wang, C.; Wu, Y. Natural products that target the NLRP3 inflammasome to treat fibrosis. *Front. Pharmacol.* **2020**, *11*, 591393. [CrossRef]
41. Du, D.; Lv, W.; Jing, X.; Ma, X.; Wuen, J.; Hasi, S. Dietary supplementation of camel whey protein attenuates heat stress-induced liver injury by inhibiting NLRP3 inflammasome activation through the HMGB1/RAGE signalling pathway. *J. Funct. Foods* **2021**, *84*, 104584. [CrossRef]
42. Liu, B.; Yu, J. Anti-NLRP3 inflammasome natural compounds: An update. *Biomedicines* **2021**, *9*, 136.
43. ZHOU, P.; Zhao, C.C.; Li, J.Y.; Zhang, M.; Shi, H.; Wang, L. A review on the role of quinones in cardiovascular disease via inhibiting nlrp3 inflammasome. *Acta Pol. Pharm.* **2021**, *78*, 743–748. [CrossRef]

44. Özenver, N.; Efferth, T. Phytochemical inhibitors of the NLRP3 inflammasome for the treatment of inflammatory diseases. *Pharmacol. Res.* **2021**, *170*, 105710. [CrossRef] [PubMed]
45. Zou, J.; Wang, S.P.; Wang, Y.T.; Wan, J.B. Regulation of the NLRP3 inflammasome with natural products against chemical-induced liver injury. *Pharmacol. Res.* **2021**, *164*, 105388. [CrossRef]
46. Honda, H.; Nagai, Y.; Matsunaga, T.; Okamoto, N.; Watanabe, Y.; Tsuneyama, K.; Hayashi, H.; Fujii, I.; Ikutani, M.; Hirai, Y.; et al. Isoliquiritigenin is a potent inhibitor of NLRP3 inflammasome activation and diet-induced adipose tissue inflammation. *J. Leukoc. Biol.* **2014**, *96*, 1087–1100.
47. Wang, W.; Pang, J.; Ha, E.H.; Zhou, M.; Li, Z.; Tian, S.; Li, H.; Hu, Q. Development of novel NLRP3-XOD dual inhibitors for the treatment of gout. *Bioorg. Med. Chem. Lett.* **2020**, *30*, 126944.
48. Jing, M.; Yang, J.; Zhang, L.; Liu, J.; Xu, S.; Wang, M.; Zhang, L.; Sun, Y.; Yan, W.; Hou, G.; et al. Celastrol inhibits rheumatoid arthritis through the ROS-NF-κB-NLRP3 inflammasome axis. *Int. Immunopharmacol.* **2021**, *98*, 107879.
49. Yu, X.; Zhao, Q.; Zhang, X.; Zhang, H.; Liu, Y.; Wu, X.; Li, M.; Li, X.; Zhang, J.; Ruan, X.; et al. Celastrol ameliorates inflammation through inhibition of NLRP3 inflammasome activation. *Oncotarget* **2017**, *8*, 67300.
50. Ay, M.; Charli, A.; Jin, H.; Anantharam, V.; Kanthasamy, A.; Kanthasamy, A.G. Quercetin. In *Nutraceuticals*; Elsevier: Amsterdam, The Netherlands, 2021; pp. 749–755.
51. Williams, C.A.; Grayer, R.J. Anthocyanins and other flavonoids. *Nat. Prod. Rep.* **2004**, *21*, 539–573.
52. Li, H.; Chen, F.J.; Yang, W.L.; Qiao, H.Z.; Zhang, S.J. Quercetin improves cognitive disorder in aging mice by inhibiting NLRP3 inflammasome activation. *Food Funct.* **2021**, *12*, 717–725. [CrossRef] [PubMed]
53. Ruiz-Miyazawa, K.W.; Staurengo-Ferrari, L.; Mizokami, S.S.; Domiciano, T.P.; Vicentini, F.T.; Camilios-Neto, D.; Pavanelli, W.R.; Pinge-Filho, P.; Amaral, F.A.; Teixeira, M.M.; et al. Quercetin inhibits gout arthritis in mice: Induction of an opioid-dependent regulation of inflammasome. *Inflammopharmacology* **2017**, *25*, 555–570. [CrossRef]
54. Nutmakul, T. A review on benefits of quercetin in hyperuricemia and gouty arthritis. *Saudi Pharm. J.* **2022**, *30*, 918–926. [CrossRef] [PubMed]
55. Rupasinghe, H.V. Application of NMR spectroscopy in plant polyphenols associated with human health. In *Applications of NMR Spectroscopy*; Elsevier: Amsterdam, The Netherlands, 2015; Volume 2, pp. 3–92.
56. Rue, E.A.; Rush, M.D.; Breemen, R.B.V. Procyanidins: A comprehensive review encompassing structure elucidation via mass spectrometry. *Phytochem. Rev.* **2018**, *17*, 1–16. [CrossRef] [PubMed]
57. Liu, H.J.; Pan, X.X.; Liu, B.Q.; Gui, X.; Hu, L.; Jiang, C.Y.; Han, Y.; Fan, Y.X.; Tang, Y.L.; Liu, W.T. Grape seed-derived procyanidins alleviate gout pain via NLRP3 inflammasome suppression. *J. Neuroinflamm.* **2017**, *14*, 1–10. [CrossRef]
58. OpenEye Scientific Software. Available online: https://www.eyesopen.com (accessed on 7 January 2022).
59. Rajan, V.K.; Muraleedharan, K. A computational investigation on the structure, global parameters and antioxidant capacity of a polyphenol, Gallic acid. *Food Chem.* **2017**, *220*, 93–99. [CrossRef] [PubMed]
60. Yang, K.; Zhang, L.; Liao, P.; Xiao, Z.; Zhang, F.; Sindaye, D.; Xin, Z.; Tan, C.; Deng, J.; Yin, Y.; et al. Impact of gallic acid on gut health: Focus on the gut microbiome, immune response, and mechanisms of action. *Front. Immunol.* **2020**, *11*, 580208. [CrossRef]
61. Lin, Y.; Luo, T.; Weng, A.; Huang, X.; Yao, Y.; Fu, Z.; Li, Y.; Liu, A.; Li, X.; Chen, D.; et al. Gallic acid alleviates gouty arthritis by inhibiting NLRP3 inflammasome activation and pyroptosis through enhancing Nrf2 signaling. *Front. Immunol.* **2020**, *11*, 580593. [CrossRef]
62. Elhemely, M.A.; Belgath, A.A.; El-Sayed, S.; Burusco, K.K.; Kadirvel, M.; Tirella, A.; Finegan, K.; Bryce, R.A.; Stratford, I.J.; Freeman, S. SAR of Novel 3-Arylisoquinolinones: Meta-Substitution on the Aryl Ring Dramatically Enhances Antiproliferative Activity through Binding to Microtubules. *J. Med. Chem.* **2022**, *65*, 4783–4797. [CrossRef]
63. Prota, A.E.; Danel, F.; Bachmann, F.; Bargsten, K.; Buey, R.M.; Pohlmann, J.; Reinelt, S.; Lane, H.; Steinmetz, M.O. The novel microtubule-destabilizing drug BAL27862 binds to the colchicine site of tubulin with distinct effects on microtubule organization. *J. Mol. Biol.* **2014**, *426*, 1848–1860. [CrossRef]
64. Paschke, S.; Weidner, A.F.; Paust, T.; Marti, O.; Beil, M.; Ben-Chetrit, E. Technical advance: Inhibition of neutrophil chemotaxis by colchicine is modulated through viscoelastic properties of subcellular compartments. *J. Leukoc. Biol.* **2013**, *94*, 1091–1096. [CrossRef] [PubMed]
65. Bonaventura, A.; Vecchié, A.; Dagna, L.; Tangianu, F.; Abbate, A.; Dentali, F. Colchicine for COVID-19: Targeting NLRP3 inflammasome to blunt hyperinflammation. *Inflamm. Res.* **2022**, *71*, 293–307. [CrossRef] [PubMed]
66. Dalbeth, N.; Lauterio, T.J.; Wolfe, H.R. Mechanism of action of colchicine in the treatment of gout. *Clin. Ther.* **2014**, *36*, 1465–1479. [CrossRef] [PubMed]
67. He, H.; Jiang, H.; Chen, Y.; Ye, J.; Wang, A.; Wang, C.; Liu, Q.; Liang, G.; Deng, X.; Jiang, W.; et al. Oridonin is a covalent NLRP3 inhibitor with strong anti-inflammasome activity. *Nat. Commun.* **2018**, *9*, 1–12. [CrossRef]
68. Coll, R.C.; Schroder, K.; Pelegrín, P. NLRP3 and pyroptosis blockers for treating inflammatory diseases. *Trends Pharmacol. Sci.* **2022**, *43*, 653–668. [CrossRef]
69. Seok, J.K.; Kang, H.C.; Cho, Y.Y.; Lee, H.S.; Lee, J.Y. Therapeutic regulation of the NLRP3 inflammasome in chronic inflammatory diseases. *Arch. Pharm. Res.* **2021**, *44*, 16–35. [CrossRef]
70. Juliana, C.; Fernandes-Alnemri, T.; Wu, J.; Datta, P.; Solorzano, L.; Yu, J.W.; Meng, R.; Quong, A.A.; Latz, E.; Scott, C.P.; et al. Anti-inflammatory compounds parthenolide and Bay 11-7082 are direct inhibitors of the inflammasome. *J. Biol. Chem.* **2010**, *285*, 9792–9802. [CrossRef]

71. Francomano, F.; Caruso, A.; Barbarossa, A.; Fazio, A.; La Torre, C.; Ceramella, J.; Mallamaci, R.; Saturnino, C.; Iacopetta, D.; Sinicropi, M.S. β-Caryophyllene: A sesquiterpene with countless biological properties. *Appl. Sci.* **2019**, *9*, 5420. [CrossRef]
72. Meeran, M.N.; Laham, F.; Azimullah, S.; Sharma, C.; Al Kaabi, A.J.; Tariq, S.; Adeghate, E.; Goyal, S.N.; Ojha, S. β-Caryophyllene, a natural bicyclic sesquiterpene attenuates β-adrenergic agonist-induced myocardial injury in a cannabinoid receptor-2 dependent and independent manner. *Free Radic. Biol. Med.* **2021**, *167*, 348–366. [CrossRef]
73. Li, W.Y.; Yang, F.; Chen, J.H.; Ren, G.F. β-Caryophyllene Ameliorates MSU-Induced Gouty Arthritis and Inflammation Through Inhibiting NLRP3 and NF-κB Signal Pathway: In Silico and In Vivo. *Front. Pharmacol.* **2021**, *12*, 651305. [CrossRef]
74. Lee, H.E.; Yang, G.; Kim, N.D.; Jeong, S.; Jung, Y.; Choi, J.Y.; Park, H.H.; Lee, J.Y. Targeting ASC in NLRP3 inflammasome by caffeic acid phenethyl ester: A novel strategy to treat acute gout. *Sci. Rep.* **2016**, *6*, 1–11. [CrossRef] [PubMed]
75. Hewlings, S.J.; Kalman, D.S. Curcumin: A review of its effects on human health. *Foods* **2017**, *6*, 92. [CrossRef]
76. Subedi, L.; Gaire, B.P. Neuroprotective effects of curcumin in cerebral ischemia: Cellular and molecular mechanisms. *ACS Chem. Neurosci.* **2021**, *12*, 2562–2572. [CrossRef] [PubMed]
77. Hasanzadeh, S.; Read, M.I.; Bland, A.R.; Majeed, M.; Jamialahmadi, T.; Sahebkar, A. Curcumin: An inflammasome silencer. *Pharmacol. Res.* **2020**, *159*, 104921. [CrossRef]
78. Zhang, M.; Zhang, X.; Tian, T.; Zhang, Q.; Wen, Y.; Zhu, J.; Xiao, D.; Cui, W.; Lin, Y. Anti-inflammatory activity of curcumin-loaded tetrahedral framework nucleic acids on acute gouty arthritis. *Bioact. Mater.* **2022**, *8*, 368–380. [CrossRef] [PubMed]
79. Schneider, C.; Gordon, O.N.; Edwards, R.L.; Luis, P.B. Degradation of curcumin: From mechanism to biological implications. *J. Agric. Food Chem.* **2015**, *63*, 7606–7614. [CrossRef] [PubMed]
80. Zhou, Z.; Gong, F.; Zhang, P.; Wang, X.; Zhang, R.; Xia, W.; Gao, X.; Zhou, X.; Cheng, L. Natural product curcumin-based coordination nanoparticles for treating osteoarthritis via targeting Nrf2 and blocking NLRP3 inflammasome. *Nano Res.* **2022**, *15*, 3338–3345. [CrossRef]
81. Yang, G.; Lee, H.E.; Moon, S.J.; Ko, K.M.; Koh, J.H.; Seok, J.K.; Min, J.K.; Heo, T.H.; Kang, H.C.; Cho, Y.Y.; et al. Direct Binding to NLRP3 Pyrin Domain as a Novel Strategy to Prevent NLRP3-Driven Inflammation and Gouty Arthritis. *Arthritis Rheumatol.* **2020**, *72*, 1192–1202. [CrossRef]
82. Yun, B.W.; Yan, Z.; Amir, R.; Hong, S.; Jin, Y.W.; Lee, E.K.; Loake, G.J. Plant natural products: History, limitations and the potential of cambial meristematic cells. *Biotechnol. Genet. Eng. Rev.* **2012**, *28*, 47–60. [CrossRef]
83. Atanasov, A.G.; Zotchev, S.B.; Dirsch, V.M.; Supuran, C.T. Natural products in drug discovery: Advances and opportunities. *Nat. Rev. Drug Discov.* **2021**, *20*, 200–216. [CrossRef]
84. Blagosklonny, M.V. Overcoming limitations of natural anticancer drugs by combining with artificial agents. *Trends Pharmacol. Sci.* **2005**, *26*, 77–81. [CrossRef] [PubMed]
85. Lahlou, M. The success of natural products in drug discovery. *Sci. Res.* **2013**, *4*, 17–31. [CrossRef]
86. Thomford, N.E.; Senthebane, D.A.; Rowe, A.; Munro, D.; Seele, P.; Maroyi, A.; Dzobo, K. Natural products for drug discovery in the 21st century: Innovations for novel drug discovery. *Int. J. Mol. Sci.* **2018**, *19*, 1578. [CrossRef] [PubMed]
87. Chen, L.Z.; Zhang, X.X.; Liu, M.M.; Wu, J.; Ma, D.; Diao, L.Z.; Li, Q.; Huang, Y.S.; Zhang, R.; Ruan, B.F.; et al. Discovery of novel pterostilbene-based derivatives as potent and orally active NLRP3 inflammasome inhibitors with inflammatory activity for colitis. *J. Med. Chem.* **2021**, *64*, 13633–13657. [CrossRef]
88. Jiang, H.; He, H.; Chen, Y.; Huang, W.; Cheng, J.; Ye, J.; Wang, A.; Tao, J.; Wang, C.; Liu, Q.; et al. Identification of a selective and direct NLRP3 inhibitor to treat inflammatory disorders. *J. Exp. Med.* **2017**, *214*, 3219–3238. [CrossRef]
89. Omar, F.; Tareq, A.M.; Alqahtani, A.M.; Dhama, K.; Sayeed, M.A.; Emran, T.B.; Simal-Gandara, J. Plant-based indole alkaloids: A comprehensive overview from a pharmacological perspective. *Molecules* **2021**, *26*, 2297. [CrossRef]
90. Kanwal, K.M.K.; Fatima, B.; Bano, B.; Salar, U. A Facile Route towards the Synthesis of 2-(1H-indol-3-yl)-acetamides Using 1, 1-Carbonyldiimidazole. *J. Chem. Soc. Pak.* **2016**, *38*, 771.
91. Jiao, Y.; Nan, J.; Mu, B.; Zhang, Y.; Zhou, N.; Yang, S.; Zhang, S.; Lin, W.; Wang, F.; Xia, A.; et al. Discovery of a novel and potent inhibitor with differential species-specific effects against NLRP3 and AIM2 inflammasome-dependent pyroptosis. *Eur. J. Med. Chem.* **2022**, *232*, 114194. [CrossRef]
92. British National Formulary (BNF). Available online: https://www.bnf.org (accessed on 15 August 2022).
93. FitzGerald, J.D.; Dalbeth, N.; Mikuls, T.; Brignardello-Petersen, R.; Guyatt, G.; Abeles, A.M.; Gelber, A.C.; Harrold, L.R.; Khanna, D.; King, C.; et al. American College of Rheumatology guideline for the management of gout. *Arthritis Care Res.* **2020**, *72*, 744–760. [CrossRef]

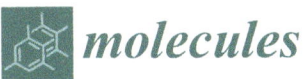

Article

A Bio-Guided Screening for Antioxidant, Anti-Inflammatory and Hypolipidemic Potential Supported by Non-Targeted Metabolomic Analysis of *Crepis* spp.

Christina Barda [1,2], Konstantina Anastasiou [3], Ariadni Tzara [3], Maria-Eleni Grafakou [1], Eleftherios Kalpoutzakis [1], Joerg Heilmann [2], Michael Rallis [4], Angeliki P. Kourounakis [3,*] and Helen Skaltsa [1,*]

[1] Department of Pharmacognosy & Chemistry of Natural Products, Faculty of Pharmacy, School of Health Sciences, National & Kapodistrian University of Athens, 15771 Athens, Greece
[2] Department of Pharmaceutical Biology, Faculty of Pharmacy and Chemistry, University of Regensburg, D-93053 Regensburg, Germany
[3] Department of Medicinal Chemistry, Faculty of Pharmacy, School of Health Sciences, National & Kapodistrian University of Athens, 15771 Athens, Greece
[4] Unity of Dermatopharmacology, Department of Pharmaceutical Technology, Faculty of Pharmacy, School of Health Sciences, National & Kapodistrian University of Athens, 15771 Athens, Greece
* Correspondence: angeliki@pharm.uoa.gr (A.P.K.); skaltsa@pharm.uoa.gr (H.S.);
Tel.: +30-697-438-8878 (A.P.K.); +30-697-262-3095 (H.S.)

Abstract: This study was designed to evaluate the chemical fingerprints and the antioxidant, anti-inflammatory and hypolipidemic activity of selected *Crepis* species collected in Greece, namely, *C. commutata*, *C. dioscoridis*, *C. foetida*, *C. heldreichiana*, *C. incana*, *C. rubra*, and *Phitosia crocifolia* (formerly known as *Crepis crocifolia*). For the phytochemical analyses, sample measurements were carried out by using nuclear magnetic resonance (NMR) spectroscopy and liquid chromatography coupled with mass spectrometry (LC-MS). The extracts were evaluated both in vitro (radical scavenging activity: DPPH assay and total phenolic content: Folin–Ciocalteu) and in vivo (paw edema reduction and hypolipidemic activity: experimental mouse protocols). Among the tested extracts, *C. incana* presented the highest gallic acid equivalents (GAE) (0.0834 mg/mL) and the highest antioxidant activity (IC$_{50}$ = 0.07 mg/mL) in vitro, as well as the highest anti-inflammatory activity with 32% edema reduction in vivo. Moreover, in the hypolipidemic protocol, the same extract increased plasma total antioxidant capacity (TAC) by 48.7%, and decreased cholesterol (41.3%) as well as triglycerides (37.2%). According to fractionation of the extract and the phytochemical results, this biological effect may be associated with the rich phenolic composition; caffeoyl tartaric acid derivatives (cichoric and caftaric acid) are regarded as the most prominent bioactive specialized metabolites. The present study contributes to the knowledge regarding the phytochemical and pharmacological profile of *Crepis* spp.

Keywords: *Crepis*; Asteraceae; LC-MS; NMR; cichoric acid; phenolic acid; biological activity; mouse paw edema; antihyperlipidemic

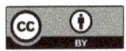

1. Introduction

The genus *Crepis* L. (Asteraceae) comprises more than 200 currently recognized species, of which less than 10% have been investigated, either from a phytochemical or bioactivity point of view [1,2]. The genus has been reported to be rich in phenolics and flavonoids, with predominant compounds being caffeoyl and luteolin derivatives, respectively [1]. Another widespread group of specialized natural products are sesquiterpene lactones and especially guaianolides, with other terpenoids also being identified, such as triterpenes and sterols [3]. The consensus view of specialized herbal metabolites as promising medicinal agents for preventing or managing oxidative stress, inflammation, hyperlipidemia and other related disorders, has been shown by maintaining good health and retarding aging processes [4]. Even though phytoconstituents of the *Crepis* genus have been documented, its pharmacological potential has not been fully explored yet. Extracts obtained from the different parts of the *Crepis* spp. and their isolated constituents have undergone only limited evaluation as antitumor, anti-inflammatory, antiviral, antimicrobial, antiulcer, antioxidant and nutritional agents [5,6]. Moreover, within the *Crepis* genus, few edible representatives appear, such as *C. bulbosa*, *C. capillaris*, *C. commutata*, *C. foetida*, *C. setosa* and *C. vesicaria* [5,6]. In Greece and Italy, many *Crepis* spp. are widely consumed together with other edible green herbs as an integral part of the traditional Mediterranean diet [6]. In this context, seven species were collected from different areas around Greece, specifically *C. commutata*, *C. dioscoridis*, *C. foetida*, *C. heldreichiana*, *C. incana*, *C. rubra*, and *Phitosiacrocifolia* (formerly known as *Crepiscrocifolia*). These samples were extracted and further investigated for their chemical profile in correlation with their biological effects. It is worth mentioning that among the selected plants, *C. heldreichiana*, *C. incana*, and *Phitosiacrocifolia* account for narrowly endemic types with limited distribution.

A non-targeted metabolomic strategy was selected to analyze and determine the differences in the phytochemical fingerprints of the abovementioned extracts. In detail, sample measurements were carried out by using both nuclear magnetic resonance (NMR) spectroscopy and liquid chromatography coupled with mass spectrometry (LC-MS). Among the under-investigation species, there are no reports in the literature except for *C. commutata*, *C. incana* and *C. dioscoridis*, which have been previously described by our group with emphasis on the non-polar and/or less polar sesquiterpene lactones [5,7,8]. In addition, we, herein, examined the polar extracts, which are more likely to contain hydrophilic compounds more relevant to their local use as edible green herbs and potentially potent antioxidant agents. Thus, the present study further includes a bio-guided approach using antioxidant, anti-inflammatory and hypolipidemic assays to unveil the most promising plant extract(s) through both in vitro and in vivo experimental procedures. Accordingly, the presented data encompass a widely applicable strategy for screening plant extracts, as well as information on the chemical and biological effects of the genus *Crepis*, regarding previously uninvestigated plant species. Moreover, to the best of our knowledge, no other comprehensive pharmacological evaluation has been reported so far.

2. Results and Discussion

2.1. Phytochemical Characterization of Selected Extracts

NMR and LC-MS analyses can be powerful tools to assess the chemical composition of specialized natural products that occur in complex mixtures. In respect to NMR, such protocols involve a "metabolomic" approach supported by a plethora of previously published papers, displaying the usefulness of both 1D and 2D NMR experiments for compound identification in complex matrix-like plant extracts, and also for comparative and qualitative analysis, as well as several other purposes and applications [9]. The relevant advantage of this approach is attributed to the unique NMR property of having the same response factor for different classes of metabolites. This can be used complementary to LC-MS analyses, as the sensitivity and selectivity with the low limit of detection (LODs) of LC-MS measurements (LODs 10^{-13} mol) are unachievable through NMR, thus, their combination is particularly advantageous. In this study, this approach was applied to different *Crepis* extracts to detect various classes of constituents by NMR and LC-MS/MS [10]. For the phytochemical analysis, the plant materials were initially extracted with MeOH:H_2O and further subjected to liquid/liquid extraction with n-butanol:H_2O, in order to achieve the elimination of sugars and obtain extracts rich in small molecules. The results provided by the phytochemical analyses were further associated with the data obtained from their biological evaluation.

2.1.1. NMR Characterization of Selected n-Butanol Extracts

An overlay of the ^{1}H-NMR spectra acquired for the selected plant n-butanol extracts is depicted in Figure 1, where the regional differentiation has been highlighted in different colors, aiming to distinguish the corresponding signals for phenolic derivatives (blue background), hydrocarbons, sugars and terpenoids (orange background), as well other signals assigned in the aliphatic region (green background). Moreover, due to many overlapping peaks, 2D NMR was utilized for further characterization of the ingredients. The 2D NMR spectroscopic data of all samples are provided in SI. Moreover, in Figure 1, ^{1}H NMR diagnostic signals for characteristic compounds (cichoric acid and/or caftaric acid) have also been indicated (arrows).

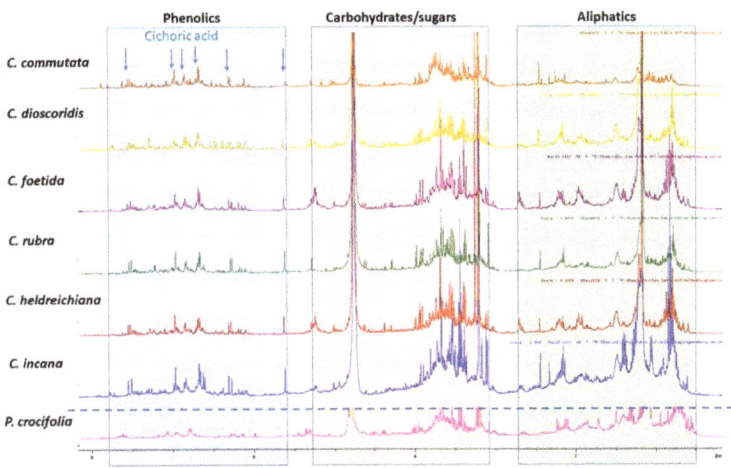

Figure 1. ^{1}H NMR comparison of plant n-butanol extracts: *Crepiscommutata*(orange), *C. dioscoridis* (yellow), *C. foetida* (purple), *C. rubra* (green), *C. heldreichiana* (red), *C. incana* (blue), *Phitosiacrocifolia* (pink) in CD$_3$OD; diagnostic signals for cichoric acid are indicated with blue arrows.

In detail, visual inspection of the 1D and 2D NMR spectra revealed the presence of different classes of metabolites. Starting with the region 5.5 to 8.5 ppm, phenolic derivatives are observed, and especially cichoric acid is predominant in all samples apart from *P. crocifolia* and *C. commutata*. Other caffeoyl derivatives, such as caffeoyl quinic isomers and flavonoids, are also detected in this region. Cichoric acid (2,3-di-O-caffeoyltartaric acid) was identified on the basis of 1D and 2D NMR spectroscopic data. Specifically, ^{1}H NMR spectra of the n-butanol extracts exhibit signals belonging to its two caffeic moieties with two trans olefinic protons at 7.47 (2H, d, J = 15.0 Hz, H-7′, 7″) and 6.27 (2H, d, J = 15.0 Hz, H-8′, 8″), and three aromatic protons of the ABX pattern at 7.05 (2H, s, H-2′, 2″), 6.94 (2H, s, H-6′, 6″) and 6.75 (2H, s, H-5′, 5″). A singlet at 5.54 ppm is attributed to the tartaric acid moiety of the compound [11]. Heteronuclear correlation experiments (HSQC and HMBC) provide additional data for structure identification (see Supplementary Material (SM)). As the extracts are complex mixtures due to the existence of other substances, the observed chemical shifts (δ_H values) in their ^{1}H NMR spectra, compared to the spectra of the pure compounds, reveal a deviation of ±0.05 ppm.

Among the measured samples, *C. commutata* possesses a lower amount of cichoric acid based on the signal of the tartaric acid moiety. Moreover, cichoric acid was not detected in *P. crocifolia*. It is worth mentioning that the main phenolics of *P. crocifolia* were inconsistent with caffeoyl quinic acid isomers and caffeic acid methyl ester (two doublets with J = 16.0 Hz at δ_H 7.53 and 6.22; ABX system with dJ = 2.1 Hz at δ_H 7.03, dJ = 8.2 Hz at 6.77 and dd J = 8.2, 2.1 Hz at 6.93; singlet at δ_H3.75) [12]. Of note, in *P. crocifolia*, sesquiterpene lactones were present in equal proportions with the phenolic derivatives, in contrast to the other samples. The NMR data permitted the identification of 2β-hydroxysantamarine-1β-D-glucopyranoside, an eudesmane-type sesquiterpene lactone previously reported by Zidorn et al. [13] from *Taraxacum linearisquameum*, as well as guaianolides with vinylic methyl at C14 andC15 (singlet at $\delta_H$ca.2.40 and ca. 2.30, respectively).

In HSQC, signals supporting the presence of flavonoid O-glycosides can be observed, such as protons of the substituted aromatic (B-) ring and several signals ascribable to H-6 and H-8, as well H-3 of the chromanone nucleus. Nevertheless, the density of the aromatic signals of flavonoids in the HSQC experiment is more distinct for the widely distributed *C. commutata*, *C. dioscoridis*, *C. rubra* and *C. foetida* (see Supplementary Materials) in comparison to the narrow endemic species (*C. incana* and *P. crocifolia*). Flavonoid accumulation can be affected by several factors, including the increase in temperature and UV-B radiation, and varies among organs within plants [14].

In higher fields, and especially in the 3–5 ppm overcrowded region, signals for different types of free sugars or sugar moieties of glucosides appear. As depicted in Figure 1, carbohydrate and glycoside substituents can be observed due to the partially overlapped doublets in the range 4.7–5.10 ppm, showing HSQC-DEPT correlations with CH carbons in the range of δ_C 90–105, that support the presence of the anomeric position of sugars.

Lastly, in the aliphatic region (0.6–2.5 ppm), the NMR analyses of all extracts confirmed the presence of fatty acid esters. The multiplets at δ_H ca. 5.34 were attributed to the olefinic protons (-CH=CH-) of the unsaturated fatty esters and the triplets at δ_H ca. 0.88 and/or 0.95 (J = 6.9) were attributed to the terminal CH_3 group of the alkyl chain; these signals were observed over a wide range of chemical shifts due to the degree of unsaturation. The nearby -CH_2 of the esters (-COOR) were distributed at δ_H ca. 2.33 (t, J = 6.8), and the intermediate -CH_2- of the double bonds were resonated at δ_H ca. 2.76 (m). The rest -CH_2 of the fatty ester chains were assigned to the intense signal at δ_H ca. 1.24.

2.1.2. LC-MS Characterization of Selected n-Butanol Extracts

To gain further insight into the chemical composition, the n-butanol extracts of the selected plants were submitted to LC-MS/MS analysis. Based on these results, the main constituents of *Crepis* spp. were confirmed to be caffeoyl tartaric acid derivatives. Moreover, the LC-MS analysis revealed the presence of more than 52 compounds, including sugars, sesquiterpene lactones and phenolics (flavonoids, phenolic acids and other phenolic derivatives). In Table 1, compounds are listed according to their retention time. The chemical characterization was in agreement with previously published data on the Cichorieae tribe and the Asteraceae family. For the identification of the compounds, the first step was performed by building an in-house database with approximately 200 molecules that have been described previously in the *Crepis* genus. In addition, all information was interpreted and correlated with mass spectra available in the literature and online databases. The molecular formulas were confirmed based on high-precision quasi-molecular ions such as [M-H]$^-$, [M+CHCOO]$^-$, [M+HCOO]$^-$, [M+H]$^+$ or [M+Na]$^+$ with a mass error of 5.0 ppm. The monitoring of phenolics and other compounds in the negative mode is reported to be more sensitive for the analysis [15]. Furthermore, the MS/MS spectra allowed an additional level of identification through the fragmentation patterns.

More specifically, the LC-MS results revealed the presence of the two main caffeoyl tartaric acid derivatives. Cichoric acid with a mass of 473.0719 [M-H]$^-$, followed by a peak at m/z 311 [M-163-H]$^-$ due to the loss of a caffeoyl- unit, a peak at m/z 293 [M-179-H]$^-$ due to the loss of a caffeic acid, followed by the fragments m/z 179 and m/z 149 of tartaric acid, which resulted from the loss of the two caffeoyl-units, is consistent with the mass spectrum for the title compound and the molecular formula $C_{22}H_{18}O_{12}$ [15,16]. In Figure 2, the fragmentation patterns and the suggested molecular structures of diagnostic ions are presented for the positive and negative ion modes. Similarly, caftaric acid ($C_{13}H_{11}O_9$) with a precursor ion of m/z 311.0405, fragmented to produce ions at m/z 149, m/z 179 and m/z 135 [179-CO_2]$^-$ which resulted from decarboxylation of the caffeic acid residue confirmed the presence of this compound [17].

Table 1. LC-MS analyses on *Crepis* spp.

Rt	Positive Ion Mode Found	Negative Ion Mode Found	Mass	Molecular Formula	Proposed Compounds	C. dioscoridis	C. incana	C. heldreichiana	C. foetida	C. communata	C. rubra	P. crocifolia
0.324	203.0530 [M+Na]+	179.0563 [M-H]-	180.0635	$C_6H_{12}O_6$	hexose	•	•	•	•	•	•	•
0.337	365.1059 [M+Na]+	341.1093 [M-H]-	342.1163	$C_{12}H_{22}O_{11}$	carbohydrates	•	•	•	•	•	•	•
0.490	349.1121 [M+Na]+	371.1189 [M+HCOO]-	326.1217	$C_{12}H_{22}O_{10}$	carbohydrates	•	•	•	•	•	•	
2.046	181.0498 [M+H]+	179.0350 [M-H]-	180.0421	$C_9H_8O_4$	caffeic acid isomer	•	•	•	•	•	•	•
2.502		311.0407 [M-H]-	312.0478	$C_{13}H_{12}O_9$	cattaric acid							•
2.610	309.0947 [M+Na]+	331.1035 [M+HCOO]-	286.1049	$C_{13}H_{18}O_7$	salicin isomer	•	•	•	•	•	•	
2.997	309.0947 [M+Na]+	331.1035 [M+HCOO]-	286.1045	$C_{13}H_{18}O_7$	salicin isomer	•	•	•	•	•	•	
3.005	343.1026 [M+H]+	339.0719 [M-H]-	342.0952	$C_{15}H_{18}O_9$	caffeic acid glycoside							•
3.050	341.0869 [M+H]+		340.0796	$C_{15}H_{16}O_9$	cichoriin	•	•	•	•	•	•	
3.210	153.0546 [M+Na]+	151.0400 [M-H]-	152.0468	$C_8H_8O_3$	methoxybenzoic acid benzyl glycoside	•						•
3.483	293.0993 [M+Na]+	315.1084 [M+HCOO]-	270.1103	$C_{13}H_{18}O_6$	caffeoylquinic acid isomer							•
3.604	355.1028 [M+H]+	353.0888 [M-H]-	354.0957	$C_{16}H_{18}O_9$	caffeoylquinic acid isomer	•	•	•	•	•	•	•
3.629	355.1028 [M+H]+	353.0879 [M-H]-	354.0953	$C_{16}H_{18}O_9$	caffeoylquinic acid isomer	•	•	•	•	•	•	•
3.772	181.0496 [M+H]+	179.0349 [M-H]-	180.0421	$C_9H_8O_4$	caffeic acid isomer	•	•	•	•	•	•	
4.246	337.0893 [M+H]+		336.0820	$C_{16}H_{16}O_8$	caffeoylshikimic acid isomer							•
4.509	337.0917 [M+H]+	335.077 [M-H]-	336.0844	$C_{16}H_{16}O_8$	caffeoylshikimic acid isomer	•	•	•	•	•	•	
4.529	449.1783 [M+Na]+	471.1868 [M+HCOO]-	426.2891	$C_{21}H_{30}O_9$	sesquiterpene lactone glycoside	•	•	•	•	•	•	
4.530	449.1783 [M+Na]+	471.1868 [M+HCOO]-	426.1890	$C_{21}H_{30}O_9$	sesquiterpene lactone glycoside	•	•	•	•	•	•	
4.580	449.1780 [M+Na]+	471.1868 [M+HCOO]-	426.1897	$C_{21}H_{30}O_9$	sesquiterpene lactone glycoside	•	•	•	•	•	•	
4.707	165.0548 [M+H]+	163.0398 [M-H]-	164.0473	$C_9H_8O_3$	coumaric acid							•
4.790	611.1607 [M+H]+	609.1458 [M-H]-	610.1535	$C_{27}H_{30}O_{16}$	luteolin diglycoside isomer	•	•	•	•	•	•	•
4.997	449.1082 [M+H]+	447.0937 [M-H]-	448.1009	$C_{21}H_{20}O_{11}$	luteolin glycoside isomer	•	•	•	•	•	•	•
5.151	465.1027 [M+H]+	463.0885 [M-H]-	464.0954	$C_{21}H_{20}O_{12}$	quercetin glycoside isomer							•
5.199	497.0688 [M+H]+	473.0732 [M-H]-	474.0794	$C_{22}H_{18}O_{12}$	cichoric acid isomer	•						•
5.216	611.1607 [M+H]+	609.1458 [M-H]-	610.153	$C_{27}H_{30}O_{16}$	luteolin diglycoside isomer							•
5.363	447.1617 [M+Na]+	469.1715 [M+HCOO]-	424.1733	$C_{21}H_{28}O_9$	sesquiterpene lactone glycoside	•	•	•	•	•	•	
5.571	611.1609 [M+H]+	609.1458 [M-H]-	610.1534	$C_{27}H_{30}O_{16}$	luteolin diglycoside isomer	•	•	•	•	•	•	
5.716	463.087 [M+H]+	461.0724 [M-H]-	462.0798	$C_{21}H_{18}O_{12}$	luteolin glucuronide	•	•	•	•	•	•	
5.733	465.1029 [M+H]+	463.0885 [M-H]-	464.0954	$C_{21}H_{20}O_{12}$	quercetin glycoside isomer							•
5.751		285.0406 [M-H]-	286.0477	$C_{15}H_{10}O_6$	luteolin isomer	•	•	•	•	•	•	
5.760	449.1081 [M+H]+	447.0939 [M-H]-	448.101	$C_{21}H_{20}O_{11}$	luteolin glycoside isomer	•	•	•	•	•	•	•
5.780	409.1859 [M+H]+		408.1784	$C_{21}H_{28}O_8$	sesquiterpene lactone glycoside	•	•	•	•	•	•	
5.890	409.1830 [M+H]+		408.1759	$C_{21}H_{28}O_8$	sesquiterpene lactone glycoside	•	•	•	•	•	•	
5.930	517.1347 [M+H]+	515.1193 [M-H]-	516.1270	$C_{25}H_{24}O_{12}$	dicaffeoylquinic acid isomer	•	•	•	•	•	•	•
5.959	265.1436 [M+H]+		264.1363	$C_{15}H_{20}O_4$	sesquiterpene lactone	•	•	•	•	•	•	
6.021	465.1029 [M+H]+	463.0880 [M-H]-	464.0957	$C_{21}H_{20}O_{12}$	luteolin glycoside isomer							•
6.029	551.1033 [M+H]+	549.0887 [M-H]-	550.0960	$C_{24}H_{22}O_{15}$	quercetin malonylglycoside isomer							•
6.116		609.1454 [M-H]-	610.1528	$C_{27}H_{30}O_{16}$	luteolin diglycoside isomer	•	•	•	•	•	•	
6.160	517.1347 [M+H]+	515.1195 [M-H]-	516.1273	$C_{25}H_{24}O_{12}$	dicaffeoylquinic acid isomer	•	•	•	•	•	•	•
6.244	195.0650 [M+H]+	193.0505 [M-H]-	194.0578	$C_{10}H_{10}O_4$	methyl caffeate	•	•	•	•	•	•	
6.253	625.1764 [M+H]+	623.1615 [M-H]-	624.1791	$C_{28}H_{32}O_{16}$	isorhamnetin-rutinoside isomer							•
6.289	287.0549 [M+H]+	285.0406 [M-H]-	286.0477	$C_{15}H_{10}O_6$	luteolin isomer	•	•	•	•	•	•	
6.296	449.1081 [M+H]+	447.0935 [M-H]-	448.1009	$C_{21}H_{20}O_{11}$	luteolin glycoside isomer	•	•	•	•	•	•	•
6.316		371.1342 [M+HCOO]-	372.1422	$C_{16}H_{20}O_7$	eugenyl glycoside isomer	•	•	•	•	•	•	
6.505	517.1343 [M+H]+	515.1193 [M-H]-	516.1268	$C_{25}H_{24}O_{12}$	dicaffeoylquinic acid isomer	•	•	•	•	•	•	•
6.436	433.1134 [M+H]+	431.0981 [M-H]-	432.1993	$C_{21}H_{20}O_{10}$	apigenin glycoside	•	•	•	•	•	•	•

Table 1. Cont.

Rt	Positive Ion Mode Found	Negative Ion Mode Found	Mass	Molecular Formula	Proposed Compounds	C. dioscoridis	C. incana	C. heldreichiana	C. foetida	C. commutata	C. rubra	P. crocifolia
7.130	449.1783 [M+Na]$^+$	471.1868 [M+HCOO]$^-$	426.2890	$C_{21}H_{30}O_9$	sesquiterpene lactone glycoside	●	●					
7.240	449.1783 [M+Na]$^+$	471.1868 [M+HCOO]$^-$	426.2891	$C_{21}H_{30}O_9$	sesquiterpene lactone glycoside	●	●	●				
7.381	492.1134 [M+NH$_4$]$^+$	473.0724 [M-H]$^-$	474.2099	$C_{22}H_{18}O_{12}$	cichoric acid isomer	●	●	●				
7.813		301.0349 [M-H]$^-$	302.0422	$C_{15}H_{10}O_7$	quercetin isomer	●	●			●	●	
7.876	287.0548 [M+H]$^+$	285.0405 [M-H]$^-$	286.0478	$C_{15}H_{10}O_6$	luteolin isomer		●	●	●	●	●	●

Shaded squares (●) indicates presence of metabolites.

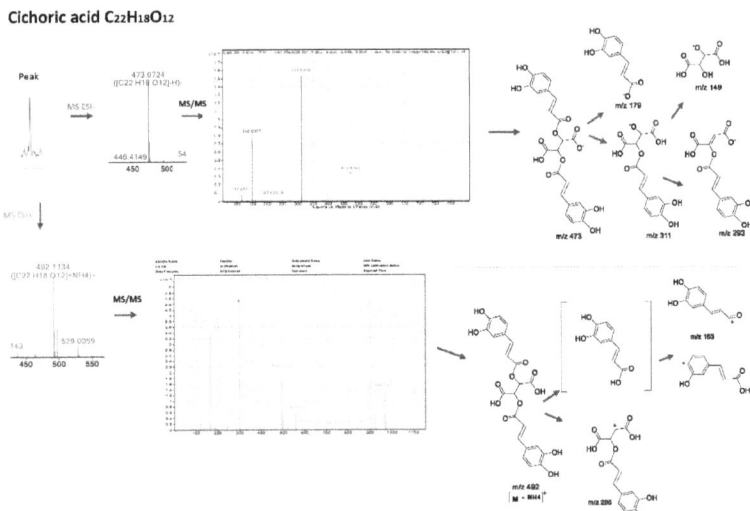

Figure 2. Mass spectra, fragmentation patterns and suggested molecular structures of diagnostic ions in positive and negative ion modes for cichoric acid.

Mono-acyl chlorogenic acid isomers matched with compounds with a molecular ion [M-H]$^-$ at m/z 353 and chemical formulas $C_{16}H_{18}O_9$, and, with respect to the literature, were attributed to 5- or 3- caffeoylquinic acids isomers (m/z 353.0870), producing fragment ions at m/z 191 [M-163-H]$^-$ due to the loss of a caffeoyl moiety [18].

Flavonoid derivatives were also present in the extracts, with luteolin isomers, as aglycones or as glycosides, such as luteolin isomers m/z 286.0478 ($C_{15}H_{10}O_6$, m/z 285.0405 [M-H]$^-$), luteolin glycoside isomers m/z 448.1009 ($C_{21}H_{20}O_{11}$, m/z 447.0935 [M-H]$^-$) and luteolin diglycoside isomers m/z 610.1528 ($C_{27}H_{30}O_{16}$, m/z 609.1454 [M-H]$^-$) being the most prominent [19].

Sesquiterpene lactones play a significant role in plants and their bioactivity and structural diversity are well studied [20]. Nevertheless, their nature limits the applicability of UV detection, as they lack chromophoric groups. Moreover, the ionization of sesquiterpene lactones has been recorded to be more effective in the positive mode in [M+H]$^+$, [M+Na]$^+$ or results in ions formed from solvent adducts and/or the loss of water or acid residues, facts that prevent their flawless detection [21]. On top of this, databases and the literature are lacking data for their fragmentation patterns, since many of them have been recorded only once. Considering the above, for the annotation of sesquiterpene lactones, ions of [M+H]$^+$ and [M+Na]$^+$ were detected and led to the chemical formulas that possessed a 15-carbon backbone or C-21 (C-15 and hexose) or C-n (C21 and various phenolic substituents) based on literature data and with the aid of the NMR spectra.

It is noteworthy that the accumulation of specialized metabolites during plant development is highly affected by many interdependent factors, such as light, photoperiod, temperature, soil water, salinity or fertility, etc. [14]. Especially, phytochemical studies for wild species feature a chemical fingerprint influenced by environmental and physiological parameters based on the time of collection. The biochemical adaptability in plants is relatively hard to discover and is still not fully understood.

2.1.3. Total Phenolic Content

For the quantification of phenolic compounds in the selected plant extracts and fractions, the Folin–Ciocalteu (F-C) method was selected, as it is a rapid method, widely applied for the determination of total polyphenol content (TPC) and it is quoted by several pharmacopoeias [22]. Polyphenols react with the F-C reagent, leading to blue-colored complexes that absorb at a specific wavelength. For this quantification, a standard solution of gallic acid was used for the reference curve, for measuring the phenolic content for each sample. TPC estimated by F-C assay ranged from 0.0359 to 0.0834 mg/mL for the hydroalcoholic and aqueous extracts, while the fractions showed similar levels from 0.1210 to 0.0937 mg/mL (Table 2).

Table 2. Total polyphenol content (TPC) of plant extracts, fractions and reference compounds, expressed as TPC or GAE values (F-C assay).

Extract (1 mg/mL)	TPC (mg/mL) or GAE (GAE/gEx) [a]	Fractions (1 mg/mL)	TPC (mg/mL) or GAE (GAE/gEx) [a]
C. commutata 5:1	0.0488	RINA	0
C. dioscoridis 5:1	0.0561	RINB	0.1282
C. foetida 5:1	0.0499	RINC	0.1712
C. foetida H_2O	0.0518	RIND	0.0796
C. heldreichiana 5:1	0.0521	RINE	0.0227
C. incana 5:1	0.0834	RINF	0.0937
C. rubra 5:1	0.0564	RINH	0.0830
C. rubra H_2O	0.0414	RINI	0.1210
P. crocifolia 5:1	0.0515	RINJ	0.0814

[a] TPC = total phenolic content, GAE = gallic acid equivalents.

2.2. In Vitro and In Vivo Activities

One of the greatest challenges concerning the chemical analysis of multiple extracts is that metabolites must be studied individually and in detail to obtain qualitative characteristics, which include time-consuming and expensive techniques. In this aspect, in vitro bio-guided tests can provide relevant information to allow the researchers to decide whether to select and intensify the fractionation and purification of established bioactive samples. This experimental approach permitted us the selection of C. incana, C. heldreichiana and C. dioscoridis based on their in vitro effects. Initially, the antioxidant activity and the determination of the phenolic content (as discussed above) were evaluated in nine complex samples, in which the most prominent was selected and relevant fractionation was conducted to diminish its complexity. The yielded fractions were similarly evaluated to unveil the active sub-fraction that demonstrates the biological effects of interest. The next step involved the in vivo assessment of the extracts and obtained fractions, on induced inflammation and hyperlipidemia in respective experimental mouse models.

The key role of free radical reactions in pathological abnormalities and their involvement in many acute and chronic inflammatory disorders, including atherosclerosis and diabetes, is well documented [23–25]. Thus, by addressing oxidative stress, inflammation and dyslipidemia with the potentially multifunctional nature of specialized natural products, we aimed to identify agents, such as extracts or compounds, that could possibly serve against various such related disorders.

2.2.1. Evaluation of Antioxidant Activity In Vitro, DPPH Assay

Using the DPPH assay, the antioxidant ability of different extracts and fractions of plants belonging to Crepis genus, expressed as IC_{50} values, compared to the reference compounds resveratrol (RSV), ascorbic acid (ASC) and di-t-butylhydroxytoluene (BHT), are shown in Table 3. MeOH:H_2O 5:1 extracts showed IC_{50} values of 0.07 to 0.26 mg/mL, while H_2O (100%) extracts possessed higher IC_{50} values of 0.30 to >1 mg/mL. As expected, the aqueous extracts rich in sugars showed the lowest activity in comparison to the hydroalcoholic extracts. Among them, the hydroalcoholic extract of C. incana showed the most potent antioxidant activity with IC_{50} 0.07 mg/mL (Table 2) and, therefore, was selected for further fractionation; the resulted fractions were evaluated in the same assay. Fractions RINH (yielded with EtoAc:MeOH:H_2O 2:8:0.8), RINI (yielded with MeOH 100%) and RINJ (yielded with MeOH:H_2O 1:1) were proven active. RINI was the most potent antioxidant fraction, with the lowest observed IC_{50} value (0.06 mg/mL), compared to the other fractions and the parent extract (*C. incana* MeOH:H$_2$O 5:1). The activity of *C. incana* 5:1 and RINI was comparable or even greater than reference compounds (RSV IC$_{50}$ 0.02 mg/mL; ASC IC$_{50}$ 0.01 mg/mL; BHT IC$_{50}$ 0.38 mg/mL). As seen, this assay demonstrated that the genus Crepis is a great source of antioxidant compounds responsible for radical scavenging ability; in particular, this effect was attributed to their phenolic content.

Table 3. Antioxidant effect of plant extracts, fractions and reference compounds, expressed as IC$_{50}$ values (DPPH assay).

Extracts	IC$_{50}$ (mg/mL)	Fractions	IC$_{50}$ (mg/mL)	Reference	IC$_{50}$ (mg/mL)
C. commutata 5:1	0.14	RINA	>1	RSV	0.02
C. dioscoridis 5:1	0.12	RINB	0.14	ASC	0.01
C. foetida 5:1	0.14	RINC	0.24	BHT	0.38
C. foetida H$_2$O	>1	RIND	0.12		
C. heldreichiana 5:1	0.10	RINE	0.35		
C. incana 5:1	0.07	RINF	>1		
C. rubra 5:1	0.19	RINH	0.12		
C. rubra H$_2$O	0.30	RINI	0.06		
P. crocifolia 5:1	0.26	RINJ	0.11		
		RINK	>1		

DPPH IC$_{50}$ values (as an indicator of in vitro antioxidant capacity) were tested for possible correlation with the TPC values for each extract/fraction. This revealed that the extracts MeOH:H$_2$O 5:1 have a higher antioxidant potency (lower IC$_{50}$ values) and higher gallic acid equivalents (GAE) or TPC. In detail, the most active was *C. incana* 5:1, bearing the highest GAE (0.0834 mg/mL) and the lowest IC$_{50}$ value (0.07 mg/mL) among the tested plant extracts. The most active fractions, RINB, RINC and RINI, showed the highest TPC values, among which RINI also had the lowest IC$_{50}$ (0.06 mg/mL), i.e., the best antioxidant activity.

2.2.2. Evaluation of Anti-Inflammatory Activity (In Vivo)

The carrageenan-induced paw edema is a well-known acute model of inflammation that is widely used for screening novel anti-inflammatory agents [25–27]. Based on the in vitro results, the most active extracts and fractions were selected and further evaluated for their anti-inflammatory activity at a dose of 3 mg/100 g of body weight i.p. using the carrageenan-induced paw edema assay. Results are shown in Figure 3 and are expressed as % edema reduction. It is worth mentioning that the extract of *C. incana* 5:1 and the fraction RINH caused a statistically significant edema reduction, with *C. incana* 5:1 bearing the highest anti-inflammatory activity (32% edema reduction) in vivo and in the activity range of known anti-inflammatory agents e.g., Indomethacin: 29%, Ibuprofen: 36% at a dose of 1.5 mmol/100 g of body weight, respectively [28,29]. It seems that the high antioxidant activity of these extracts/fractions (combined with an apparently optimum bioavailability) may be contributing to their anti-inflammatory effect [25,28,30].

2.2.3. Evaluation of (In Vivo) Antioxidant and Anti-Hyperlipidemic Activity

The extracts/fractions studied in this protocol were administered to mice i.p. (dose: 0.3 mg/kg body weight) after tyloxapol i.p. administration, which caused acute hyperlipidemia. The total antioxidant capacity (TAC), total cholesterol (TC) and triglyceride levels (TG) in plasma were measured and compared to control and untreated groups, 24 h after tyloxapol administration. Results are shown in Tables 4–6, while representative graphs of the effect of the most active extract *C. incana* 5:1 are shown in Figure 4.

The most active extract that increased total antioxidant capacity (TAC) by 49%, compared to (the hyperlipidemic) Control, was *C. incana* 5:1 (Figure 4a). In specific, it almost restored TAC levels to normal (6% lower than the Untreated group). At the same time, it was one of the two most active extracts in lowering TC levels (53%), together with *C.*

dioscoridis 5:1 (57%) (Figure 4b). Regarding TG levels, *C. incana* 5:1 showed again the highest potency, decreasing TG levels by 37% (Figure 4c). Thus, the antioxidant profile of *C. incana* 5:1 was superior to the other extracts/fractions. Even though *C. dioscoridis* 5:1 was successful at lowering TC levels, it did not show such a similar potency in TAC or TG levels. It is concluded that *C. incana* 5:1 caused a significant decrease in TC and TG levels, as well as the greatest antioxidant (TAC) and anti-inflammatory (edema) activity in vivo, proving the most promising extract for further studies.

Table 4. Effect of extract *C. incana* 5:1, *C. dioscoridis* 5:1 and fractions RINH and RINI on TAC.

Groups	TAC [a]	% TAC Increase (vs. Control)	% TAC Decrease (vs. Untreated)
Untreated	100% (±11.8) ***	-	-
Control	63.3% (±12.2)	-	36.7
C. incana 5:1	94.1% (±12.2) ***	48.7	5.9
C. dioscoridis 5:1	84.6% (±7.1) * #	33.6	15.4
RINH	83.7% (±5.4) ** ##	32.2	16.3
RINI	71.9% (±7.7) ###	13.6	28.1

[a] Total antioxidant capacity (TAC) is measured as % reduction of a solution of DPPH. The TAC value of the Untreated group is considered 100%. The effect of other groups (extracts/fractions) is expressed as a percentage of TAC increase compared to Control and TAC decrease compared to Untreated. Each value represents the mean ± SD obtained from eight animals. Significant difference of Control group from Untreated group: *** p = 0.0001, *C. incana* 5:1 from Control group: *** p = 0.0001, *C. dioscoridis* from Control group: * p = 0.0004 and from Untreated group: # p = 0.0035, and RINH from Control group: ** p = 0.0003 and from Untreated group: ## p = 0.0016, RINI from Untreated group: ### p = 0.0001.

Table 5. Effect of extract *C. incana* 5:1, *C. dioscoridis* 5:1 and fractions RINH, RINI on total cholesterol plasma levels (TC).

Groups	TC (mg/dL)	% TC Decrease (vs. Control)	% TC Increase (vs. Untreated)
Untreated	96.4 (±6.7) *	-	-
Control	124.0 (±12.7)	-	28.6
C. incana 5:1	58.4 (±8.9) ** ##	52.9	−39.4
C. dioscoridis 5:1	53.0 (±16.2)	57.3	−45.0
RINH	77.2 (±16.3)	37.7	−19.9
RINI	74.3 (±7.1)	40.1	−22.9

The effect is expressed as a percentage of reduction in total cholesterol levels in plasma, compared to Control and Untreated. Each value represents the mean ± SD obtained from eight animals. Significant difference of Control from Untreated group: * p = 0.045. *C. incana* 5:1 from Control: ** p = 0.001, from Untreated group: ## p = 0.0045.

Table 6. Effect of extract *C. incana* 5:1, *C. dioscoridis* 5:1 and fractions RINH, RINI on triglyceride plasma levels (TG).

Groups	TG (mg/dL)	% TG Decrease (vs. Control)	% TG Increase (vs. Untreated)
Untreated	59.0 (±6.1)	-	-
Control	123.5 (±37.9)	-	109.3
C. incana 5:1	77.5 (±15.1)	37.2	31.4
C. dioscoridis 5:1	110.4 (±11.5) *	10.6	87.1
RINH	99.5 (±12.7)	19.4	68.6
RINI	89.0 (±22.7)	27.9	50.8

The effect is expressed as a percentage of reduction in total triglyceride levels in plasma, compared to Control and Untreated group. Each value represents the mean ± SD obtained from eight animals. Significant difference of *C. dioscoridis* 5:1 from Control group: * p = 0.02.

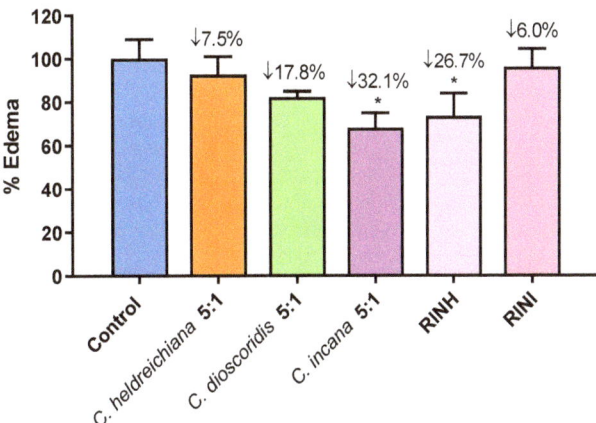

Figure 3. Effect of extracts *C. heldreichiana* 5:1, *C. dioscoridis* 5:1, *C. incana* 5:1 and fractions RINH and RINI on carrageenan-induced mouse paw edema. Each value represents the mean obtained from 6 animals. Significant difference of Control from *C. incana* group: * $p = 0.05$ and from RINH: * $p = 0.05$. [The average weight difference between the injected and un-injected paws for the Control group (100%) is 0.058 g (mean weight of injected/uninjected paw is 0.210 vs. 0.146 g)].

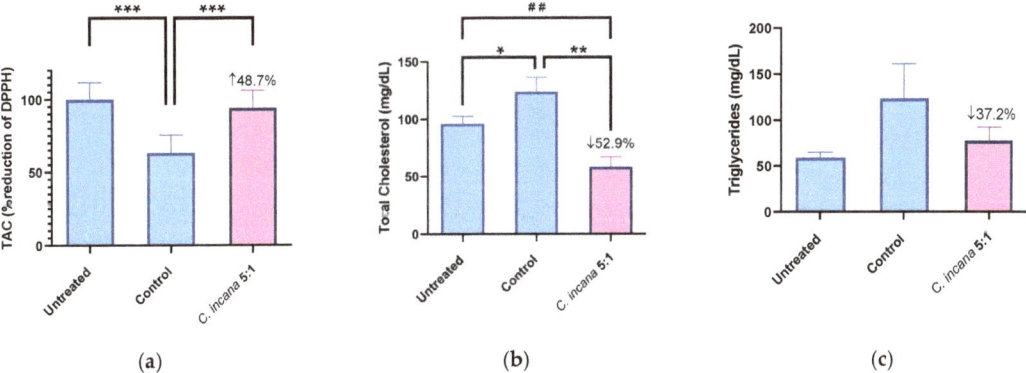

Figure 4. Representative graphs for TAC (**a**), TC (**b**) and TG (**c**) of the most active extract *C. incana* 5:1, compared to Untreated and Control group. Significant difference in (**a**) of Control group from Untreated group: *** $p = 0.0001$, *C. incana* 5:1 from Control group: *** $p = 0.0001$. Statistical difference in (**b**) of Control from Untreated group: * $p = 0.045$. *C. incana* 5:1 from Control: ** $p = 0.001$, from Untreated group: ## $p = 0.0045$.

2.3. Pharmacological Profile of Crepis spp.

The genus *Crepis* belongs to the tribe Cichorieae, which encompasses many well-known taxa such as *Taraxacum* spp. and *Cichorium* spp. [1]. According to the literature, a plethora of records illustrate their significant pharmacological interest [31,32]. Nevertheless, the biological potential of the genus *Crepis* is untapped. As described previously, the chemical compositions of the *Crepis* taxa mainly includes phenolics and flavonoids as well as lignans, sterols, volatile constituents, triterpenesand sesquiterpene lactones, of which phenolics andsesquiterpene lactones are generally considered the major active components [6,33].Contemporary pharmacological studies aim at evaluating *Crepis* extracts or their isolated compounds with in vitro assays, while in vivo experiments related to this genus are more or less absent.Limited records for antibacterial, antifungal, antiviral, cytotoxic and antiulcer activitiesand toxicity, as well as (relevant to our study) antioxidant, anti-inflammatoryandantidiabetic potential can be found for the *Crepis* taxa [6]. In detail, a previous study showed the antioxidant activity of the aerial parts from *C. foetida* L. subsp. *rhoeadifolia* using DPPH (IC_{50} = 0.26 mg/mL) and TBARS assays (MDA level = 4.54 nmol/mL) [34]. The methanolic extract of *C. sancta* [35] was evaluated for its antioxidant capacity with the ABTS decolorization assay and alsoshowed promising results, while the infusion fromaerial parts of *C. foetida* L. [35] showed moderate activity (DPPH method). Lastly, the hydro–alcoholic extract of *C. vesicaria* subsp. *taraxacifolia* exhibited antioxidant activity in DPPH (IC_{50} = 26.20 μg/mL), ABTS (IC_{50} = 18.92 μg/mL) and FRAP (0.68 μg/mL of Trolox Equivalent) [36].

Based on our biological evaluation by use of the DPPH methodregarding *C. commutata*, *C. dioscoridis*, *C. foetida*, *C. heldreichiana*, *C. incana*, *C. rubra*, *C. commutata*, and *Phitosia crocifolia*, the aqueous extract possessed lower activity, in accordance with the literature, while the tested methanol–water extracts possessed higher DPPH inhibition in the range of IC_{50}= 0.07 to 0.26 mg/mL. According to our phytochemical findings, these antioxidant effects can be associated with the rich phenolic composition, i.e., caffeoyl tartaric acid derivatives (cichoric and caftaric acid), other caffeoyl derivatives and flavonoids. *C. incana* revealed the most prominent activity, while its bio-active subfractions suggested the compounds responsible for the observed effects. Fractions RINI with IC_{50} value 0.06 mg/mL, characterized by cichoric acid, while fractions RINB-RINE with IC_{50} values ranging from 0.12 to 0.35 mg/mL showed high amounts of flavonoid glucosides (luteolin–quercetin derivatives), along with free sugars and minor levels of sesquiterpene lactones.Based on the literature, several phenolics, including caftaric acid, chlorogenic acid, caffeic acid, cichoric acid, 3,5-di-O-caffeoylquinic acid and luteolin, isolated from *Taraxacum mongolicum*, have been reported to exert IC_{50} values of 7.3, 12.7, 7.1, 9.6, 10.1, 5.3 μg/mL, respectively (DPPH method) [37].

To the best of our knowledge, one study showed the anti-inflammatory activity of *C. vesicaria* subsp. *taraxacifolia* (ethanolic extract) in vitro (using macrophage cell cultures) by means of inhibition of NO production in a dose-dependent manner with an IC_{50} of 0.43 mg/mL [36]. In our findings, the in vivo anti-inflammatory activity at a dose of 0.3 mg/kg of body weight i.p. via the reduction in carrageenan-induced paw edema of the methanol:water extract of *C. incana* and the fraction RINH showed statistically significant results, exerting up to 32% edema reduction. For comparison purposes, it is worth noting that in another study, *Taraxacum officinale*, administered orally (100 mg/kg bodyweight) 1 h before edema, elicited inhibition of carrageenan-induced rat paw edema by 25% [31]. The different administration routes (gastrointestinal or intraperitoneal) may give rise to the argument of bioavailability of cichoric acid and similar phenolic derivatives [16], which may hamper their clinical application. Contradictory reports show low permeability per os and the possibility of transfer across the blood-brain barrier [16,17,38]. Additional in vivo research demonstrated that cichoric acid was partly metabolized through Phase I to caffeic acid and caftaric acid by cytochrome P450s in rat liver [17].

Cardiovascular diseases and diabetes are related to metabolic disorders that include hyperglycemia, hyperlipidemia, hyperuricemia, hypertension, atherosclerosis, etc. [38]. Many studies have been performed on species from the tribe Cichorieae, whichare widely consumed as salads or in traditional remedies and contributebeneficiallyto human health [6,32,36]. Specifically, studies have demonstrated that obesity, diabetes or renal tubular injury induced by a high-fat diet caused a significant increase in the body weight, fasting blood glucose, serum TC and TG and uric acid levels in mice. Treatment with cichoric acid demonstrated positive effects on the above metabolic parameters by decreasing body weight, fasting blood glucose and serum TC and TG levels. Similarly, based on our work hereby, the anti-hyperlipidemic activity of *C. incana* indicates that such plants may play a key role as a rich source of cichoric acid with desirable effects on human health.

Nevertheless, despite the demonstrated promising results, it should be noted that plant extracts are exceedingly complex multicomponent mixtures that may influence biological processes by either playing an important role by acting synergetically, or else potentially negatively (due to antagonistic interactions of the molecules) or without any significant consequences.

3. Materials and Methods

3.1. Plant Material

The plant material (aerial) parts of the selected plants were collected during the flowering stage and identified by Dr. E. Kalpoutzakis (Faculty of Pharmacy, National and Kapodistrian University of Athens) and Associate Prof. Th. Constantinidis (Faculty of Biology, National and Kapodistrian University of Athens). The voucher specimens were deposited at the Herbarium of Laboratory of Natural Products Chemistry, NKUA. The detailed information is presented in Table 7.

Table 7. Collection data of the investigated *Crepis* spp.

Taxon	Locality	Latitude	Longitude	Altitude	Date	Voucher
C. commutata (Spreng.) Greuter	Anabyssos	37°43″ N	23°55″ E	1400–2400 m	4-2016	Skaltsaand Barda 001
C. dioscoridis L.	Boumistos mountain	38°70657′ N	21°04338′ E	487 m	6-2016	Skaltsaand Tsoukalas 001
C. foetida L.	Phaleron	37°56′23.24″ N	23°40′ 55.83″ E	4 m	5-2019 6-2016	Kalpoutzakis5122/ 5-5-2019
C. heldreichiana (Kuntze) Greuter	Taygetos mountain	36°56′43.3″ N	22°21′16.4″ E	1450–2300 m	6-2017	Skaltsaand Grafakou 004
C. incana Sm.	Dirphys mountain	38°61″ N	23°85″ E	1100–1200 m	6-2012	Skaltsaand Tsoukalas 002
C. rubra L.	Cithaeron mountain	38°10′11.25″ N	23°18′31.75″ E	647 m	6-10-2018	Kalpoutzakis5115/ 2-5-2019
Phitosiacrocifolia Kamari andGreuter	Parnonas mountain	37°16.897′ N	22°36.760′ E	1860 m	6-10-2018	Kalpoutzakis5036/ 6-10-2018

3.2. Extraction and Isolation

The air-dried aerial parts were finely ground and extracted at room temperature successively with cyclohexane (cHex): diethyl ether (Et_2O): methanol (MeOH) [(1:1:1; 3 × 1 L, for 2 days each (non-polar extracts)] and MeOH: H_2O [5:1; 3 × 1 L, for 1 day each (polar extracts)]. Amounts of 80–120 mg from the polar extract of each plant were extracted with n-butanol and the organic phase, after evaporation, was analyzed by LC-MS. The same residues were used for the NMR-metabolomic analysis. *C. incana* was selected for further analysis andpart of its MeOH: H_2O (5:1) (9.0 g) extract was fractionated by VLC over silica gel (6.5 cm × 10.0 cm) using mixtures of increasing polarity (cHex: ethyl acetate: MeOH: H_2O) with gradient elution and afforded ten fractions of 500 mL each (fractions RINA–RINJ) [5,7,8].

Vacuum liquid chromatography (VLC) was performed on a silica gel (Merck, Art. 7736). Fractionation was always monitored by TLC silica gel 60 F-254 (Merck, Art. 5554) and cellulose (Merck, Art. 5552) and visualized under UV (254 and 365 nm) and/or spraying with vanillin–sulfuric acid solution (Merck, Art. S26047 841) and with Neu's reagent for phenolics (Alfa Aesar A16606). All obtained extracts and fractions were evaporated to dryness in a vacuum under low temperature and then placed in desiccators activated with P_2O_5 until their weights were stable.

3.3. Nuclear Magnetic Resonance (NMR) Spectroscopy

NMR spectra were measured in an AVANCE III 600 instrument equipped with a 5 mm TBI CryoProbe (^{1}H-NMR 600 MHz, ^{13}C-NMR 150 MHz) or a Bruker DRX 400 (^{1}H-NMR 400 MHz, Bruker BioSpin) at 298 K. Chemical shifts are given in ppm (δ) and were referenced to the solvent signals at 3.31/49.0 ppm for methanol-d4 (CD$_3$OD) and 7.24/77.0 ppm for CDCl$_3$. COSY (correlation spectroscopy), HSQC (heteronuclear single-quantum correlation) and HMBC (heteronuclear multiple-bond correlation) experiments were performed using standard Bruker microprograms.

During the whole analysis, all extracts and obtained subfractions were continuously monitored and traced down using an NMR metabolomic strategy, which permitted in-detail characterization of their chemical profiles. Furthermore, the 1D and 2D NMR spectra of the BuOH residues were measured (see SM) [15,39,40]. The metabolites were identified using NMR experiments, by comparing the obtained chemical shifts and coupling constant values with standards, as well as with the aid of LC-MS. All candidate structures were compared with those previously published in the literature.

3.4. Liquid Chromatography High-Resolution Quadrupole Time-of-Flight Mass Spectrometry (LC-Q-TOF-MS/MS)

Analyses of the butanol residues of each plant were performed with UHPLC Agilent 1290 infinity system with a DAD G4212A and MS Agilent G6540A Q-TOF with Agilent Jet Stream technology electrospray ionization. Separation was performed on a Phenomenex Luna Omega column (C18, 1.9 u, 90 A°, 75 × 2.0 mm) using gradient mixtures of 0.1% formic acid (solvent A) and MeCN supplemented with 0.1% formic acid (solvent B). Gradient: 0.0–8.0 min, 0→30% B; 8.0–8.1 min, 30→98% B; 8.1–9.1 min, 98% B; 9.1–9.2 min, 98→5% B; 9.2–10.0 min, 5% B; flow rate, 0.6 mL/min; injection volume, 1 µL; oven temperature, 40 °C. Data analysis was performed by MassHunter Workstation Software Qualitative Analysis (B.07.00, B.10.00, Agilent) using automatic mass spectrum integration. LC-Q-TOF-MS/MS analyses were performed in positive and negative ionization modes to obtain maximum information on its composition. The metabolites were characterized based on their mass spectra, using the precursor ion and comparison of the fragmentation patterns with molecules described in the literature [15]. The putative identification of these compounds is summarized in Table 1, where the compounds are listed according to their retention times in the total ion chromatogram (TIC).

3.5. In Vitro Activity

3.5.1. DPPH (2,2-Diphenyl-1-Picrylhydrazyl) Radical Scavenging Assay

The free-radical scavenging capacity of *C. commutata*, *C. dioscoridis*, *C. foetida*, *C. heldreichiana*, *C. incana*, *C. rubra*, and *Phitosiacrocifolia* extracts and *Crepisincana* fractions RINA–RINK were evaluated using the DPPH radicalsscavenging assay. Briefly, solid extracts dissolved in absolute methanol (at final concentrations of 0.01–0.5 mg/mL) were added to an equal volume of a methanolic solution of DPPH (Sigma-Aldrich) (final concentration 200 µM) at room temperature (22 ± 2 °C). The contents were mixed and incubated in the dark for 30 min and the absorbance measured at 517 nm by a Tecan Sunrise Microplate reader (Biodirect). In order to compare the radical scavenging efficiency of the extracts, the results were expressed as IC$_{50}$ (mg/mL), i.e., the concentration that caused 50% scavenging of the DPPH radical [25,41].

3.5.2. Total Phenolic Content-Folin–Ciocalteu(F-C) Protocol

Briefly, the same fractions as mentioned in paragraph 3.5.1 were used to quantifying the total phenolic content. Solid extracts were dissolved in methanol (1 mg/mL). F-C reagent (Sigma-Aldrich) was diluted 1:10 in water and was used together with a solution of sodium carbonate 7.5% *w/v* in water. Finally, solutions of gallic acid in methanol in various concentrations (0.02–0.1 mg/mL) were used for the reference curve. After 30 min of incubation, the absorbance (765 nm) was recorded by Tecan Infinite 200 Pro Microplate Reader using ELISA 96-wellplates. Each measurement was performed in triplicate [22,42].

3.6. In Vivo Activity

3.6.1. Animals

Animal care was performed according to the guidelines established by the European Council Directive 2010/63/EU. The experimental procedures were approved by the National Peripheral Veterinary Authority Animal Ethics Committee after the affirmative opinion by the Animal Protocols Evaluation Committee. Male (hypolipidemic assay) and female (paw edema assay) C57BL/6 mice (3–6 months old) were used in this study. All mice originated from the breeding stock of the Small Animal Laboratory of the Section of Pharmaceutical Technology, Department of Pharmacy (EL 25 BIO 06). The animal's room temperature and humidity were maintained at 24 ± 1 °C and 45%, respectively. The room was illuminated by yellow fluorescent tubes in a 12h cycle of light and dark (switched on at 8:00 and off at 20:00); these lamps do not emit any measurable UV radiation. The mice had unrestricted continuous access to standard solid pellets (Nuevo SA-Farma-Efyra Industrial & Commercial SA, Greece) and fresh water.

3.6.2. Carrageenan-Induced Paw Edema Reduction Assay

For the in vivo anti-inflammatory activity, C57BL/6 female mice (6 per group, 5–6 months old, 20–34 g) were injected with 0.025 mL carrageenan (Merck KGaA, Darmstadt, Germany) (2% w/v solution in saline) i.d. into the right hind paw, with the left paw serving as the control. The test extracts *C. incana* 5:1, *C. heldreichiana* 5:1, *C. dioscoridis* 5:1 and fractions RINH and RINI, dissolved in saline with a few drops of Tween-80, were administered i.p. (0.3 mg/kg body weight) after the carrageenan injection. After 3.5 h, mice were sacrificed, hind legs were removed, and their weights measured in a precision analytical balance. The produced edema was estimated as the difference in weight (g) between the challenged right paw and the left paw. Results were expressed as the percentage of reduction in paw edema (mean from six animals per extract) [24,25,43].

3.6.3. Hypolipidemic Activity Assay

For the in vivo hypolipidemic activity, C57BL/6 male mice (8 per group, 3–4 months old) were used. An aqueous solution of Triton WR 1339 (tyloxapol) was given i.p. to all mice (except the untreated group) at a dose of 30 mg/kg body weight and one hour later the test extracts (0.3 mg/kg body weight) of *C. incana* 5:1, *C. dioscoridis* 5:1 or fractions RINH and RINI, dissolved in saline or saline alone (for the control groups), were administered i.p. After 24 h, blood was drawn from the aorta/heart, the plasma was separated by centrifugation (15 min, 3000 rpm, 4 °C) and used for the determination of plasma total antioxidant capacity (TAC), total cholesterol (TC) and triglyceride (TG) levels, using commercially diagnostic kits [Biosis Biotechnological applications L.T.D., Athens, Greece]. Levels in plasma were determined in duplicate while the values presented are the mean from eight animals (per extract) [44,45]. For TAC, the average value of % reduction in DPPH which is considered 100% is 22.1%.

3.7. Statistical Analysis

All results are presented as means ± SD. The data were tested for normality of distribution. Data were evaluated by Student's t-test. The p-value ≤ 0.05 was set as significance level for all data. Graphs were generated using GraphPad Prism 8.4.2 (GraphPad Software, Inc., San Diego, CA, USA).

4. Conclusions

Crepis is a widely distributed genus that can be found in different types of habitats around the globe, with the Mediterranean area being the most important center of its diversification. This study investigated the antioxidant, anti-inflammatory and antihyperlipidemic properties of *Crepis* spp. According to our findings, *Crepis* spp. is a rich source of phenolic compounds and, specifically, polyphenolic and flavonoid derivatives. In particular, the *Crepis* species may play a key role as an alternative source of caffeoyl tartaric acid derivatives, such as cichoric and caftaric acid. These promising secondary metabolites attract the interest of the scientific community due to their numerous biological activities, including antioxidant, anti-diabetic and anti-inflammatory potential. The specific pharmacological profile exhibited by the studied hereby *C. incana* extract justifies its further investigation and renders it attractive for use as a potential beneficial nutritional supplement. However, other important aspects of the genus, such as the analysis of new promising bioactivities, including the elucidation of their mechanisms of action and potential toxicity in higher doses, should be further investigated.

Supplementary Materials: The following supporting information can be downloaded at: https://www.mdpi.com/article/10.3390/molecules27196173/s1, S1.1–S1.8:LC-MS chromatograms; S2.1–S2.5: MS-MS spectrum of selected compounds; S3.1–S3.28: NMR data.

Author Contributions: Conceptualization, H.S. and A.P.K.; plant material: E.K. and M.-E.G.; phytochemical investigation, C.B. and M.-E.G.; biological investigation, K.A., A.T. and A.P.K.; writing—original draft preparation, C.B., M.-E.G., A.T. and A.P.K.; writing—review and editing, H.S. and A.P.K.; supervision, A.P.K., H.S., M.R. and J.H. All authors have read and agreed to the published version of the manuscript.

Funding: The research work was supported by the Hellenic Foundation for Research and Innovation (HFRI) under the HFRI PhD Fellowship grant (Fellowship Number: 16274).

Institutional Review Board Statement: The protocols of the animal studies were approved by the National Peripheral Veterinary Authority Animal Ethics Committee after the affirmative opinion of the Animal Protocols Evaluation Committee (Ethics approval numbers: 77659/29-01-2020 and 77645/29-01-2020, respectively).

Data Availability Statement: Not applicable.

Acknowledgments: The authors wish to express their gratitude to Fritz Kastner for measuring the 1D and 2D NMR spectra and to Josef Kiermaier and Wolfgang Söllner for recording the MS data (Faculty of Chemistry and Pharmacy, University of Regensburg).

Conflicts of Interest: The authors declare no conflict of interest.

References

1. Zidorn, C. Sesquiterpene lactones and their precursors as chemosystematic markers in the tribe Cichorieae of the Asteraceae. *Phytochemistry* **2008**, *69*, 2270–2296. [CrossRef] [PubMed]
2. Shulha, O.; Zidorn, C. Sesquiterpene lactones and their precursors as chemosystematic markers in the tribe Cichorieae of the Asteraceae revisited: An update (2008–2017). *Phytochemistry* **2019**, *163*, 149–177. [CrossRef] [PubMed]
3. Zidorn, C. Bioprospecting of plant natural products in Schleswig-Holstein (Germany) I: Chemodiversity of the Cichorieae tribe (Asteraceae) in Schleswig-Holstein. *Phytochem. Rev.* **2019**, *18*, 1223–1253. [CrossRef]
4. Salehi, B.; Azzini, E.; Zucca, P.; Maria Varoni, E.V.; Anil Kumar, N.; Dini, L.; Panzarini, E.; Rajkovic, J.; ValereTsouhFokou, P.; Peluso, I.; et al. Plant-Derived Bioactives and Oxidative Stress-Related Disorders: A Key Trend towards Healthy Aging and Longevity Promotion. *Appl. Sci.* **2020**, *10*, 947. [CrossRef]
5. Barda, C.; Ciric, A.; Soković, M.; Tsoukalas, M.; Skaltsa, H. Phytochemical investigation of Crepisincana Sm. (Asteraceae) endemic to southern Greece. *Biochem. System. Ecol.* **2018**, *80*, 59–62. [CrossRef]
6. Badalamenti, N.; Sottile, F.; Bruno, M. Ethnobotany, Phytochemistry, Biological, and Nutritional Properties of Genus *Crepis*—A Review. *Plants* **2022**, *11*, 519. [CrossRef] [PubMed]
7. Kotti, I.; Barda, C.; Karioti, A.; Skaltsa, H. Sesquiterpene lactones and other secondary metabolites from *Crepiscommutata* (Spreng.) Greuter–Asteraceae. *Biochem. Syst. Ecol.* **2019**, *86*, 103917. [CrossRef]
8. Tsoukalas, M.; Gousiadou, C.; Skaltsa, H. Sesquiterpene lactones and phenolics from *Crepisdioscoridis* L., growing wild in Greece. *Phytochem. Lett.* **2014**, *7*, 202–206. [CrossRef]
9. Sut, S.; Tahmasebi, A.; Ferri, N.; Ferrarese, I.; Rossi, I.; Panighel, G.; Lupo, M.G.; Maggi, F.; Karami, A.; Dall'Acqua, S. NMR, LC-MS Characterization of Rydingiamichauxii Extracts, Identification of Natural Products Acting as Modulators of LDLR and PCSK9. *Molecules* **2022**, *27*, 2256. [CrossRef]
10. Gathungu, R.M.; Kautz, R.; Kristal, B.S.; Bird, S.S.; Vouros, P. The integration of LC-MS and NMR for the analysis of low molecular weight trace analytes in complex matrices. *Mass Spectrom. Rev.* **2020**, *39*, 35–54. [CrossRef]
11. Luo, Z.; Gao, G.; Ma, Z.; Liu, Q.; Gao, X.; Tang, X.; Gao, Z.; Li, C.; Sun, T. Cichoric Acid from Witloof Inhibit Misfolding Aggregation and Fibrillation of HIAPP. *Int. J. Biol. Macromol.* **2020**, *148*, 1272–1279. [CrossRef] [PubMed]

12. Saleem, M.; Kim, H.J.; Jin, C.; Lee, Y.S. Antioxidant caffeic acid derivatives from leaves of *Parthenocissus tricuspidata*. *Arch. Pharm. Res.* **2004**, *27*, 300–304. [CrossRef] [PubMed]
13. Zidorn, C.; Ellmerer-Müller, E.P.; Stuppner, H. Eudesmanolides and inositol derivatives from *Taraxacum linearisquameum*. *Phytochemistry* **1999**, *51*, 991–994. [CrossRef]
14. Yang, L.; Wen, K.S.; Ruan, X.; Zhao, Y.X.; Wei, F.; Wang, Q. Response of Plant Secondary Metabolites to Environmental Factors. *Molecules* **2018**, *23*, 762. [CrossRef]
15. Tsami, K.; Barda, C.; Ladopoulos, G.; Didaras, N.A.; Grafakou, M.E.; Heilmann, J.; Mossialos, D.; Rallis, M.C.; Skaltsa, H. Chemical Profile and *In Vitro* Evaluation of the Antibacterial Activity of *Dioscorea communis* Berry Juice. *Sci* **2022**, *4*, 21. [CrossRef]
16. Wang, Y.; Xie, G.; Liu, Q.; Duan, X.; Liu, Z.; Liu, X. Pharmacokinetics, tissue distribution, and plasma protein binding study of chicoric acid by HPLC–MS/MS. *J. Chromatogr. B Analyt. Technol. Biomed. Life Sci.* **2016**, *1031*, 139–145. [CrossRef]
17. Liu, Q.; Wang, Y.; Xiao, C.; Wu, W.; Liu, X. Metabolism of chicoric acid by rat liver microsomes and bioactivity comparisons of chicoric acid and its metabolites. *Food Funct.* **2015**, *6*, 1928–1935. [CrossRef]
18. Yang, L.; Wenzhao, T.; Jing, C.; Ru, J.; Lianjie, M.; Shaoli, W.; Jiao, W.; Xiangling, S.; Zhaohui, C.; Changxiang, Z.; et al. Development of Marker-Free Transgenic Potato Tubers Enriched in Caffeoylquinic Acids and Flavonols. *J. Agric. Food Chem.* **2016**, *64*, 2932–2940.
19. Zidorn, C.; Schubert, B.; Stuppner, H. Phenolics as Chemosystematic Markers in and for the Genus *Crepis* (Asteraceae, Cichorieae). *Sci. Pharm.* **2008**, *76*, 743–750. [CrossRef]
20. Paço, A.; Brás, T.; Santos, J.O.; Sampaio, P.; Gomes, A.C.; Duarte, M.F. Anti-Inflammatory and Immunoregulatory Action of Sesquiterpene Lactones. *Molecules* **2022**, *27*, 1142. [CrossRef]
21. Merfort, I. Review of the analytical techniques for sesquiterpenes and sesquiterpene lactones. *J. Chromatogr. A* **2002**, *967*, 115–130. [CrossRef]
22. Tzara, A.; Lambrinidis, G.; Kourounakis, A. Design of Multifaceted Antioxidants: Shifting towards Anti-Inflammatory and Atihyperlipidemic Activity. *Molecules* **2021**, *26*, 4928. [CrossRef] [PubMed]
23. Matralis, A.N.; Kourounakis, A.P. Optimizing the pharmacological profile of new bifunctional antihyperlipidemic/antioxidant morpholine derivatives. *ACS Med. Chem. Lett.* **2018**, *10*, 98–104. [CrossRef]
24. Aswad, M.; Rayan, M.; Abu-Lafi, S.; Falah, M.; Raiyn, J.; Abdallah, Z.; Rayan, A. Nature is the best source of anti-inflammatory drugs: Indexing natural products for their anti-inflammatory bioactivity. *Inflamm. Res.* **2018**, *67*, 67–75. [CrossRef]
25. Blainski, A.; Lopes, G.C.; de Mello, J.C. Application and analysis of the folinciocalteu method for the determination of the total phenolic content from *Limonium brasiliense* L. *Molecules* **2013**, *18*, 6852–6865. [CrossRef]
26. Sadeghi, H.; Hajhashemi, V.; Minaiyan, M.; Movahedian, A.; Talebi, A. A study on the mechanisms involving the anti-inflammatory effect of amitriptyline in carrageenan-induced paw edema in rats. *Eur. J. Pharmacol.* **2011**, *667*, 369–401. [CrossRef]
27. Necas, J.; Bartosikova, L. Carrageenan: A Review. *Vet. Med.* **2013**, *58*, 187–205. [CrossRef]
28. Kourounakis, A.P.; Galanakis, D.; Tsiakitzis, K.; Rekka, E.A.; Kourounakis, P.N. Synthesis and pharmacological evaluation of novel derivatives of anti-inflammatory drugs with increased antioxidant and anti-inflammatory activities. *Drug Dev. Res.* **1999**, *47*, 9–16. [CrossRef]
29. Theodosis-Nobelos, P.; Kourti, M.; Gavalas, A.; Rekka, E.A. Amides of non-steroidal anti-inflammatory drugs with thiomorpholine can yield hypolipidemic agents with improved anti-inflammatory activity. *Bioorg. Med. Chem. Lett.* **2016**, *26*, 910–913. [CrossRef]
30. Chatterjee, S. Oxidative stress, Inflammation, and disease. In *Oxidative Stress and Biomaterials*; Chapter 2; Academic Press: Cambridge, MA, USA, 2016; pp. 35–58.
31. Schütz, K.; Carle, R.; Schieber, A. *Taraxacum*—A review on its phytochemical and pharmacological profile. *J. Ethnopharmacol.* **2006**, *107*, 323. [CrossRef]
32. Janda, K.; Gutowska, I.; Geszke-Moritz, M.; Jakubczyk, K. The Common Cichory (*Cichorium intybus* L.) as a Source of Extracts with Health-Promoting Properties—A Review. *Molecules* **2021**, *26*, 1814. [CrossRef]
33. Barda, C.; Grafakou, M.E.; Kalpoutzakis, E.; Heilmann, J.; Skaltsa, H. Chemical composition of *Crepis foetida* L. and *C. rubra* L. volatile constituents and evaluation of the in vitro anti-inflammatory activity of salicylaldehyde rich volatile fraction. *Biochem. Syst. Ecol.* **2021**, *96*, 104256. [CrossRef]
34. Gokhan, Z.; Cengiz, S.; Pembegul, U.; Abdurrahman, A.; Sengul, U.; Mehmet, S.M.; Ramazan, C. *Crepis foetida* L. subsp. *rhoeadifolia* (Bieb.) Celak. as a source of multifunctional agents: Cytotoxic and phytochemical evaluation. *J. Funct. Food* **2015**, *17*, 698–708.
35. Okmen, A.S. Antioxidant and antibacterial activities of different plants extracts against *Staphylococcus aureus* isolated from soccerplayer's shoes and knowledge and applications about foot hygiene of the soccer players. *Afr. J. Tradit. Complement. Altern. Med.* **2015**, *12*, 143–149. [CrossRef]
36. Pedreiro, S.; da Ressurreição, S.; Lopes, M.; Cruz, M.T.; Batista, T.; Figueirinha, A.; Ramos, F. *Crepis vesicaria* L. subsp. *taraxacifolia* Leaves: NutritionalProfile, Phenolic Composition andBiological Properties. *Int. J. Environ. Res. Public Health* **2021**, *18*, 151. [CrossRef]
37. Duan, L.; Zhang, C.; Zhao, Y.; Chang, Y.; Guo, L. Comparison of Bioactive Phenolic Compounds and Antioxidant Activities of Different Parts of *Taraxacum mongolicum*. *Molecules* **2020**, *25*, 3260. [CrossRef]
38. Lv, C.; Huang, S.; Wang, Y.; Hu, Z.; Zhao, G.; Ma, C.; Cao, X. Chicoric acid encapsulated within ferritin inhibits tau phosphorylation by regulating AMPK and GluT1 signaling cascade. *J. Funct. Food* **2021**, *86*, 104681. [CrossRef]

39. Ding, X.Q.; Jian, T.Y.; Gai, Y.N.; Niu, G.T.; Liu, Y.; Meng, X.H.; Li, J.; Lyu, H.; Ren, B.R.; Chen, J. Chicoric Acid Attenuated Renal Tubular Injury in HFD-Induced Chronic Kidney Disease Mice through the Promotion of Mitophagy via the Nrf2/PINK/Parkin Pathway. *J. Agric. Food Chem.* **2022**, *70*, 2923–2935. [CrossRef]
40. Grafakou, M.E.; Barda, C.; Karikas, G.A.; Heilmann, J.; Skaltsa, H. Cajamolides A-N: Cytotoxic and anti-inflammatory sesquiterpene lactones from *Caleajamaicensis*. *Bioorg. Chem.* **2021**, *116*, 105351. [CrossRef]
41. Katselou, M.G.; Matralis, A.N.; Kourounakis, A.P. Developing potential agents against atherosclerosis: Design, synthesis and pharmacological evaluation of novel dual inhibitors of oxidative stress and Squalene Synthase activity. *Eur. J. Med. Chem.* **2017**, *138*, 748–760. [CrossRef]
42. Naz, S.; Ahmad, S.; Rasool, S.; Sayeed, S.; Siddiqi, R. Antibacterial activity directed isolation of compounds from *Onosmahispidum*. *Microbiol. Res.* **2006**, *161*, 43–48. [CrossRef]
43. Di Rossa, M. Biological properties of carrageenan. *J. Pharm. Pharmacol.* **1972**, *24*, 89–102. [CrossRef]
44. Kourounakis, A.P.; Victoratos, P.; Peroulis, N.; Stefanou, N.; Yiangou, M.; Hadjipetrou, L.; Kourounakis, P.N. Experimental hyperlipidemia and the effect of NSAIDs. *Exp. Mol. Pathol.* **2002**, *73*, 135–138. [CrossRef]
45. Matralis, A.N.; Kourounakis, A.P. Design of Novel Potent Antihyperlipidemic Agents with Antioxidant/Anti-inflammatory Properties: Exploiting Phenothiazine's Strong Antioxidant Activity. *J. Med. Chem.* **2014**, *57*, 2568–2581. [CrossRef]

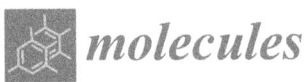

Article

Ameliorative Effect of Citropten Isolated from *Citrus aurantifolia* Peel Extract as a Modulator of T Cell and Intestinal Epithelial Cell Activity in DSS-Induced Colitis

Hyun-Su Lee [1], Eun-Nam Kim [2] and Gil-Saeng Jeong [2,*]

[1] Department of Physiology, School of Medicine, Daegu Catholic University, Daegu 42472, Korea; lhs6858@cu.ac.kr
[2] College of Pharmacy, Chungnam National University, Daejeon 34134, Korea; enkim@cnu.ac.kr
* Correspondence: gsjeong@cnu.ac.kr

Abstract: Citropten is a coumarin that is mainly found in fruits of Rutaceae trees, but its anti-inflammatory activities in colitis is still unknown. In this study, we investigated its attenuating effect of citropten isolated from *Citrus aurantifolia* extract on DSS-induced colitis through the modulation of the activity of T cells and intestinal epithelial cells. We found that pre-treatment with citropten downregulates the activity of T cells and intestinal epithelial cells without a negative effect on the viability of Jurkat and HT-29 cells. The results from the Western blot analysis revealed that pre-treatment with citropten reduces the NFκB and MAPK signaling pathway in activated T cells and intestinal epithelial cells. We elucidated that the oral administration of citropten alleviates the colonic inflammation and activity of effector T cells in DSS-induced colitis by measuring changes in body weight, histological scoring from H&E-stained sections, mRNA levels of pro-inflammatory cytokines and the phosphorylation level of the MAPK signaling pathway.

Keywords: citropten; colitis; T cell activation; intestinal cell activation; anti-inflammation; MAPK

1. Introduction

Colitis has been investigated as an inflammatory disorder provoked by several factors including infection, allergic reactions and inflammatory bowel disease (IBD) [1]. IBD is a chronic disease of the digestive tract, mainly ulcerative colitis (UC) and Crohn's disease (CD), characterized by the chronic and spontaneous recurrence of inflammation. The symptoms of IBD include abdominal pain, cramping and diarrhea with blood in the stool [2]. The accurate etiology of IBD is still unknown, but accumulated evidence shows that it is correlated with uncontrolled excessive immune responses [3,4]. It has been elucidated that the uncontrolled activation of mucosal T cells causes mucosal damage during IBD which results in functional changes as well as tissue destructions [5]. Since intestinal epithelial cells play a pivotal role as a first barrier that defends against pathogens, it is important to maintain immunological homeostasis, including the activity of intestinal epithelial cells, during IBD [6]. Even though the inhibition or interruption of immunopathogenic responses including T cells and intestinal epithelial cells can be a potential therapeutic strategy, this still needs to be properly proven.

The engagement of T cell receptor (TCR) and major histocompatibility complex (MHC) molecules with antigenic peptides is one of the critical events that provokes a T-cell-mediated immune response [7]. CD28 is also involved as a costimulatory molecule in T cell activation which leads to the activation of the nuclear kappa-light-chain-enhancer of activated B cells (NFκB) pathway through the NFκB binding site on the CD28 response element (CD28RE) [8]. It has been well studied as one of most important transcription factors that translocates into the nucleus in an active state [9]. It has been also reported that the NFκB pathway in intestinal epithelial cells plays a crucial role in the maintenance of immune homeostasis during inflammatory colitis [10,11]. Nevertheless, considering the fact that the activation of the NFκB pathway is involved in disease activity in IBD patients, efforts to develop treatments targeting the NFκB pathway remain insufficient.

Citropten (5,7-dimethoxycoumarin or limettin, $C_{11}H_{10}O_4$) is one of coumarin derivatives that possesses a variety of biological properties including antioxidant and anti-cancer activities [12,13]. Several studies in the literature have reported that it is isolated from *Citrus limon*, *Carica papaya* and *Citrus bergamia* [14–16]. It has been also elucidated that it has diverse biological functions, including an anti-proliferating effect on B16 melanoma cells, an inhibitory effect on MAPK in carcinoma tissues and a preventive effect on chronic-depression-induced mild stress in rats [17–19]. Though various activities of citropten have been well established, little is known as to whether citropten has an anti-inflammatory effect on inflammatory colitis.

In the current study, we investigated the ameliorative effect of citropten isolated from *Citrus aurantifolia* extract on inflammatory colitis using a DSS-induced colitis animal model. The modulation of activities of T cells and intestinal epithelial cells through the suppression of the nuclear translocation of p65 in the NFκB pathway and the phosphorylation of MAPK signaling molecules through pre-treatment with citropten was presented as the underlying mechanism.

2. Results

2.1. Isolation of Citropten from C. aurantifolia Peel Extract and Its Chemical Structure

Liquid chromatography–mass spectrometry analysis was performed on the 70% EtOH extract of *C. aurantifolia* peel, and the MS spectrum for compound **1** detected at 26.2 min was obtained. Compound **1** isolated in the positive ion mode of MS spectrum showed a mass to charge ratio of 207.2 (Figure 1A). In addition, the purity of the isolated citropten was evaluated using HPLC-DAD, and the purity of citropten was confirmed to be about 98.65% (Figure 1B).

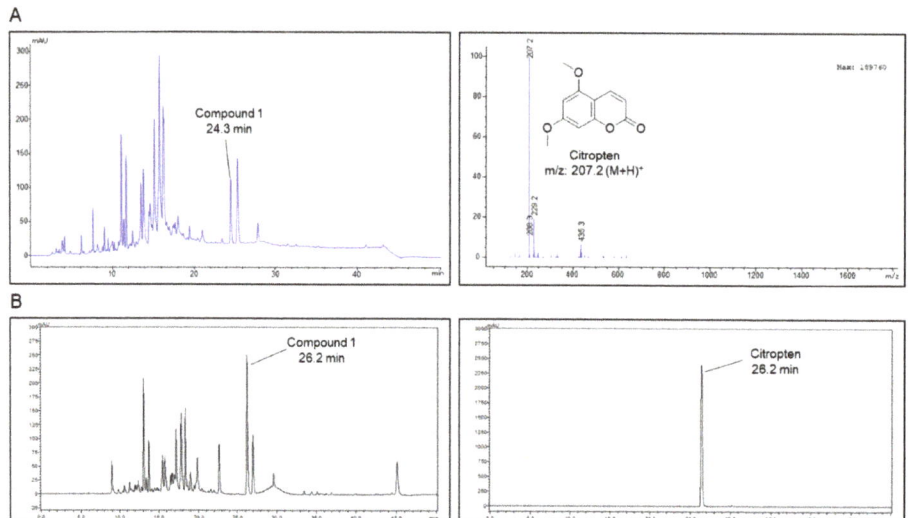

Figure 1. Isolation of citropten from *C. aurantifolia* peel extract and its chemical structure. (**A**) High-performance liquid chromatography (HPLC)-mass spectrum of *C. aurantifolia* peel 70% EtOH extract, and ESI-MS spectra of the [M + H]$^+$ ion of citropten. (**B**) Purity evaluation of isolated citropten using HPLC-DAD (330 nm).

2.2. Citropten Has No Negative Effect on the Viability of Jurkat and HT-29 Cells

Since the cytotoxicity of compounds has been mainly reported as an underlying mechanism of the inhibitory effect on the activity, first, we explored whether citropten leads to cytotoxicity in T cells and epithelial intestinal cells. For the in vitro assay, Jurkat T cells and HT-29 cells were used in the present study. Figure 2A shows that the confluency of both cells is not affected by treatment with citropten up to 40 μM. To estimate the cellular viability in the presence of citropten, an MTT viability assay was performed using Jurkat cells and HT-29 cells. Comparable viability was revealed in Jurkat and HT-29 cells incubated with citropten for 24 h up to 40 μM (Figure 2B). To confirm whether treatment with citropten induces apoptosis-related cell death in Jurkat and HT-29 cells, an AnnexinV/PI apoptosis assay was performed. The population of AnnexinV/PI double-positive cells was measured via flow cytometry. Figure 2C shows that treatment with citropten up to 40 μM did not change the percentage of Jurkat and HT-29 cells expressing AnnexinV and PI. These results suggest that citropten treatment up to 40 μM does not have a negative effect on the viability of Jurkat and HT-29 cells.

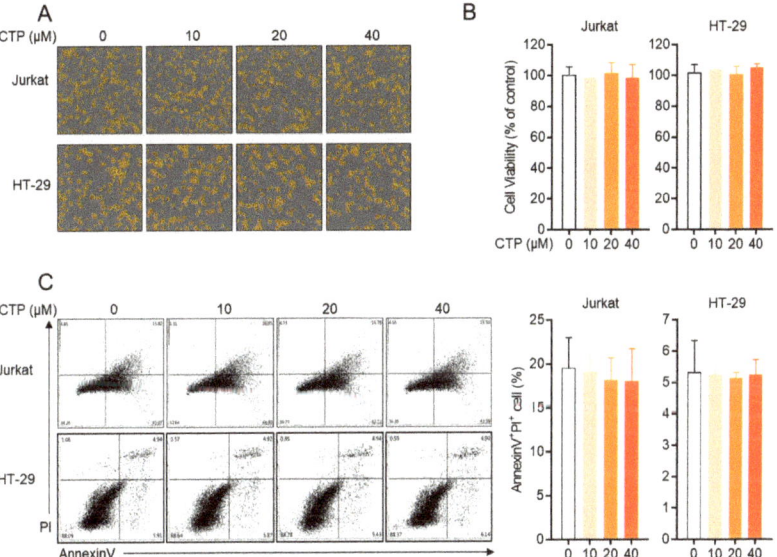

Figure 2. Citropten has no negative effect on the viability of Jurkat and HT-29 cells. (**A,B**) Jurkat cells (1×10^4/well) and HT-29 cells (1×10^4/well) were treated with indicated concentration (0 to 40 μM) of citropten for 24 h; then, cells were marked in orange using IncuCyte imaging system (**A**). Cell viability was determined by performing MTT assay (**B**). Cell viability was presented in % of control (0 μM). (**C**) Jurkat cells (5×10^5/well) and HT-29 cells (5×10^5/well) were treated with indicated concentrations (0 to 40 μM) of citropten for 24 h; then, AnnexinV$^+$PI$^+$ double-positive cells were detected by performing AnnexinV/PI apoptosis assay. Results are expressed as mean ± SD of three independent experiments.

2.3. Activity of Jurkat T Cells Is Downregulated by Pre-Treatment with Citropten

Since the activation of T cells in the inflammatory response plays a pivotal role in the pathogenesis of colitis, we investigated whether citropten affects T cell activity in vitro. Three in vitro models of stimulating T cells were used in the present study, including TCR-mediated stimulation using anti-CD3 and anti-CD28 antibodies, treatment with PMA and A23187 and a co-culture system with superantigen-loaded Raji B cells. Figure 3A shows that pre-treatment with citropten inhibited the mRNA level of IL-2 from activated Jurkat T cells in a dose-dependent manner. It was confirmed that released IL-2 from activated

T cells is suppressed by citropten (Figure 3B). To examine whether citropten blocks IL-2 production from stimulated T cells, cytosolic IL-2 was detected using a Western blot assay. Figure 3C shows that pre-treatment with citropten downregulated IL-2 production in activated T cells. The expression of CD69, which is one of the specific markers of T cell activation, on the surface of activated T cells was monitored using flow cytometry. As shown in Figure 3D, the intensity of CD69 was significantly decreased by pre-treatment with citropten. These results suggest that citropten effectively abrogates T cell activation, including IL-2 production as well as CD69 expression, from activated T cells.

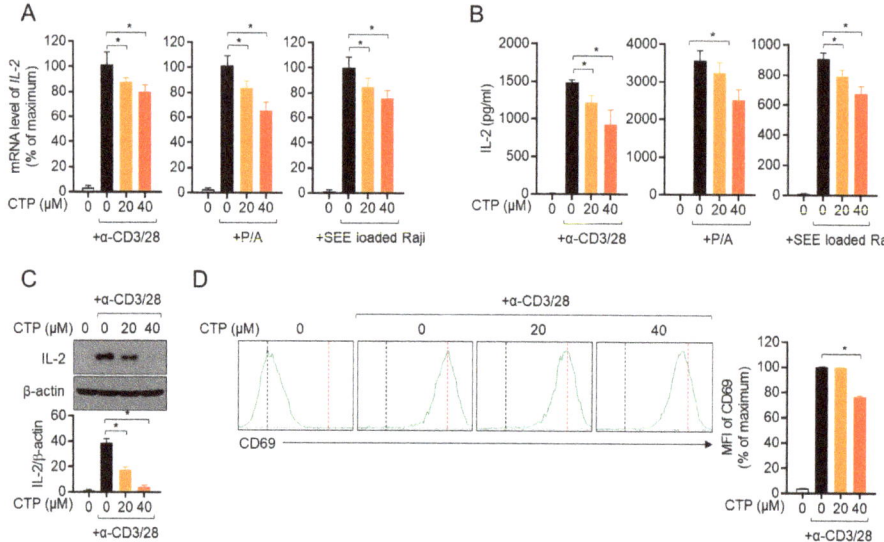

Figure 3. Activity of Jurkat T cells is downregulated by pre-treatment with citropten. (**A,B**) Jurkat T cells (5×10^5/well) were pre-treated with the indicated concentration (0 to 40 µM) of citropten for 1 h and stimulated with anti-CD3 antibodies (20 µg/mL) and anti-CD28 antibodies (7 µg/mL, left), PMA (100 nM) and A23187- (1 µM, middle) or SEE-loaded Raji B cells (right) for 6 h (**A**) or 24 h (**B**). mRNA level of IL-2 was detected via real-time quantitative PCR (**A**), and released IL-2 was measured using ELISA (**B**). (**C**) Jurkat T cells (1×10^6/well) were pre-treated with the indicated concentration (0 to 40 µM) of citropten for 1 h and stimulated with anti-CD3 antibodies (20 µg/mL) and anti-CD28 antibodies (7 µg/mL) for 6 h. Cells were harvested and lysed in RIPA buffer. Produced IL-2 was detected via Western blot analysis. Detected IL-2 was normalized with the intensity of β-actin and is shown in bar graph below. (**D**) Pre-treated Jurkat cells (5×10^5) with 40 µM of citropten were stimulated with anti-CD3 antibodies (20 µg/mL) and anti-CD28 antibodies (7 µg/mL) for 16 h. After stimulation, cells were stained with anti-CD69 antibodies conjugated with APC and acquired for detection of fluorescence via flow cytometry. Each plot is presented, and mean fluorescence intensity is shown in bar graph. Results are expressed as mean ± SD of three independent experiments (*, $p < 0.05$).

2.4. Citropten Suppresses the Production of Inflammatory Cytokines in Activated HT-29 Cells

We further investigated whether citropten has a modulatory effect on the production of inflammatory cytokines from activated HT-29 by treatment with recombinant TNFα. The mRNA levels of pro-inflammatory cytokines including TNFα, IL-1β and IL-8 were explored in the presence or absence of pre-treatment with citropten of HT-29 cells via real-time quantitative PCR. Figure 4A shows that pre-treatment with dose-dependent citropten reduced the mRNA levels of pro-inflammatory cytokines. To elucidate whether pre-treatment with citropten modulated the expression of surface molecules on activated cells by recombinant TNFα, we checked the mRNA levels of ICAM1 and VCAM1 via real-time quantitative PCR. A downregulated mRNA level of ICAM1 and VCAM1 was observed on activated HT-29 cells pre-treated with citropten in a dose-dependent manner. These data suggest that pre-treatment with citropten effectively regulates the activity of HT-29 cells in terms of the production of pro-inflammatory cytokines and the expression of surface molecules.

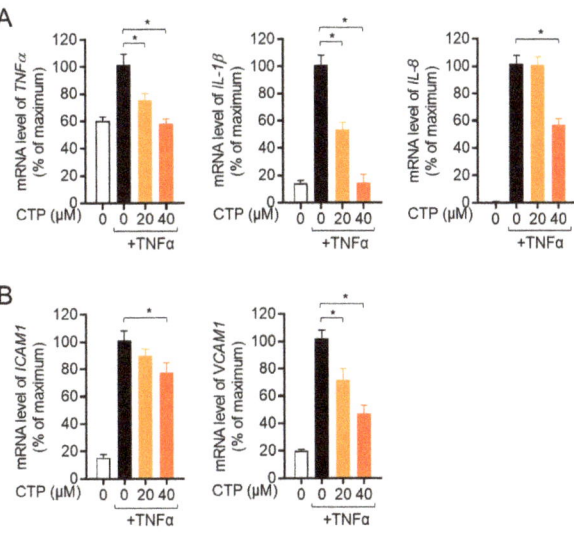

Figure 4. Citropten suppresses the production of inflammatory cytokines in activated HT-29 cells. (**A**, **B**) HT-29 cells were pre-treated with the indicated concentration (0 to 40 µM) for 1 h and stimulated with recombinant TNFα (10 ng/mL) for 6 h. mRNA levels of TNFα, IL-1β and IL-8 (**A**) or ICAM1 and VCAM1 (**B**) were measured via real-time quantitative PCR analysis. The value was presented in % of maximum by normalization with GAPDH. Results are expressed as mean ± SD of three independent experiments (*, $p < 0.05$).

2.5. Pre-Treatment with Citropten Reduces NFκB and MAPK Signaling Pathway in Activated Jurkat and HT-29

It has been well reported that NFκB is a one of the main transcription factors that is involved in T cell activation. To investigate whether pre-treatment with citropten affects to the NFκB signaling pathway in TCR-mediated activation, the nuclear translation of p65 was assessed via Western blot analysis. Activated T cells showed the increased translocation of nuclear p65, but pre-treatment with citropten slightly reduced it, and simultaneously, the remaining p65 in cytosol was increased in activated T cells pre-treated with citropten (Figure 5A). To explore how the activity of IκBα is affected by pre-treatment with citropten in activated T cells, the degradation and phosphorylation of IκBα was examined. Figure 5A shows that the enhanced degradation and phosphorylation of IκBα in activated T cells were significantly suppressed by pre-treatment with citropten. We further examined whether the MAPK signaling pathway is affected by pre-treatment with citropten in activated T cells. Figure 5B shows that the phosphorylation levels of ERK, p38 and JNK were augmented by TCR-mediated stimulation, but pre-treatment with citropten inhibited them in a dose-dependent manner. We aimed to confirm whether the modulatory effect of citropten through the NFκB and MAPK signaling pathway is also shown in activated HT-29 cells by TNFα. Figure 5C,D reveals that citropten pre-treatment had a negative effect on the NFκB and MAPK signaling pathway in activated HT-29 cells. These data suggest that pre-treatment with citropten suppresses the activity of T cells and epithelial intestinal cells through the NFκB and MAPK signaling pathway in vitro.

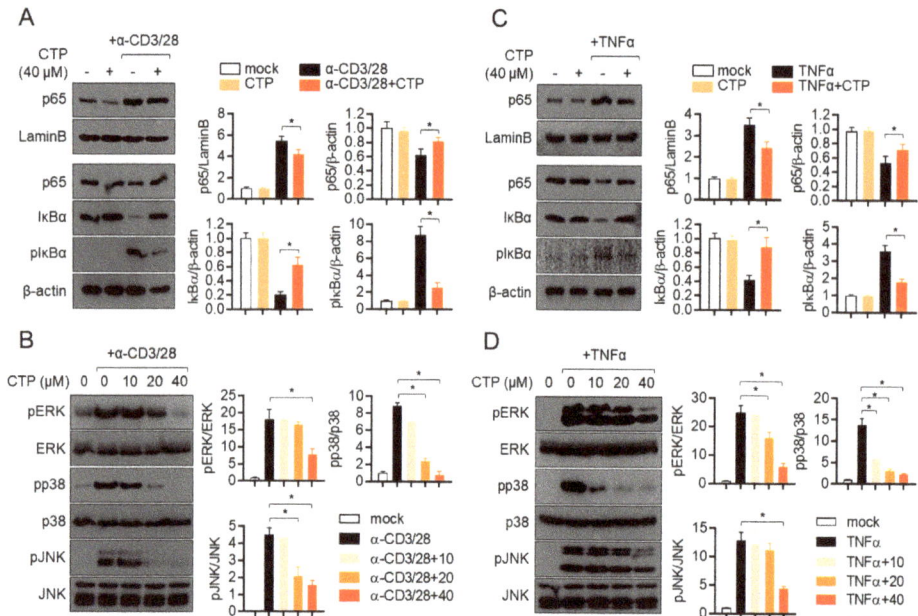

Figure 5. Pre-treatment with citropten reduces NFκB and MAPK signaling pathway in activated Jurkat and HT-29. (**A**,**B**) Jurkat cells were pre-treated with 40 µM (**A**) or the indicated concentration (0 to 40 µM, (**B**)) of citropten and were stimulated with anti-CD3 antibodies (20 µg/mL) and anti-CD28 antibodies (7 µg/mL) for 1 h (**A**) or 30 min (**B**). For separation of nucleic extract (**A**), cells were lysed by using NE-PER kit. Nuclear transported p65 was detected in nuclear extract and cytosolic extract. Degraded and phosphorylated IκBα were detected in cytosolic extract. Detected proteins were normalized with the intensity of loading control proteins (LaminB for nuclear extract and β-actin for cytosolic extract). For the detection of phosphorylated level (**B**), harvested cells were lysed in RIPA buffer. Phosphorylated and total protein of ERK, p38 and JNK were determined via Western blot analysis. Phosphorylated levels were normalized with the intensity of total proteins and are presented in bar graphs. (**C**,**D**) HT-29 cells were pre-treated with 40 µM (**C**) or the indicated concentration (0 to 40 µM, (**D**)) of citropten and were stimulated with recombinant TNFα (10 ng/mL) for 1 h (**C**) or 30 min (**D**). For separation of nucleic extract (**C**), cells were lysed by using NE-PER kit. Nuclear transported p65 was detected in nuclear extract and cytosolic extract, respectively. Degraded and phosphorylated IκBα were detected in cytosolic extract. Detected proteins were normalized with the intensity of loading control proteins (LaminB for nuclear extract and β-actin for cytosolic extract). For the detection of phosphorylated level (**D**), harvested cells were lysed in RIPA buffer. Phosphorylated and total protein of ERK, p38 and JNK were determined via Western blot analysis. Phosphorylated levels were normalized with the intensity of total proteins and are presented in bar graphs. Results are expressed as mean ± SD of three independent experiments (*, $p < 0.05$).

2.6. Oral Administration of Citropten Attenuates DSS-Induced Colitis in Mice Model

To explore whether citropten has an ameliorative effect on inflammatory colitis in vivo, a DSS-induced colitis model was used. An inflammatory colitis model was used by feeding mice water containing 2.5% DSS for 7 days in the presence of the daily oral administration of citropten. To obtain more accurate results, two doses of citropten (10 mg/kg and 40 mg/kg) were used in animal model experiments (Figure 6A). Feeding water containing 2.5% DSS significantly reduced the body weight of mice due to severe inflammatory responses, but the oral administration of citropten protected weight loss caused by the feeding of DSS-containing water (Figure 6B). To measure how severely the colitis lesion progressed, a daily stool score was measured according to the pathological criteria. Figure 6C reveals that mice with colitis who underwent the oral administration of citropten exhibited a downregulated stool score. Pictures of the anuses of mice which were taken on day 7 showed improved manifestation in the mouse group with the oral administration of citropten (Figure 6D). The assessed disease activity index (DAI) also confirmed that the oral administration of citropten decreased various disease levels in the colitis model (Figure 6E). These data suggest that the oral administration of citropten ameliorates the manifestations of inflammatory colitis.

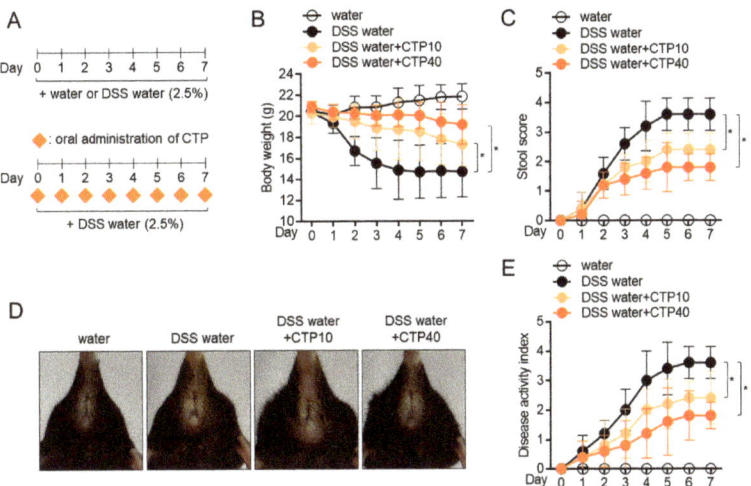

Figure 6. Oral administration of citropten attenuates DSS-induced colitis in mice model. (**A**) Experimental scheme of IBD induction. (**B**) Transition of body weight during 7 days of IBD induction. (**C**) Transition of stool score during 7 days of IBD induction. (**D**) Representative pictures of mice anus on day 7 post-induction. (**E**) Transition of disease activity index during 7 days of IBD induction. Data are expressed as mean ± SD ($n = 5$/group) (*, $p < 0.05$). Water: mouse group fed with fresh water, DSS water: mouse group fed with water containing 2.5% DSS, DSS water + CTP10; mouse group fed with water containing 2.5% DSS and orally administered with 10 mg/kg citropten, DSS water + CTP40, mouse group fed with water containing 2.5% DSS and orally administered with 40 mg/kg citropten.

2.7. Oral Administration of Citropten Alleviates the Colonic Inflammation in DSS-Induced Colitis Model

To elucidate whether the oral administration of citropten leads to alteration in colons, colons tissues were removed, and the colonic length was measured. Figure 7A,B shows that colons from mice fed with 2.5% DSS water were shrunken in length due to inflammation, but the oral administration of citropten prevented the inflammatory shrinkage in a dose-dependent manner. The results obtained from tissue section staining with H&E revealed that the collapse of intestinal structures was restored by the oral administration of citropten (Figure 7C). In particular, the infiltration of inflammatory cells, the epithelial damages and crypt lesions were improved in a dose-dependent manner. The measurement of histological scores from obtained H&E tissue staining also confirmed that the oral administration of citropten ameliorated the severity of inflammation in colon tissue (Figure 7D). The mRNA levels of TNFα, IL-1β and IL-8 were determined using a real-time quantitative PCR to confirm whether the oral administration of citropten decreased to produce pro-inflammatory cytokines on colonic tissues. Figure 7E shows that elevated mRNA levels of TNFα, IL-1β and IL-8 were reduced by the oral administration of citropten in a dose-dependent manner. To prove the connection with the in vitro results and how the oral administration of citropten suppresses inflammatory responses in the colitis model, a Western blot analysis was performed using colonic tissues. Figure 7F shows that the MAPK signaling pathway, including the phosphorylation of ERK, p38 and JNK, was slightly affected by the oral administration of citropten. These data suggest that the oral administration of citropten modulated the inflammatory responses on colonic tissue in the colitis model.

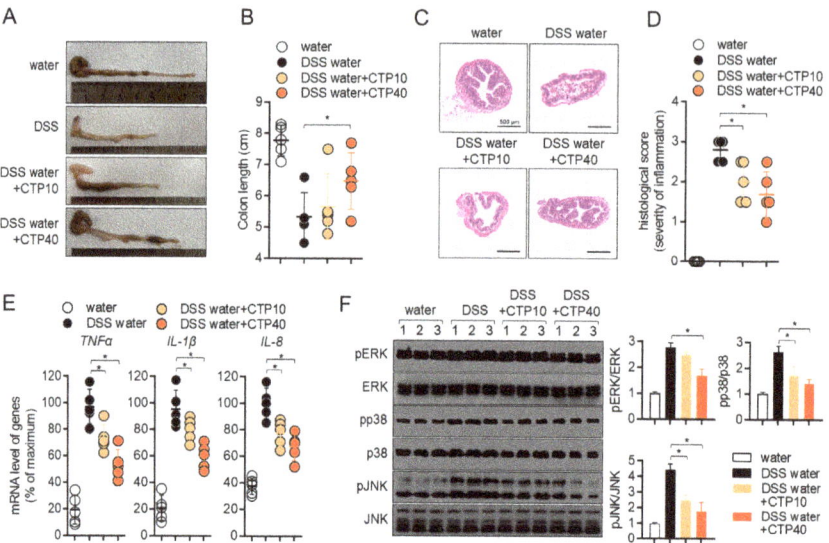

Figure 7. Oral application of citropten alleviates the colonic inflammation in DSS-induced colitis. (**A**) Representative photographs of colons from each group of mice at day 7. (**B**) Length of colons from (**A**). (**C**) Colons were removed on day 7 post-IBD induction, and sections were stained with H&E. Bars, 500 μm. (**D**) Histological scores of sections staining with H&E from (**C**). (**E**) mRNA levels of pro-inflammatory cytokines in colon tissues from each group of mice were measured via real-time quantitative PCR. The levels were normalized with GAPDH and presented in % of maximum. (**F**) Phosphorylated levels of ERK, p38 and JNK were detected via Western blot analysis on lysed colon tissues. Phosphorylated levels were normalized with the intensity of total proteins and are presented in bar graphs. Data are presented as mean ± SD ($n = 5$/group) (*, $p < 0.05$). Water: mouse group fed with fresh water, DSS water: mouse group fed with water containing 2.5% DSS, DSS water + CTP10: mouse group fed with water containing 2.5% DSS and orally administered with 10 mg/kg citropten, DSS water + CTP40: mouse group fed with water containing 2.5% DSS and orally administered with 40 mg/kg citropten.

2.8. Oral Treatment with Citropten Ameliorates T Cell Activity in DSS-Induced Colitis Model

Since the activity of T cells has been investigated as a major player in colonic inflammation, we collected information regarding mesenteric lymph nodes at day 7 post-induction to compare the T cell activation in different groups. Figure 8A,B shows elevations in the length and weight of mesenteric lymph nodes, but the oral administration of citropten decreased them. To explore whether the oral application of citropten suppressed the activity of effector T cells in the colitis model, the mRNA levels of IL-2, IFNγ and IL-17 were measured via real-time quantitative PCR. Increased mRNA levels of IL-2, IFNγ and IL-17 in colons from DSS mice were significantly decreased via the oral administration of citropten in vivo. The phosphorylation level of ERK, p38 and JNK was also confirmed via Western blot analysis to find the relationship between in vitro results and in vivo manifestations. Figure 8D shows that ERK and JNK phosphorylation were slightly affected by the oral administration of citropten on mesenteric lymph nodes. These data suggest that the oral administration of citropten attenuates the activity of effector T cells in DSS-induced colitis in vivo.

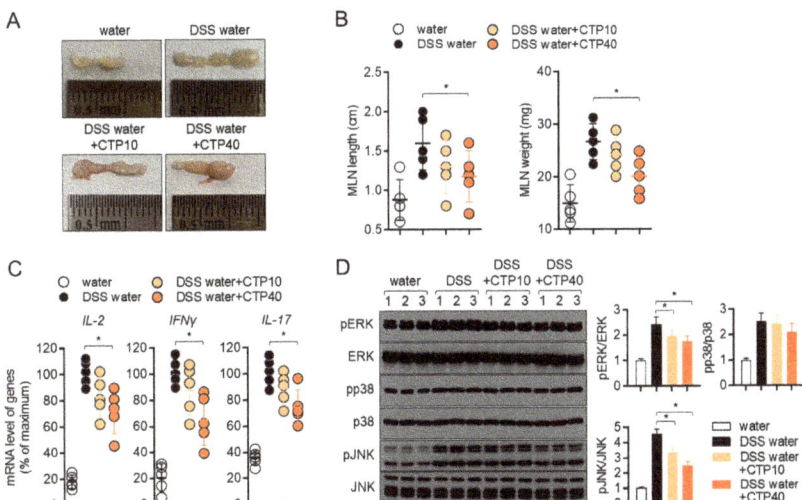

Figure 8. Oral treatment with citropten ameliorates T cell activity in DSS-induced colitis model. (**A**) Representative photographs of mesenteric lymph nodes from each group of mice at day 7. (**B**) Length and weight of mesenteric lymph nodes from (**A**). (**C**) mRNA levels of effector cytokines in mesenteric lymph nodes from each group of mice were measured via real-time quantitative PCR. The levels were normalized with *GAPDH* and presented in % of maximum. (**D**) Phosphorylated levels of ERK, p38 and JNK were detected via Western blot analysis on lysed lymph nodes. Phosphorylated levels were normalized with the intensity of total proteins and are presented in bar graphs. Data are presented as mean ± SD (n = 5/group) (*, $p < 0.05$). Water: mouse group fed with fresh water, DSS water: mouse group fed with water containing 2.5% DSS, DSS water + CTP10: mouse group fed with water containing 2.5% DSS and orally administered with 10 mg/kg citropten, DSS water + CTP40: mouse group fed with water containing 2.5% DSS and orally administered with 40 mg/kg citropten.

3. Discussion

In the current study, we found that citropten isolated from *Poncirus trifoliate* extract attenuates the manifestations of DSS-induced colitis in vivo. We showed that pre-treatment with citropten effectively modulates the activity of T cells and intestinal epithelial cells through the NFκB and MAPK signaling pathway in vitro without cytotoxicity. These findings suggest that citropten has promising potential as an ingredient in therapeutic drugs for inflammatory colitis.

Traditionally, citrus plants have been considered to have abundant flavonoids and coumarins which show beneficial bioactivities such as antioxidant and anti-inflammation [20]. *C. aurantifolia* has been widely used in edible fruits that have unique flavors, and it contains a lot of vitamin C [21]. In particular, even though several reports have determined that vitamin C itself exerts the therapeutic effect on colitis, the protective effect of citropten on inflammatory colitis still elusive [22,23]. Our findings have scientific significance considering the traditional use of *C. aurantifolia*, which we used to isolate citropten for this study.

Since effector cytokines from activated T cells including IL-2 have been determined to be involved in endocrine, paracrine or autocrine proliferation in soluble forms [24], the amount of released IL-2 after stimulation is important. Several studies in the literature have elucidated that produced cytokines undergo a secretion process that is tightly controlled by vesicle trafficking molecules including the VAMPs family or SNAP molecules [25,26]. To understand whether the inhibitory effect of citropten on T cell activation is associated with the vesicle trafficking of cytokine release, we detected the cytosolic IL-2 that is produced after TCR-mediated stimulation. Figure 3C reveals that the modulatory effect of citropten on T cell activity is through an intrinsic mechanism including the downregulation of signaling pathways. The result that shows the expression of CD69, which is the marker of T cell activity on the surface, also supports the concept that citropten may induce intrinsic suppression on T cell activation.

It has been shown that lymphocytes including T cells and B cells migrate into mesenteric lymph nodes to encounter antigens, be primed and proliferate during inflammatory colitis [27]. As the number of cells migrating into mesenteric lymph nodes during colitis increased, the enhanced size and weight of mesenteric lymph nodes were observed [28]. Lymphadenopathy has been defined as the swelling of localized lymph nodes during inflammatory responses including infections or allergic responses [29]. In the results obtained from the present animal experiment, changes in the length and weight of mesenteric lymph nodes were found; the oral administration of citropten significantly reduced the length and weight of mesenteric lymph nodes (Figure 8B). These results suggest that the oral administration of citropten ameliorates the manifestation of lymphadenopathy by the modulation of inflammatory responses during DSS-induced colitis.

The NFκB signaling pathway is one of the most critical transcription factors in T cell activation and differentiation. It has been elucidated to be involved in polarization into Th1 via the induction of the required cytokines, including IL-12 [30]. Several reports have revealed that NFκB plays a critical role in Th17 differentiation from naïve T cells by positively affecting the gene expression of RORγt, which is the master transcription factor of Th17 differentiation [31,32]. In the current study, we showed that pre-treatment with citropten controls T cell activation through the NFκB signaling pathway in vitro (Figure 5A). We also determined that the mRNA levels of IFNγ and IL-17 on mesenteric lymph nodes were regulated by the oral administration of citropten in a DSS-induced colitis model (Figure 8C). These findings suggest that the oral administration of citropten may have an influence on T cell differentiation into Th1 and Th17 effector T cells, which are the most important subunits in the pathogenesis of inflammatory colitis through the modulation of the NFκB signaling pathway.

It was shown that MAPK involves several inflammatory disorders, including colitis, after it was discovered more than 25 years ago [33]. Among MAPK, the ERK1/2 pathway, the most evaluated subunit in inflammatory responses, has been determined to play a critical role in the progression and development of IBD and the generation of pro-inflammatory cytokines such as IL-1 and IL-21 [34,35]. Results from inhibitor studies of p38 have shown that the phosphorylation of p38 is dramatically enhanced in IBD tissues [36,37]. In addition, several publications have demonstrated that an elevated phosphorylation level of JNK was detected in IBD patients, and results from an inhibitor assay of JNK have revealed that the expression of proinflammatory cytokines was significantly downregulated in an inhibitor-administrated group in an animal model [37–39]. In the present study, we found that the phosphorylation levels of ERK, p38 and JNK were remarkably reduced in the colon tissues of the DSS group with the oral administration of citropten (Figure 7F). These results are highly relevant to in vitro data showing the modulatory effect of citropten on epithelial intestinal cells' activation (Figure 5D).

ICAM1 and VCAM1 have been studied as adhesion molecules; their expressions are upregulated on intestinal epithelial cells in inflammatory colitis patients [40,41]. Since enhanced expressions of ICAM and VCAM1 play a critical role in the transmigration of leukocytes into the lesion of inflammatory colitis, several studies have shown their possibility as therapeutic targets of inflammatory colitis by blocking the activity of ICAM1 and VCAM1 [42,43]. These findings suggest that the transmigration of leukocytes and the interaction between inflammatory leukocytes and intestinal epithelial cells are pivotal for the development of inflammatory colitis. In the present study, we elucidated that pre-treatment with citropten mitigates the mRNA levels of ICAM1 and VCAM1 on activated intestinal epithelial cells via TNFα treatment (Figure 4B). In addition, we also revealed that the expression of IL-8 is downregulated by pre-treatment with citropten, which acts as a chemoattractant for leukocytes in colitis pathogenesis. The regulatory effects of citropten on the expression of ICAM1, VCAM1 and IL-8 can be applied to the development of new drugs for inflammatory colitis.

4. Materials and Methods

4.1. Cell Culture

Jurkat T cells (KCLB number: 40152) and HT-29 cells (KCLB number: 30038) were purchased from the Korean Cell Line Bank (Seoul, Korea), and Raji B (ATCC cat#. CCL-86) cells were obtained from ATCC (Manassas, VA, USA). Cells were cultured in RPMI (Jurkat cells and Raji cells) or DMEM (HT-29 cells) medium (Welgene, Gyeongsan, Korea) supplemented with penicillin G (100 units/mL), streptomycin (100 µg/mL), 10% fetal bovine serum (FBS) and L-glutamine (2 mM). Both cell lines were maintained within 10 passages and grown at 37 °C in a humidified incubator containing 5% CO_2 and 95% air.

4.2. Animals

Six- to eight-week-old C57BL/6J female mice were purchased from Samtako Bio (Osan, Korea) and housed under specific pathogen-free (SPF) conditions. All experiments were approved by the Animal Care and Use Committee of the College of Pharmacy, Keimyung University (approval number: KM2020-004).

4.3. Plant Material

C. aurantifolia was purchased at the Daegu Yangnyeong Herbal Medicine Market in 2020, and a plant voucher specimen (KMU-2020-04-08) was deposited at Keimyung University College of Pharmacy.

4.4. Isolation of Citropten from C. aurantifolia Peel Extract

The *C. aurantifolia* the peels were manually separated, the pulp was deseeded and the separated peel was dried. The dried *C. aurantifolia* peels (265.0 g) were extracted with 70% EtOH (1 L) at room temperature for 1 day, and extraction was performed at a temperature of 60 degrees for 2 h. The alcoholic extract was evaporated in vacuo to yield a residue (41.2 g) and was partitioned with *n*-hexane, EtOAc, and *n*-butanol successively. Among them, the n-hexane fraction (16.00 g, Fr.1) was partitioned with silica gel column chromatography with a gradient elution of hexane–EtOAc (0–100 hexane/EtOAc v/v%), affording 14 fractions (Fr. 1–1~14). A white precipitate of Fr. 1–8 (87.6 mg) in the separated fraction was recrystallized in chloroform to obtain compound **1** (11.6 mg). The ^1H and ^{13}C nuclear magnetic resonance and liquid chromatography–mass spectrometry analysis was performed on the isolated compound **1**, and compound **1** was identified as citropten by comparing the analysis results with the previously reported literature [44].

Compound **1** (citropten): ^1H NMR data (500 MHz, $CDCl_3$) δ: 8.00 (d, J = 9.7 Hz, 1H, H-4), 6.40 (d, J = 1.7, 1H, H-8), 6.67 (d, J = 2.3, 1H, H-8), 6.27 (d, J = 2.0 Hz, 1H, H-6), 6.20 (d, J = 9.0 Hz, 1H, H-6), 6.15 (d, J = 9.2 Hz, 1H, H-3), 3.89 (s, 3H, OCH_3), 3.73 (s, 3H, OCH_3). ^{13}C NMR data (500 MHz, $CDCl_3$) δ: 163.8 (C-7), 161.7 (C-2), 157.0 (C-5), 156.9 (C-8a), 138.9 (C-4), 110.0 (C-3), 104.1 (C-4a), 94.9 (C-6), 92.9 (C-8), 56.0 (OCH_3), 55.9 (OCH_3).

4.5. Condition of Liquid Chromatography–Mass Spectrometry Analysis

Analyses were performed using a reversed-phase high-performance liquid chromatography (HPLC) system (Agilent model 1260 series, Santa Clara, CA, USA) with a Capcell pak C18 column (5 µm × 4.6 mm × 250 mm; Shiseido, Japan) and Agilent 6120 (Santa Clara, CA, USA) in the single-quadrupole positive ion mode. Chromatography was performed at room temperature at a flow rate of 1 mL/min, and 10 µL was analyzed for 50 min. The mobile phase consisted of 0.1% formic acid in water (A) and 0.1% formic acid in acetonitrile (B) in a ratio specified by the following binary gradient with linear interpolation: 0 min 5% B, 40 min 80% B and 50 min 5% B.

4.6. Reagents and Antibodies

Stimulatory antibodies against human CD3 and CD28 for the stimulation of T cells were obtained from BioXcell (West Lebanon, NH, USA). Recombinant human TNFα was purchased from PeproTech EC Ltd. (London, UK). MTT powder (1-(4,5-dimethylthiazol-2-yl)-3,5-diphenylformazan), TRIZOL reagent and radioimmunoprecipitation assay (RIPA) buffer for Western blot analysis, phorbol 12-myristate 13-acetate (PMA) and A23187 were provided by Sigma Chemical Co. (St. Louis, MO, USA). *Staphylococcus aureus* enterotoxin E (SEE) was obtained from Toxin Technology (Sarasota, FL, USA). ECL Western blotting detection reagents and an apoptosis AnnexinV/PI assay kit was purchased from Thermo Fisher Scientific (Waltham, MA, USA). SYBR Premix Ex Taq was provided by TaKaRa (Shiga, Japan). Anti-IL-2 antibodies, anti-β-actin and anti-ERK antibodies were obtained from Santa Cruz Biotechnology (Dallas, TX, USA). Antibodies against p65, LaminB, IκBα, phosphorylated IκBα, phosphorylated ERK, phosphorylated p38, p38, phosphorylated JNK and JNK were purchased from Cell Signaling Technology (Danvers, MA, USA). Anti-CD69 conjugated with APC were provided by eBiosciences. The RT PreMix kit was obtained from Enzynomics (Daejeon, Korea). DSS (molecular weight: 36,000–50,000 Da) was purchased from MP Biomedicals (Irvine, CA, USA).

4.7. Cell Confluency Check by IncuCyte Imaging System

Jurkat cells (1×10^4/well) and HT-29 cells (1×10^4/well) were treated with the indicated concentrations (0 to 40 μM) of citropten for 24 h; then, the cells were automatically marked in orange using the IncuCyte imaging system.

4.8. Cell Viability Check by MTT Assay

Cell viability was determined by performing an MTT assay. Jurkat cells (1×10^4/well) and HT-29 cells (1×10^4/well) were treated with the indicated concentrations (0 to 40 μM) of citropten for 24 h; then, MTT (500 μg/mL) was added for 2 h. After incubation, the supernatants were discarded, and formazan crystals at the bottom were dissolved with 200 μL of dimethyl sulfoxide (DMSO). To obtain the OD value, the plate was read at 540 nm. Cell viability was calculated using the obtained OD value and presented in % of control (0 μM).

4.9. AnnexinV/PI Apoptosis Assay

For the determination of apoptosis after treatment with citropten, an AnnexinV/PI apoptosis kit was used. Jurkat cells (5×10^5/well) and HT-29 cells (5×10^5/well) were treated with the indicated concentrations (0 to 40 μM) of citropten for 24 h and then stained with AnnexinV and PI following the manufacturer's instructions. Cells were acquired through flow cytometry, and all single cells were gated by using BD software. AnnexinV and PI double-positive cells were obtained from double plots.

4.10. T Cell Stimulation

For T cell stimulation, three methods were used in the present study. For TCR-mediated stimulation, Jurkat T cells were replaced on the plate coated with anti-CD3 antibodies (20 μg/mL) and anti-CD28 soluble antibodies (7 μg/mL). For PMA/A23187 stimulation, Jurkat T cells were treated with 100 nM PMA and 1 μM A23187. Jurkat T cells were also stimulated by co-culturing them with same number of Raji B cells that were previously pulsed with SEE superantigen (1 μg/mL) for 1 h.

4.11. Determination of mRNA Levels by Real-Time Quantitative PCR

For the determination of mRNA levels via real-time quantitative PCR, harvested cells or colon tissues were lysed in TRIZOL reagents for total RNA isolation. The reverse transcription of the RNA was performed using an RT PreMix kit (Enzynomics, Daejeon, Korea). In addition, RNA was obtained after the colon tissue was washed with PBS 3 times to remove DSS. The primers used in the present study were as follows (forward and reverse primers): human *IL-2*, 5′-CAC GTC TTG CAC TTG TCA C-3′ and 5′-CCT TCT TGG GCA TGT AAA ACT-3′; human *TNFα*, 5′-CCT ACC AGA CCA AGG TCA AC-3′ and 5′-AGG GGG TAA TAA AGG GAT TG-3′; human *IL-1β*, 5′-GGA TAT GGA GCA ACA AGT GG-3′ and 5′-ATG TAC CAG TTG GGG AAC TG-3′; human *IL-8*, 5′-GTG CAG TTT TGC CAA GGA GT-3′ and 5′-TTA TGA ATT CTC AGC CCT CTT CAA AAA-3′; human *ICAM1*, 5′-AGC GGC TGA CGT GTG CAG TAA T-3′ and 5′-TCT GAG ACC TCT GGC TTC GTC A-3′; human *VCAM1*, 5′-GAT TCT GTG CCC ACA GTA AGG C-3′ and 5′-TGG TCA CAG AGC CAC CTT CTT G-3′; human *GAPDH*, 5′-CGG AGT CAA CGG ATT TGG TCG TAT-3′ and 5′-AGC CTT CTC CAT GGT GGT GAA GAC-3′; mouse *TNFα*, 5′-GGC AGG TCT ACT TTG GAG TCA TTG C-3′ and 5′-ACA TTC GAG GCT CCA GTG AAT TCG G-3′; mouse *IL-1β*, 5′-ATA ACC TGC TGG TGT GTG AC-3′ and 5′-AGG TGC TGA TGT ACC AGT TG-3′; mouse *IL-8*, 5′-ATG CTG CTG CAA GGC TGG TC-3′ and 5′-AGG CTT TTC ATG CTC AAC ACT AT-3′; mouse *Il-2*, 5′-TGA GCA GGA TGG AGA ATT ACA GG-3′ and 5′- GTC CAA GTT CAT CTT CTA GGC AC-3′; mouse *Ifng*, 5′-TCA AGT GGC ATA GAT GTG GAA GAA-3′ and 5′-TGG CTC TGC AGG ATT TTC ATG-3′; mouse *Il17*, 5′-TCC CCT CTG TCA TCT GGG AAG-3′ and 5′-CTC GAC CCT GAA AGT GAA GG-3′; mouse *GAPDH*, 5′–GCA CAG TCA AGG CCG AGA AT–3′ and 5′–GCC TTC TCC ATG GTG GTG AA–3′. PCR amplification was performed in a DNA Engine Opticon 1 continuous fluorescence detection system (MJ Research, Waltham, MA, USA) using SYBR Premix Ex Taq. It contained 1 μL of cDNA/control and gene-specific primers. Each PCR reaction was performed using the following conditions: 95 °C 30 s, 60 °C 30 s, 72 °C 30 s and plate read (detection of fluorescent product) for 40 cycles followed by 7 min of extension at 72 °C. Melting curve analysis was performed to characterize the dsDNA product by slowly raising the temperature (0.1 °C/s) from 60 °C to 95 °C with fluorescence data collected at 0.2 °C intervals. The mRNA levels of the genes were normalized to *GAPDH*. The gene expression was calculated using the following equation: Gene expression = $2^{-\Delta\Delta CT}$, where $\Delta\Delta CT$ = (CT Target−CT *GAPDH*).

4.12. ELISA

For the detection of released IL-2 from activated Jurkat cells, ELISA was used following the manufacturer's instructions (DuoSet® ELISA kit, R&D Systems, Minneapolis, MN, USA).

4.13. Western Blot Analysis

For the detection of protein levels, Western blot analysis was performed. Harvested cells or colon tissues were lysed in RIPA buffer for 30 min on ice and centrifuged at 14,000 rpm for 20 min at 4 °C. For the separation of the nuclear extract, lysis was performed using NE-PER Nuclear and Cytoplasmic Extraction Reagents (Thermo fisher scientific, Waltham, MA, USA). Approximately 30 to 40 μg of the lysate was loaded for separation on 8–12% SDS–PAGE gels. Proteins were transferred onto PVDF membranes (Bio-Rad, Hercules, CA, USA), and membranes were blocked in 5% skim milk (1 h). After being rinsed, membranes were incubated with the indicated primary antibodies in TBS containing 0.1% Tween 20 (TBS-T) and 3% skim milk overnight. Excess primary antibodies were discarded by washing the membrane three times with TBS-T. The membranes were then incubated with 0.1 μg/mL peroxidase-labeled secondary antibodies (against rabbit or mouse) for 2 h. After three washes in TBS-T, bands were visualized with ECL Western blotting detection reagents (Thermo Fisher Scientific, Waltham, MA, USA) with an ImageQuant LAS 4000 (GE healthcare, Chicago, IL, USA). All detected bands were normalized with the intensity of the loading control proteins, and the ratio was calculated between experimental proteins and loading control proteins to be considered as 1 X. All normalized ratios were presented as fold changes compared to the 'control' group.

4.14. Determination of CD69 Expression by Flow Cytometry

For the detection of CD69 in activated Jurkat T cells, fluorescence was used after staining with flow cytometry. After stimulation, Jurkat T cells were stained with anti-CD69 antibodies conjugated with APC and acquired via flow cytometry. All live single cells were gated, and the mean fluorescence intensity was obtained by using BD flow cytometry software. Each mean fluorescence intensity is presented in a bar graph.

4.15. Induction of Colitis by Using DSS

The inflammatory colitis model was induced by feeding mice water containing DSS. Twenty mice were grouped into four groups, as follows: mice fed fresh water (water), mice fed water containing 2.5% DSS for seven days (DSS water), mice fed water containing 2.5% DSS and received oral administration of 10 mg/kg citropten every day for seven days (DSS water + CTP10) and mice fed water containing 2.5% DSS and received oral administration of 40 mg/kg citropten every day for seven days (DSS water + CTP40). Changes in body weight were examined for seven days.

4.16. Determination of Stool Scoring

Changes in the shape of stool were checked daily to examine the progress of inflammatory colitis as follows: 0 (normal), 2 (loose stool) and 4 (diarrhea).

4.17. Determination of Disease Activity Index

The disease activity index was monitored to evaluate the progression of inflammatory colitis according to the published criteria, and it involves the relative loss of body weight, shape of stool and bleeding on the stool and anus area. The scoring criteria were as follows: weight loss: 0 (no loss), 1 (1–5%), 2 (5–10%), 3 (10–20%) and 4 (more than 20%); stool form: 0 (normal), 2 (loose stool) and 4 (diarrhea); and bleeding: 0 (no blood), 1 (Hemoccult positive), 2 (Hemoccult positive and visual pellet bleeding) and 4 (bleeding around the anus).

4.18. H&E Staining and Determination of Histological Score

At day 7 post-induction of colitis, colon tissues were removed and prepared for histological analysis. The collected colons (0.5 cm) were fixed in 10% paraformaldehyde and embedded using paraffin. Embedded tissues were cut (5-μm-thick axial sections) and put on slide glass to be deparaffinized. Deparaffinized tissues were stained with H&E for histological analysis. The histological scores were evaluated according to previously reported methods [45].

4.19. Statistics

The mean values ± SD were calculated from the data collected from three independent experiments performed on separate days and are presented in bar graphs. For mice experiments, the mean values ± SD were calculated from the data obtained from five mice experiments and are presented in bar or dot graphs. One-way ANOVA was used to determine significance (p value), and Tukey's post hoc test was used after one-way ANOVA. * indicates differences between the two indicated groups considered significant at $p < 0.05$.

Author Contributions: Conceptualization, H.-S.L.; methodology, H.-S.L.; formal analysis, E.-N.K.; writing—original draft preparation, H.-S.L.; supervision, G.-S.J.; project administration, G.-S.J. All authors have read and agreed to the published version of the manuscript.

Funding: This work was supported by the National Research Foundation grants (2021R1I1A3051395).

Institutional Review Board Statement: Not applicable.

Informed Consent Statement: Not applicable.

Data Availability Statement: Not applicable.

Conflicts of Interest: The authors declare no conflict of interest.

References

1. Wedro, B. Colitis: Symptoms, Causes, Diet, and Treatment. MedicineNet 2021. Available online: https://www.medicinenet.com/colitis/article.htm (accessed on 23 March 2022).
2. Ordás, I.; Eckmann, L.; Talamini, M.; Baumgart, D.C.; Sandborn, W.J. Ulcerative colitis. *Lancet* 2012, *380*, 1606–1619. [CrossRef]
3. Fiocchi, C. Inflammatory bowel disease: Etiology and pathogenesis. *Gastroenterology* 1998, *115*, 182–205. [CrossRef]
4. Ko, J.; Auyeung, K. Inflammatory Bowel Disease: Etiology, Pathogenesis and Current Therapy. *Curr. Pharm. Des.* 2014, *20*, 1082–1096. [CrossRef] [PubMed]
5. Neurath, M.F.; Finotto, S.; Fuss, I.; Boirivant, M.; Galle, P.R.; Strober, W. Regulation of T-cell apoptosis in inflammatory bowel disease: To die or not to die, that is the mucosal question. *Trends Immunol.* 2001, *22*, 21–26. [CrossRef]
6. Coskun, M. Intestinal epithelium in inflammatory bowel disease. *Front. Med.* 2014, *1*, 24. [CrossRef]
7. Weiss, A. TCR Signal Transduction: Opening the Black Box. *J. Immunol.* 2009, *183*, 4821–4827. [CrossRef]
8. Shapiro, V.S.; Truitt, K.E.; Imboden, J.B.; Weiss, A. CD28 mediates transcriptional upregulation of the interleukin-2 (IL-2) promoter through a composite element containing the CD28RE and NF-IL-2B AP-1 sites. *Mol. Cell. Biol.* 1997, *17*, 4051–4058. [CrossRef]
9. Cheng, J.; Montecalvo, A.; Kane, L.P. Regulation of NF-κB induction by TCR/CD28. *Immunol. Res.* 2011, *50*, 113–117. [CrossRef]
10. Bonizzi, G.; Karin, M. The two NF-κB activation pathways and their role in innate and adaptive immunity. *Trends Immunol.* 2004, *25*, 280–288. [CrossRef]
11. Hayden, M.S.; Ghosh, S. Signaling to NF-κB. *Genes Dev.* 2004, *18*, 2195–2224. [CrossRef]
12. Hayes, J.D.; Pulford, D.J.; Ellis, E.M.; McLeod, R.; James, R.F.L.; Seidegård, J.; Mosialou, E.; Jernström, B.; Neal, G.E. Regulation of rat glutathione S-transferase A5 by cancer chemopreventive agents: Mechanisms of inducible resistance to aflatoxin B1. *Chem. Biol. Interact.* 1998, *111*, 51–67. [CrossRef]
13. Sharma, S.; Stutzman, J.D.; Kelloff, G.J.; Steele, V.E. Screening of Potential Chemopreventive Agents Using Biochemical Markers of Carcinogenesis. *Cancer Res.* 1994, *54*, 5848–5855. [PubMed]
14. Borgatti, M.; Mancini, I.; Bianchi, N.; Guerrini, A.; Lampronti, I.; Rossi, D.; Sacchetti, G.; Gambari, R. Bergamot (*Citrus bergamia* Risso) fruit extracts and identified components alter expression of interleukin 8 gene in cystic fibrosis bronchial epithelial cell lines. *BMC Biochem.* 2011, *12*, 15. [CrossRef] [PubMed]
15. Canini, A.; Alesiani, D.; D'Arcangelo, G.; Tagliatesta, P. Gas chromatography-mass spectrometry analysis of phenolic compounds from *Carica papaya* L. leaf. *J. Food Compos. Anal.* 2007, *20*, 584–590. [CrossRef]
16. Salvatore, A.; Borkosky, S.; Willink, E.; Bardón, A. Toxic effects of lemon peel constituents on Ceratitis capitata. *J. Chem. Ecol.* 2004, *30*, 323–333. [CrossRef]
17. Alesiani, D.; Cicconi, R.; Mattei, M.; Montesano, C.; Bei, R.; Canini, A. Cell cycle arrest and differentiation induction by 5,7-dimethoxycoumarin in melanoma cell lines. *Int. J. Oncol.* 2008, *32*, 425–434. [CrossRef]
18. Fang, J.Y.; Richardson, B.C. The MAPK signalling pathways and colorectal cancer. *Lancet Oncol.* 2005, *6*, 322–327. [CrossRef]
19. Yang, W.; Wang, H. 5,7-Dimethoxycoumarin prevents chronic mild stress induced depression in rats through increase in the expression of heat shock protein-70 and inhibition of monoamine oxidase-A levels. *Saudi J. Biol. Sci.* 2018, *25*, 253–258. [CrossRef]
20. Musumeci, L.; Maugeri, A.; Cirmi, S.; Lombardo, G.E.; Russo, C.; Gangemi, S.; Calapai, G.; Navarra, M. Citrus fruits and their flavonoids in inflammatory bowel disease: An overview. *Nat. Prod. Res.* 2020, *34*, 122–136. [CrossRef]
21. Patil, J.R.; Jayaprakasha, G.K.; Chidambara Murthy, K.N.; Chetti, M.B.; Patil, B.S. Characterization of Citrus aurantifolia bioactive compounds and their inhibition of human pancreatic cancer cells through apoptosis. *Microchem. J.* 2009, *94*, 108–117. [CrossRef]
22. Dunleavy, K.A.; Ungaro, R.C.; Manning, L.; Gold, S.; Novak, J.; Colombel, J.F. Vitamin C Deficiency: The Forgotten Micronutrient. *Crohn's Colitis 360* 2021, *3*, 1.
23. Kondo, K.; Hiramoto, K.; Yamate, Y.; Goto, K.; Sekijima, H.; Ooi, K. Ameliorative Effect of High-Dose Vitamin C Administration on Dextran Sulfate Sodium-Induced Colitis Mouse Model. *Biol. Pharm. Bull.* 2019, *42*, 954–959. [CrossRef] [PubMed]
24. Toribio, M.L.; Gutiérrez-Ramos, J.C.; Pezzi, L.; Marcos, M.A.R.; Martínez-A, C. Interleukin-2-dependent autocrine proliferation in T-cell development. *Nature* 1989, *342*, 82–85. [CrossRef] [PubMed]
25. Lacy, P.; Stow, J.L. Cytokine release from innate immune cells: Association with diverse membrane trafficking pathways. *Blood* 2011, *118*, 9–18. [CrossRef] [PubMed]
26. Stanley, A.C.; Lacy, P. Pathways for cytokine secretion. *Physiology* 2010, *25*, 218–229. [CrossRef] [PubMed]
27. Marsal, J.; Agace, W.W. Targeting T-cell migration in inflammatory bowel disease. *J. Intern. Med.* 2012, *272*, 411–429. [CrossRef] [PubMed]
28. Stephens, M.; Liao, S.; Von Der Weid, P.Y. Mesenteric lymphatic alterations observed during DSS induced intestinal inflammation are driven in a TLR4-PAMP/DAMP discriminative manner. *Front. Immunol.* 2019, *10*, 557. [CrossRef] [PubMed]
29. Heitman, B.; Irizarry, A. Infectious disease causes of lymphadenopathy: Localized versus diffuse. *Lippincott's Prim. Care Pract.* 1999, *3*, 19–38.
30. Oh, H.; Ghosh, S. NF-κB: Roles and regulation in different CD4+ T-cell subsets. *Immunol. Rev.* 2013, *252*, 41–51. [CrossRef]
31. Park, S.-H.; Cho, G.; Park, S.-G. NF-κB Activation in T Helper 17 Cell Differentiation. *Immune Netw.* 2014, *14*, 14. [CrossRef]

32. Ruan, Q.; Kameswaran, V.; Zhang, Y.; Zheng, S.; Sun, J.; Wang, J.; DeVirgiliis, J.; Liou, H.C.; Beg, A.A.; Chen, Y.H. The Th17 immune response is controlled by the Rel-RORγ-RORγT transcriptional axis. *J. Exp. Med.* **2011**, *208*, 2321–2333. [CrossRef] [PubMed]
33. Broom, O.J.; Widjaya, B.; Troelsen, J.; Olsen, J.; Nielsen, O.H. Mitogen Activated Protein Kinases: A Role in Inflammatory Bowel Disease? *Clin. Exp. Immunol.* **2009**, *158*, 272–280. [CrossRef] [PubMed]
34. Kwon, K.H.; Ohigashi, H.; Murakami, A. Dextran Sulfate Sodium Enhances Interleukin-1β Release via Activation of P38 MAPK and ERK1/2 Pathways in Murine Peritoneal Macrophages. *Life Sci.* **2007**, *81*, 362–371. [CrossRef] [PubMed]
35. Caruso, R.; Fina, D.; Peluso, I.; Stolfi, C.; Fantini, M.C.; Gioia, V.; Caprioli, F.; del Vecchio Blanco, G.; Paoluzi, O.A.; MacDonald, T.T.; et al. A Functional Role for Interleukin-21 in Promoting the Synthesis of the T-Cell Chemoattractant, MIP-3alpha, by Gut Epithelial Cells. *Gastroenterology* **2007**, *132*, 166–175. [CrossRef] [PubMed]
36. Waetzig, G.H.; Seegert, D.; Rosenstiel, P.; Nikolaus, S.; Schreiber, S. P38 Mitogen-Activated Protein Kinase Is Activated and Linked to TNF-α Signaling in Inflammatory Bowel Disease. *J. Immunol.* **2002**, *168*, 5342–5351. [CrossRef] [PubMed]
37. Dahan, S.; Roda, G.; Pinn, D.; Roth-Walter, F.; Kamalu, O.; Martin, A.P.; Mayer, L. Epithelial: Lamina Propria Lymphocyte Interactions Promote Epithelial Cell Differentiation. *Gastroenterology* **2008**, *134*, 192. [CrossRef]
38. Assi, K.; Pillai, R.; Gómez-Muñoz, A.; Owen, D.; Salh, B. The Specific JNK Inhibitor SP600125 Targets Tumour Necrosis Factor-Alpha Production and Epithelial Cell Apoptosis in Acute Murine Colitis. *Immunology* **2006**, *118*, 112–121. [CrossRef]
39. Mitsuyama, K.; Suzuki, A.; Tomiyasu, N.; Tsuruta, O.; Kitazaki, S.; Takeda, T.; Satoh, Y.; Bennett, B.L.; Toyonaga, A.; Sata, M. Pro-Inflammatory Signaling by Jun-N-Terminal Kinase in Inflammatory Bowel Disease. *Int. J. Mol. Med.* **2006**, *17*, 449–455. [CrossRef]
40. Reinisch, W.; Hung, K.; Hassan-Zahraee, M.; Cataldi, F. Targeting endothelial ligands: ICAM-1/alicaforsen, MAdCAM-1. *J. Crohn's Colitis* **2018**, *12*, S669–S677. [CrossRef]
41. Soriano, A.; Salas, A.; Sans, M.; Gironella, M.; Elena, M.; Anderson, D.C.; Piqué, J.M.; Panés, J. VCAM-1, but not ICAM-1 or MAdCAM-1, immunoblockade ameliorates DSS-induced colitis in mice. *Lab. Investig.* **2000**, *80*, 1541–1551. [CrossRef]
42. Burns, R.C.; Rivera-Nieves, J.; Moskaluk, C.A.; Matsumoto, S.; Cominelli, F.; Ley, K. Antibody blockade of ICAM-1 and VCAM-1 ameliorates inflammation in the SAMP-1/Yit adoptive transfer model of Crohn's disease in mice. *Gastroenterology* **2001**, *121*, 1428–1436. [CrossRef]
43. Villablanca, E.J.; Cassani, B.; Von Andrian, U.H.; Mora, J.R. Blocking lymphocyte localization to the gastrointestinal mucosa as a therapeutic strategy for inflammatory bowel diseases. *Gastroenterology* **2011**, *140*, 1776–1784. [CrossRef] [PubMed]
44. Henrique, D.M.; Ana, C.P.; Guilherme, T.P.B.; Helton, C.L.; Nelson, S.M.J.; Luciano, B.; Mark, W.; Jairo, K.B.; Gilberto, U.L.B. Furocoumarins and coumarins photoinactivate *Colletotrichum acutatum* and *Aspergillus* nidulans fungi under solar radiation. *J. Photochem. Photobiol. B* **2014**, *131*, 74–83.
45. Koelink, P.J.; Wildenberg, M.E.; Stitt, L.W.; Feagan, B.G.; Koldijk, M.; van't Wout, A.B.; Atreya, R.; Vieth, M.; Brandse, J.F.; Duijst, S.; et al. Development of reliable, valid and responsive scoring systems for endoscopy and histology in animal models for inflammatory bowel disease. *J. Crohn's Colitis* **2018**, *12*, 794–803. [CrossRef] [PubMed]

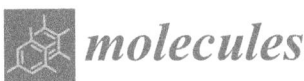

Article

Protective Effects of Baicalin on Peritoneal Tight Junctions in Piglets Challenged with *Glaesserella parasuis*

Jiacheng Zhang [1,†], Zhaoran Zhang [1,†], Jianfeng Xu [1], Chun Ye [1], Shulin Fu [1], Chien-An Andy Hu [2], Yinsheng Qiu [1,*] and Yu Liu [1,*]

[1] Hubei Key Laboratory of Animal Nutrition and Feed Science, School of Animal Science and Nutritional Engineering, Wuhan Polytechnic University, Wuhan 430023, China; zhangjiacheng0826@163.com (J.Z.); 15893715001@163.com (Z.Z.); xujianfeng2017@163.com (J.X.); yechun@whpu.edu.cn (C.Y.); shulinfu@whpu.edu.cn (S.F.)
[2] Biochemistry and Molecular Biology, University of New Mexico School of Medicine, Albuquerque, NM 87131, USA; AHU@salud.unm.edu
* Correspondence: Qiuyinsheng6405@whpu.edu.cn (Y.Q.); lyywfy@whpu.edu.cn (Y.L.); Tel./Fax: +86-27-83956175 (Y.Q. &Y.L.)
† These authors contributed equally to this work.

Citation: Zhang, J.; Zhang, Z.; Xu, J.; Ye, C.; Fu, S.; Hu, C.-A.A.; Qiu, Y.; Liu, Y. Protective Effects of Baicalin on Peritoneal Tight Junctions in Piglets Challenged with *Glaesserella parasuis*. *Molecules* 2021, 26, 1268. https://doi.org/10.3390/molecules26051268

Academic Editor: Francesco Maione

Received: 31 January 2021
Accepted: 18 February 2021
Published: 26 February 2021

Publisher's Note: MDPI stays neutral with regard to jurisdictional claims in published maps and institutional affiliations.

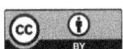

Copyright: © 2021 by the authors. Licensee MDPI, Basel, Switzerland. This article is an open access article distributed under the terms and conditions of the Creative Commons Attribution (CC BY) license (https://creativecommons.org/licenses/by/4.0/).

Abstract: *Glaesserella parasuis* (*G. parasuis*) causes inflammation and damage to piglets. Whether polyserositis caused by *G. parasuis* is due to tight junctions damage and the protective effect of baicalin on it have not been examined. Therefore, this study aims to investigate the effects of baicalin on peritoneal tight junctions of piglets challenged with *G. parasuis* and its underlying molecular mechanisms. Piglets were challenged with *G. parasuis* and treated with or without baicalin. RT-PCR was performed to examine the expression of peritoneal tight junctions genes. Immunofluorescence was carried out to detect the distribution patterns of tight junctions proteins. Western blot assays were carried out to determine the involved signaling pathways. Our data showed that *G. parasuis* infection can down-regulate the tight junctions expression and disrupt the distribution of tight junctions proteins. Baicalin can alleviate the down-regulation of tight junctions mRNA in peritoneum, prevent the abnormalities and maintain the continuous organization of tight junctions. Our results provide novel evidence to support that baicalin has the capacity to protect peritoneal tight junctions from *G. parasuis*-induced inflammation. The protective mechanisms of baicalin could be associated with inhibition of the activation of PKC and MLCK/MLC signaling pathway. Taken together, these data demonstrated that baicalin is a promising natural agent for the prevention and treatment of *G. parasuis* infection.

Keywords: baicalin; *Glaesserella parasuis*; tight junctions; peritoneum; piglets

1. Introduction

Glaesserella parasuis (*G. parasuis*), previously named *Haemophilus parasuis*, is a Gram-negative bacterium and one of the most important bacteria affecting pigs as an early commensal colonizer in the upper respiratory tract of weaning pigs [1]. The disease caused by this pathogen is characterized by polyserositis and it is known as Glässer's disease [2]. It can result in high mortality and morbidity, with significant economic losses for pig producers [3]. Because of the incomplete efficacy of current vaccines, antimicrobials are commonly used to treat *G. parasuis* infections [4]. However, the phenomenon of bacterial resistance has become more and more serious. Therefore, exploring the pathogenesis and finding alternative feasible ways of preventing and controlling *G. parasuis* infections has become very urgent.

Peritonitis, a common clinical symptom of *G. parasuis* infections, might stem from damage to peritoneal tight junctions [5]. The peritoneum is a membranous tissue mainly composed of mesothelial cells, which has a coating effect on most organs in the abdominal cavity, and can secrete mucus to alleviate the friction between organs [6]. The molecular correlation between the paracellular channel and this barrier function have been discovered, namely tight junctions, which show a tissue-specific expression of tight junction proteins determining the functional properties of the tissues [7]. Tight junctions are complex structure of different proteins, including integral membrane proteins (claudins, occludin, junctional adhesion molecules "JAMs") and peripheral membrane proteins (zonula occludins or ZOs, such as ZO-1, ZO-2, and ZO-3) [8]. The stability of its function requires the coordination of multiple proteins [9]. An indispensable role of tight junctions involved in pathogen infection has been widely demonstrated since disruption of tight junctions leads to a distinct increase in paracellular permeability and polarity defects which facilitate viral or bacterial entry and spread [10]. Changes in the peritoneal mesothelial cell phenotype, including loss of tight junctions, may allow ectopic cells to bind to, or early lesions invade into, the extracellular matrix. Signaling pathways involved in the assembly, disassembly, and maintenance of tight junctions are controlled by a number of signaling molecules, such as protein kinase C (PKC), mitogen-activated protein kinases (MAPK), myosin light chain kinase (MLCK), and myosion light chain 2 (MLC-2) [11–14].

Many natural compounds such as flavonoids have been demonstrated to exhibit a broad spectrum of biological activities such as anti–inflammatory properties [15,16]. The available reports reveal that flavonoids such as baicalin, naringin, and hesperidin (Figure 1), have promotive and protective effects on tight junctions barrier functions [17–20]. Baicalin (7-glucuronic acid-5,6-dihydroxy-flavone), is one of the primary bioactive flavonoid compounds extracted from the roots of *Scutellaria baicalensis* Georgi. Baicalin is used clinically in humans and animals because of its antimicrobial, anti-inflammatory, antitumor and antioxidant properties [21–24]. Our previously work demonstrated that baicalin has anti–inflammatory effects in *G. parasuis*-challenged piglets in vivo and in vitro by suppressing inflammatory cytokines and HMGB1 via NF-κB and NLRP3 signaling and reversing apoptosis by altering PKC–MAPK signaling cells [25–28]. Baicalin is prominent in the literature on protection of tight junction in epithelial and endothelial cells [17,29,30], although high doses of baicalin can reduce tight junction integrity by partly targeting the first PDZ domain of ZO-1 [31]. However, whether an appropriate dose of baicalin can protect tight junctions to inhibit inflammation in piglets against *G. parasuis* challenge has not been investigated.

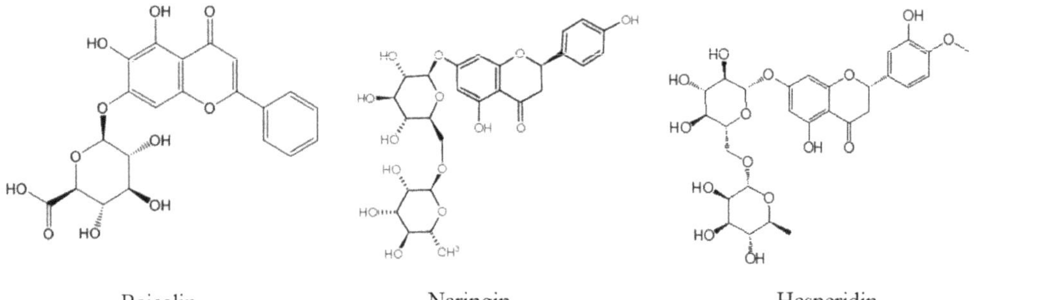

Baicalin　　　　　　　　　　Naringin　　　　　　　　　　Hesperidin

Figure 1. Chemical structures of flavonoids, baicalin, naringin, and hesperidin.

In this study, we attempted to investigate the protection effects of baicalin on tight junctions in the peritoneum of piglets challenged with *G. parasuis* and its underlying molecular mechanisms.

2. Results

2.1. Effects of Baicalin on the Expression of Tight Junctions Genes in Peritoneum of G. parasuis Challenged Piglets

Figure 2 shows the regulation of tight junction genes in peritoneum in all groups. Challenged with *G. parasuis* resulted in a significant decrease in the mRNA expressions of occludin, ZO-1, claudin-1, and JAM-1, compared with control group ($p < 0.01$). Ethyl pyruvate (EP) and flunixin meglumine (FM) were used as positive controls in the experiments. EP and FM could significantly up-regulate the gene expressions of ZO-1 and JAM-1 in piglets' peritoneum ($p < 0.01$). FM could significantly up-regulate the gene expression of occludin in peritoneum ($p < 0.01$). EP could significantly up-regulate the gene expression of blaudin-1 ($p < 0.01$). Baicalin at 25, 50 and 100 mg/kg could significantly restore the expressions of occludin and ZO-1 in the peritoneum of piglets infected with G. parasuis ($p < 0.01, p < 0.05$). Baicalin at 50 mg/kg could significantly up-regulate the gene expression of claudin-1 ($p < 0.01$). Baicalin at 100 mg/kg could significantly up-regulate the gene expression of JAM-1 ($p < 0.05$).

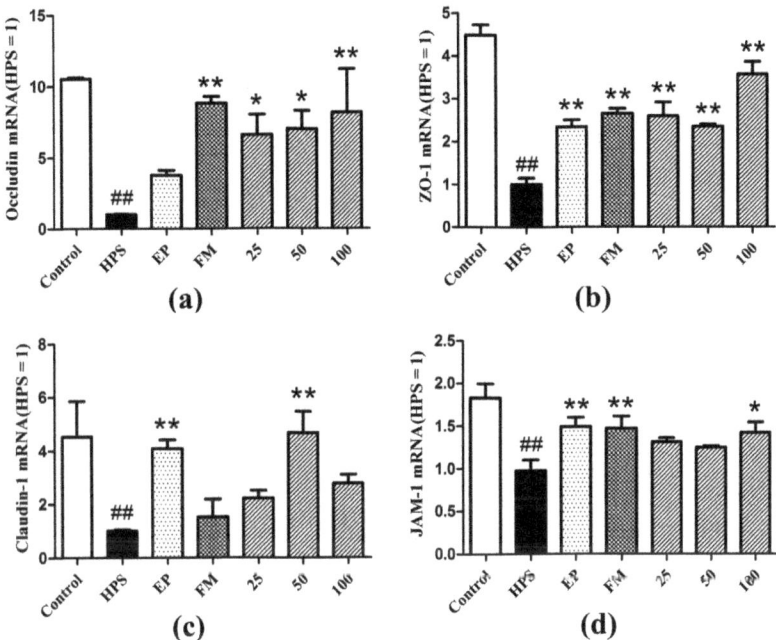

Figure 2. Expressions of tight junctions genes (**a**) Occludin, (**b**) ZO-1, (**c**) Claudin-1, (**d**) JAM-1 in the peritoneum of piglets challenged with G. parasuis (Mean ± SD, $n = 3$). HPS: G. parasuis group, EP:EP + G. parasuis group, FM:FM + G. parasuis group, 25:25 mg/kg baicalin + G. parasuis group, 50:50 mg/kg baicalin + G. parasuis group, 100:100 mg/kg baicalin + G. parasuis group. ## $p < 0.01$ vs control. * $p < 0.05$ vs G. parasuis group, and ** $p < 0.01$ vs G. parasuis group.

2.2. Effect of Baicalin on the Distibution Patterns of Tight Junctions in Peritoneum of G. parasuis Challenged Piglets

In addition to appropriate expression, proper organization and distribution of the tight junction proteins is critical for the maintenance of a permeability barrier. The G. parasuis mediated disruption of the distribution results of tight junctions proteins in peritoneum and the effect of each drug are shown in Figures 3–6. As expected, G. parasuis infection alters the distribution of occludin, ZO-1, claudin-1 and JAM-1 in the peritoneum. We observed that occludin, ZO-1, claudin-1 and JAM-1 protein staining appeared to be reduced and more fragmented in the G. parasuis group. Administration with EP or FM could significantly prevent these abnormalities and maintain the continuous organization of tight junctions ($p < 0.01$). Treatment with 25, 50 and 100 mg/kg baicalin could significantly attenuate this disorganization ($p < 0.01$). Among all drug treatment groups, 50 mg/kg baicalin was demonstrated the best protection effect on the disruption of the distribution of tight junction proteins. These findings identify a *G. parasuis*-induced global impairment of tight junction integrity, a process largely prevented by baicalin supplementation.

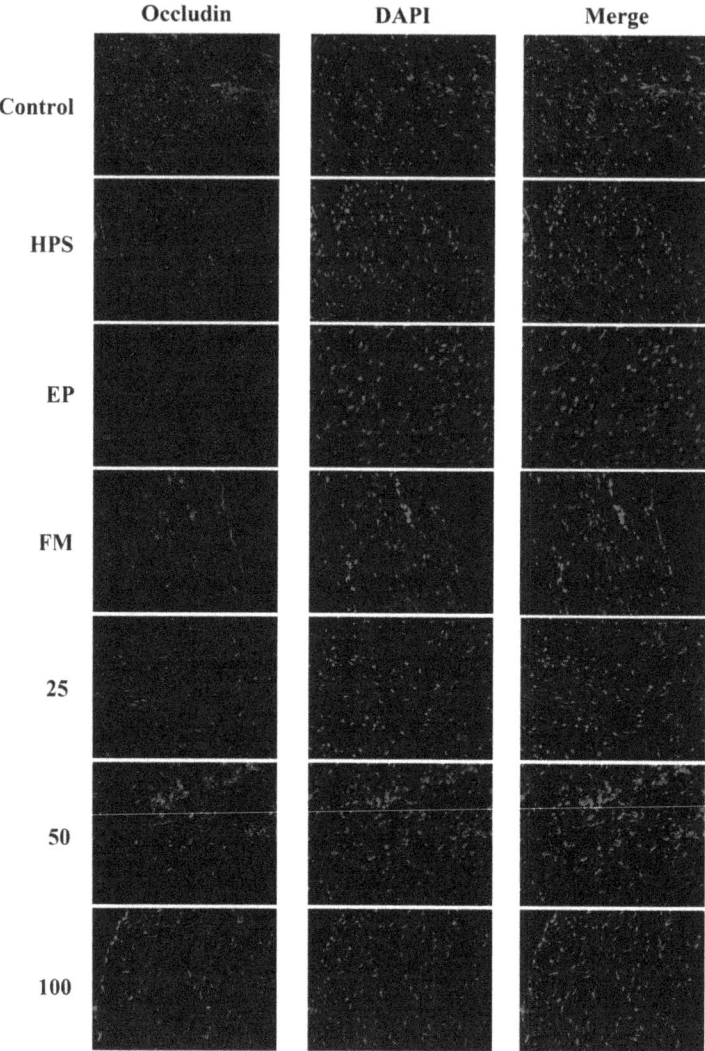

Figure 3. Effect of baicalin on the distribution patterns of Occludin in the peritoneum of piglets challenged with *G. parasuis* (magnification 10×40). HPS: *G. parasuis* group, EP:EP + *G. parasuis* group, FM:FM + *G. parasuis* group, 25:25 mg/kg baicalin + *G. parasuis* group, 50:50 mg/kg baicalin + *G. parasuis* group, 100:100 mg/kg baicalin + *G. parasuis* group.

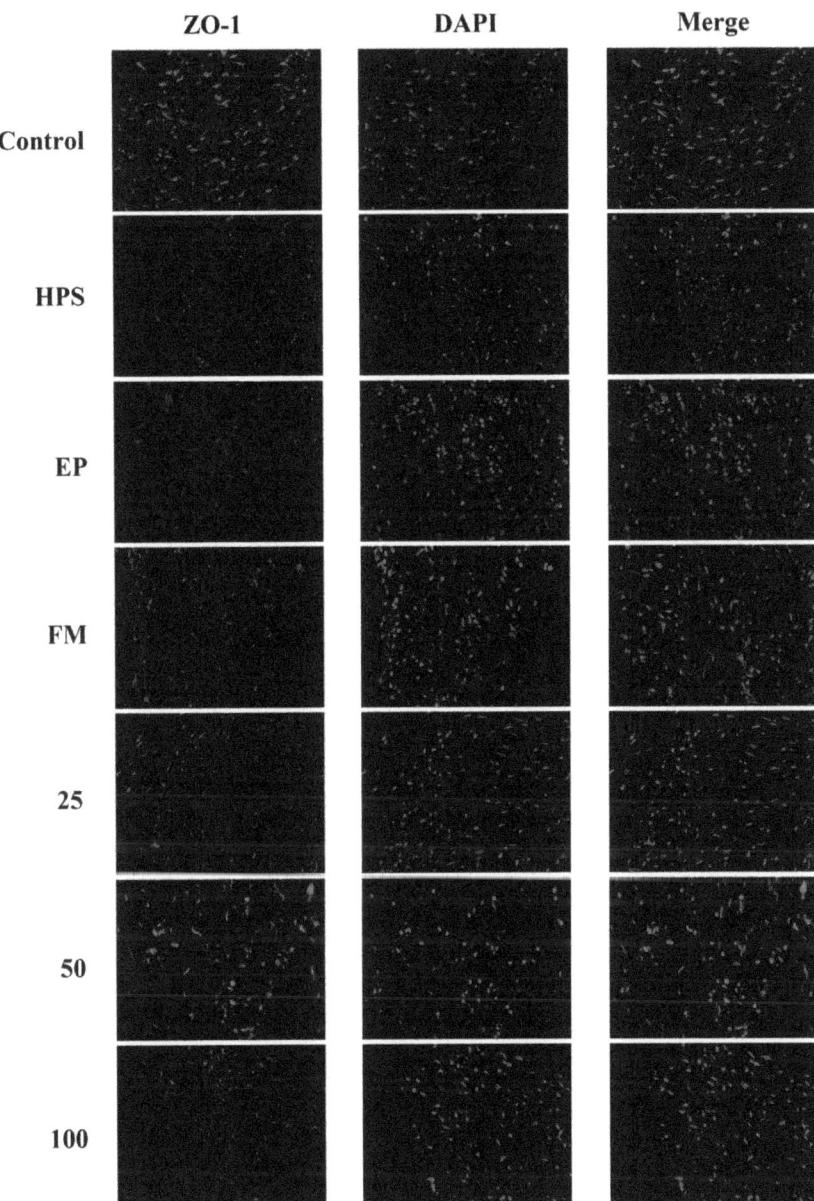

Figure 4. Effect of baicalin on the distribution patterns of ZO-1 in the peritoneum of piglets challenged with *G. parasuis* (magnification 10 × 40). HPS: *G. parasuis* group, EP:EP + *G. parasuis* group, FM:FM + *G. parasuis* group, 25:25 mg/kg baicalin + *G. parasuis* group, 50:50 mg/kg baicalin + *G. parasuis* group, 100:100 mg/kg baicalin + *G. parasuis* group.

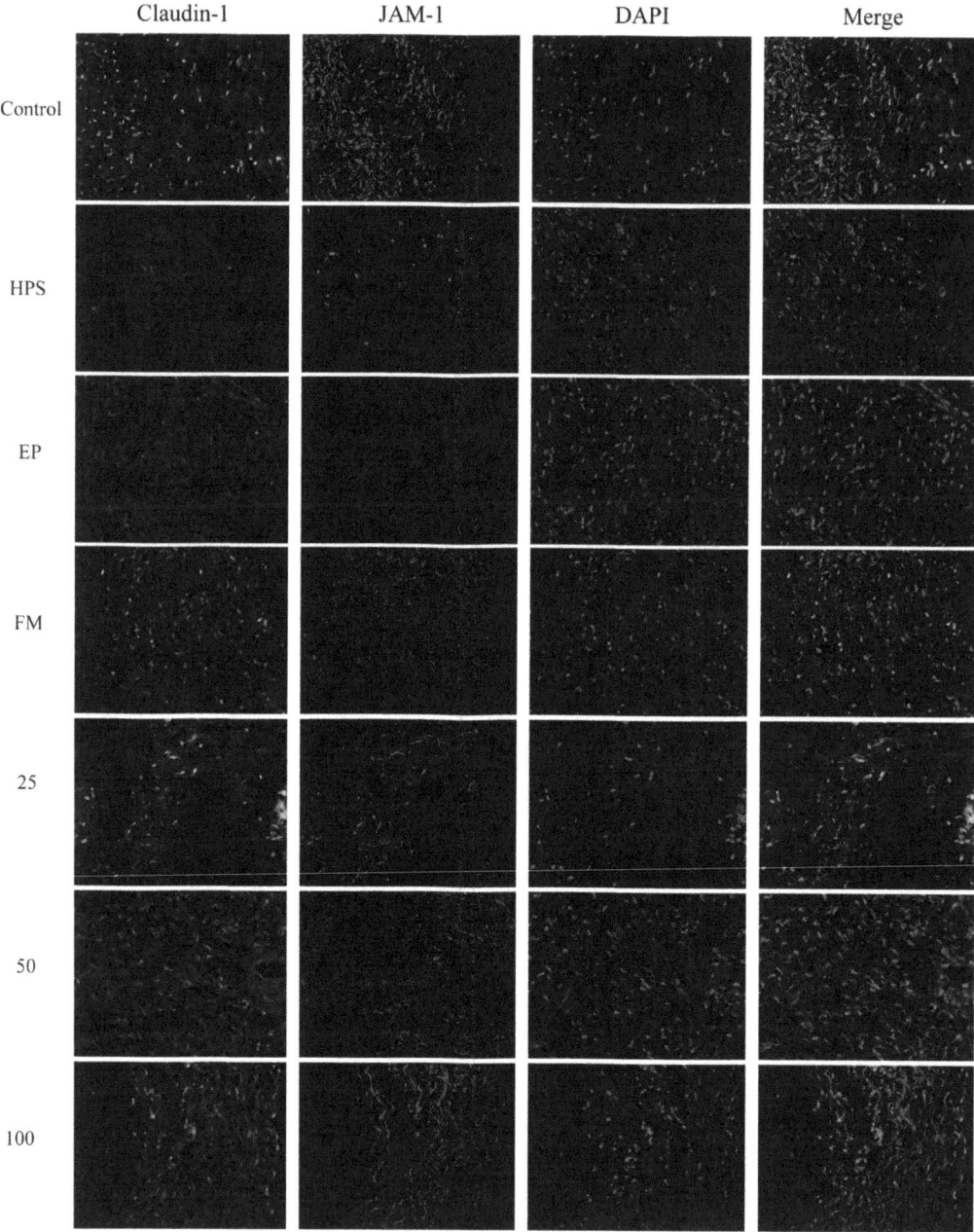

Figure 5. Effect of baicalin on the distribution patterns of claudin-1 and JAM-1 in the peritoneum of piglets challenged with *G. parasuis* (magnification 10 × 40). HPS: *G. parasuis* group, EP:EP + *G. parasuis* group, FM:FM + *G. parasuis* group, 25:25 mg/kg baicalin + *G. parasuis* group, 50:50 mg/kg baicalin + *G. parasuis* group, 100:100 mg/kg baicalin + *G. parasuis* group.

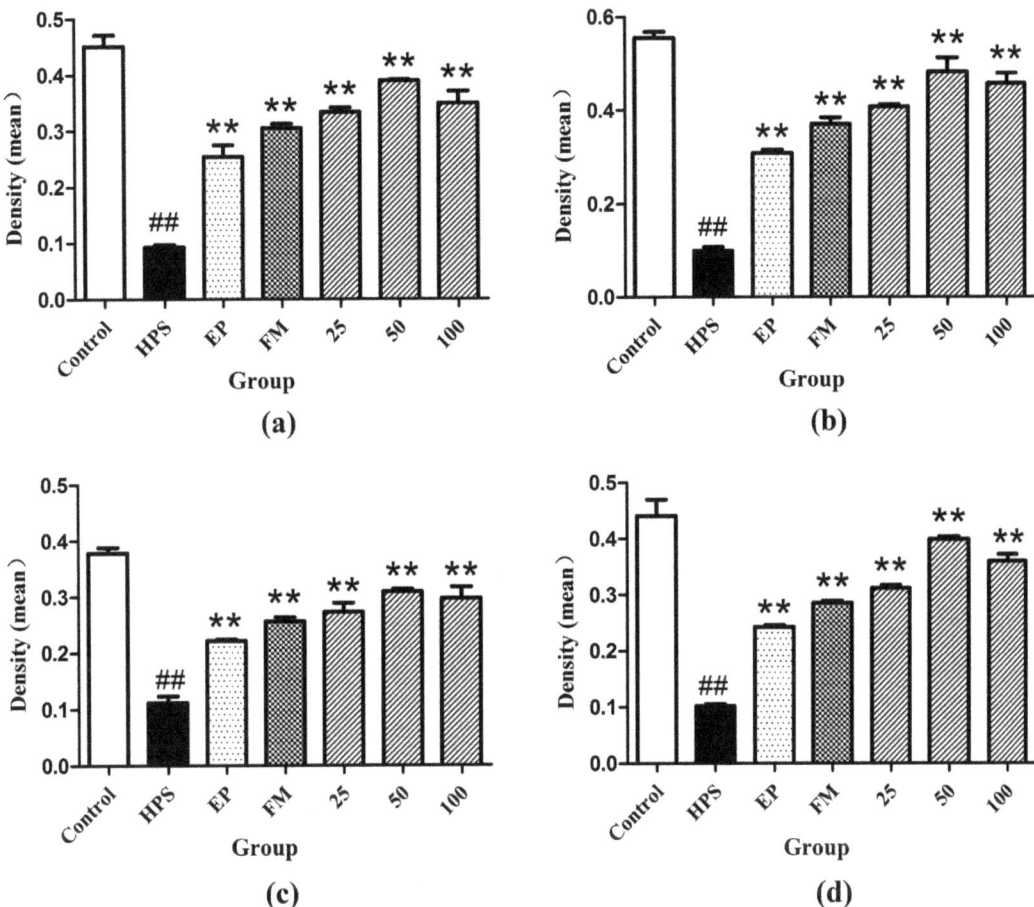

Figure 6. Fluorescence of (**a**) occludin, (**b**) ZO-1, (**c**) claudin-1 and (**d**) JAM-1 in peritoneum were measured by densitometric analysis using the software Image J. HPS: *G. parasuis* group, EP:EP + *G. parasuis* group, FM:FM + *G. parasuis* group, 25:25 mg/kg baicalin + *G. parasuis* group, 50:50 mg/kg baicalin + *G. parasuis* group, 100:100 mg/kg baicalin + *G. parasuis* group. ## $p < 0.01$ vs. control. and ** $p < 0.01$ vs. *G. parasuis* group.

2.3. Effect of Baicalin on PKC and MLCK/MLC Signaling Pathways in Peritoneum of G. parasuis Infected Piglets

Western blot assays were carried out to determine whether the protective mechanism of baicalin on tight junctions of *G. parasuis*-infected piglets acts through the PKC and MLCK/MLC pathways. As shown in Figure 7a,b, *G. parasuis* infection significantly increased the phosphorylation level of PKC-α ($p < 0.01$), while the protein level of PKC-α remained unchanged ($p > 0.05$). EP, FM, and baicalin could down-regulate the expression of p-PKC-α induced by *G. parasuis* and have no effect on the expression of PKC-α.

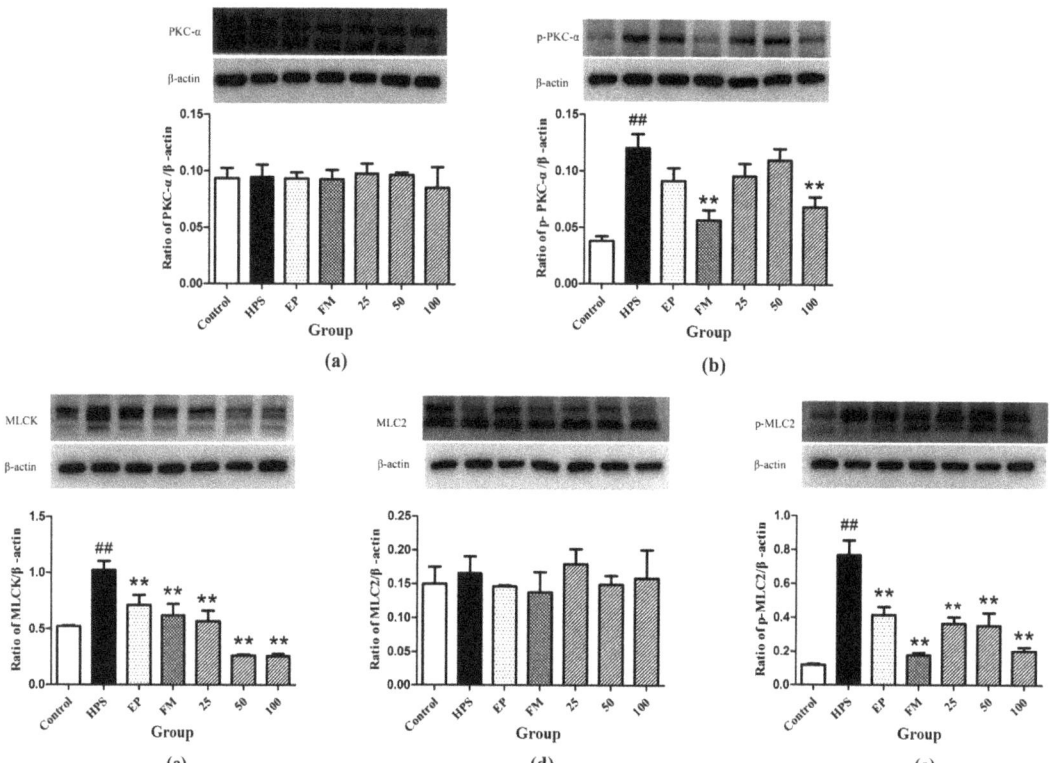

Figure 7. Inhibition effects of baicalin on PKC and MLCK/MLC signaling pathway in peritoneum activated by *G. parasuis* (**a**) PKC-α, (**b**) p-PKC-α, (**c**) MLCK, (**d**) MLC-2, (**e**) p-MLC-2 (Mean ± SD, n = 3). HPS: *G. parasuis* group, EP:EP + *G. parasuis* group, FM:FM + *G. parasuis* group, 25:25 mg/kg baicalin + *G. parasuis* group, 50:50 mg/kg baicalin + *G. parasuis* group, 100:100 mg/kg baicalin + *G. parasuis* group. ## $p < 0.01$ vs. control and ** $p < 0.01$ vs. *G. parasuis* group.

Compared to control group, the MLCK protein was significantly increased in the peritoneum in *G. parasuis* group ($p < 0.01$) (Figure 7c). EP and FM could significantly inhibit the expression of MLCK protein. Baicalin at 25, 50 and 100 mg/kg significantly altered the increasing effect of *G. parasuis* on the expression of MLCK ($p < 0.01$) (Figure 7c).

G. parasuis infection markedly elevated the phosphorylation level of MLC-2 ($p < 0.01$), yet the protein level of MLC-2 remained almost unified between the control and *G. parasuis* group ($p > 0.05$). Administration of EP, FM and baicalin could significantly down-regulated the expression of p-MLC-2 and have no effect on the expression of MLC-2 (Figure 7d,e).

2.4. Histopathological Analysis

Many fibrotic exudates and abdominal organs adhesion were observed in the abdominal cavity in the *G. parasuis* group piglets. Fibrotic lesions were found in peritoneum in *G. parasuis* group. The histopathological analysis was performed to estimate the extent of damage of peritoneum tissues. As shown in Figure 8a, the result of histopathologic analysis displayed no histopathologic changes in control group. The piglets from the *G. parasuis* infection group displayed severe pathological damage as inflammatory cell infiltration and aggregation to their peritoneum tissues (Figure 8b). Moderate inflammatory cell infiltration and aggregation was found in peritoneum in EP treatment group (Figure 8c). Only mild tissue damage was detected in the surviving piglets of the FM treatment group (Figure 8d).

The inflammatory cells infiltration was reduced, and the structure of the peritoneum was comparatively complete in the baicalin treatment groups.

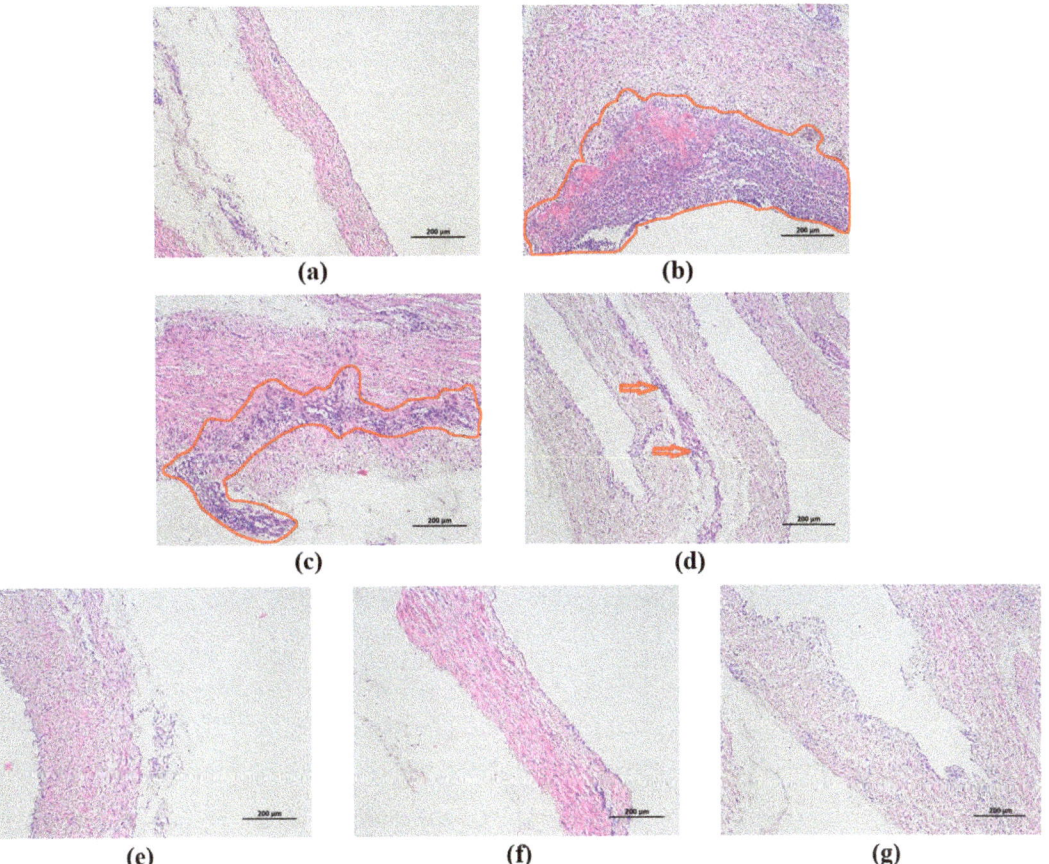

Figure 8. Histopathological change in the piglet peritoneum after G. parasuis infection (H&E, ×100). (**a**) control group, (**b**) G. parasuis group, (**c**) EP + G. parasuis group, (**d**) FM + G. parasuis group, (**e**) 25 mg/kg baicalin + G. parasuis group, (**f**) 50 mg/kg baicalin + G. parasuis group, (**g**) 100 mg/kg baicalin + G. parasuis group. Severe and moderate lesions were circled with red line. Mild lesions were pointed by red arrow.

3. Discussion

G. parasuis is the main pathogen of Glässer's disease, characterized by polyserositis [2]. The fibrotic inflammation caused by G. parasuis mainly occurs in serosa. It is originated from tight junction destruction and serosa damage, which triggers a damaged barrier function and eventually leads to fibrotic exudation [32]. Autopsy results after G. parasuis infection show that the organs of piglets are seriously adhered and there are fibrotic exudates on the surface of the pleura and peritoneum. A large number of inflammatory cells are infiltrated into the peritoneum, containing a small number of necrotic cells, which were filamentous, which is consistent with the characteristic lesions of G. parasuis. EP and FM were used as positive control drugs in the experiment derived from their anti-inflammatory effects to control inflammation-related diseases, such as G. parasuis infection [28]. Under the action of baicalin, the peritoneum lesions were alleviated to a certain degree, which showed the protective effects of baicalin on the damage of peritoneal tight junctions structures in piglets infected with G. parasuis, and provided the basis for exploring its mechanism of action on tight junctions.

Tight junctions are closed complexes at the top of the lateral membrane interface of adjacent epithelial and mesothelial cells. Occludin, claudin and JAMs form a tight junctions skeleton. ZOs are the bridge between cytoskeleton and transmembrane proteins [33]. ZOs proteins interact directly with most transmembrane proteins located at tight junctions. Occludin is involved in the regulation of cell surface receptor signal transduction. In vivo and in vitro studies have shown that occludin is a key regulator of the tight junctions barrier, and multiple domains of occludin are involved in regulating cell bypass permeability [34]. Lack of occludin can cause moderate dysfunction of tight junctions or dysfunction of other cellular signaling pathways related to occludin [35]. Inflammatory injury can cause abnormal distribution, reduce the expression and dissolution of ZO-1 protein, damage the tight junctions structures between cells, widen the intercellular space, and increase the permeability of intestinal epithelial cells [36]. Studies have shown that LPS can reduce the content of ZO-1 in intestinal epithelial cells, and baicalin can protect the ZO-1 damage caused by LPS, which is consistent with the results of our experiment [17].

To our knowledge, this is the first study where tight junctions proteins alterations in G. parasuis infected piglets were explored. The mRNA expressions of occludin, ZO-1, claudin-1, and JAM-1 in peritoneum of G. parasuis infected piglets were significantly down-regulated. The distributions of each protein in the peritoneum of G. parasuis-infected piglets were significantly disrupted. Baicalin can attenuate the down-regulation of each mRNA in peritoneum, prevent these abnormalities and maintain the continuous organization of tight junctions. These results demonstrated that baicalin can alleviate peritoneal tight junction alterations caused by G. parasuis infection. The protective effects of baicalin on tight junctions are superior to EP and FM.

The PKC family is a phospholipid dependent serine/threonine protein kinase activated by calcium, which is widely distributed in the body and plays an important role in the regulation of tight junctions [12,37–40]. Activation of PKC will increase cell permeability, which is critical for tight junction regulation. Studies have shown that PKC mediates the phosphorylation of occludin and its regulation in cell distribution. PKC regulates the assembly of tight junction complex through the phosphorylation of connexin 43 and closure protein to coordinate the formation of functional active barrier and the function of intercellular channel [41]. PKC plays a key role in the translocation of ZO-1 from the cell interior to cell membranes, which can affect the regulation and formation of tight junctions. At the same time, ZO-1 is also the existence of cytoskeleton in PKC signal transduction pathway on cell membrane junction surface [42]. In the process of tight junction decomposition, ZO-2 is phosphorylated by the atypical PKC serine located at tight junctions and combined with ZO-2 [43,44]. The isotypes of PKC and ZO-1 are co-located on the side of plasma membrane, and ZO-1 may be directly phosphorylated by PKC during tight junction assembly [37].

In this study, the protein change of PKC-α in the peritoneum of piglets infected with G. parasuis was detected. Compared with the control group, the expression of phosphorylation of PKC-α in peritoneum of G. parasuis-infected piglets was significantly increased and no significant change was found in non-phosphorylated PKC-α, indicating that PKC–α in peritoneum was activated by G. parasuis. Baicalin can attenuate the phosphorylation of PKC-α, which in consistent with our previous work and the results of other studies of the regulation effects of baicalin on PKC [27,45–47]. The protection effect of baicalin on tight junction abnormalities may relate directly on inhibition of PKC and/or the downstream signaling pathways such as MLCK/MLC.

MLCK is a serine/threonine protein kinase that has an important role in the reorganization of the cytoskeleton leading to disruption of barrier integrity [48]. MLCK catalyzes the phosphorylation of MLC proteins to stimulate the contraction of actin/myosin perijunctional filaments and consequent tight junctions permeabilization [49]. There is sufficient evidence that tight junctions proteins are regulated by MLC-2, which principally depends upon the activation of MLCK [13,14,50,51]. The increased MLCK is indicative of tight junction barrier disruption induced by pro-inflammatory cytokines. Our results showed that the MLCK and p-MLC-2 proteins were significantly increased in the peritoneum in *G. parasuis* challenged piglets, suggesting that *G. parasuis* infection could cause tight junctions barrier disruption. Baicalin can inhibit the increasing protein levels of MLCK and p-MLC-2 induced by *G. parasuis*. These results suggest that the protective effects of baicalin on tight junctions in peritoneum are derived from inhibiting MLCK/MLC pathway.

4. Materials and Methods

The study was carried out at Animal Experimental Base (Wuhan, Hubei, China) in Sinopharm Animal Health Corporation Ltd. All the experimental procedure and operations used in the management and care of piglets were in agreement with the Wuhan Polytechnic University Laboratory Animals Welfare and Animal Experimental Ethical Inspection (reference number WP20100501).

4.1. Bacterial Strains

Glaesserella parasuis strain SH0165 serovar 5 was used, which was isolated from the lung of a commercially produced pig with the typical characteristics of Glässer's disease. The SH0165 isolate was cultured at 37 °C for 12 h in tryptic soy broth (Difco, Lawrence, KS, USA) or grown for 24 h in tryptic soy agar (Difco) supplemented with nicotinamide adenine dinucleotide (Sigma, St. Louis, MO, USA) and foetal bovine serum (Gibco, Gaithersburg, MD, USA).

4.2. Experimental Products

Baicalin was purchased from National Institutes for Food and Drug Control (B110715-201318, Beijing, China). Sodium baicalin was prepared at the Hubei Key Laboratory of Animal Nutrition and Feed Science (Wuhan, China) and was >95% pure [52]. Ethyl pyruvate (EP) and flunixin meglumine (FM) were purchased from Shanghai Macklin Biochemical Co., Ltd. (Shanghai, China) and Guangdong WenS Dahuanong Biotechnology Co., Ltd. (Yunfu, China), respectively.

4.3. Experimental Animals, Management, and Design

A total of 56 weaned healthy piglets (Duroc × Landrace × Large White, 23-d weaned) weighing 8 to 10 kg were purchased from Wuhan Wannianqing Animal Husbandry Co., Ltd. (Wuhan, China). The piglets were confirmed negative for antibodies directed against *G. parasuis* using INgezim Haemophilus 11.HPS.K.1 (Ingezim, Madrid, Spain).

The 56 piglets were randomly divided into seven groups, each group consisting of eight piglets. They were: control group, *G. parasuis* group, EP + *G. parasuis* group, FM + *G. parasuis* group, and 3 baicalin + *G. parasuis* groups (dose 25, 50 and 100 mg/kg b.w., respectively). Drug treatment and challenge: The piglets in EP + *G. parasuis* group were injected intraperitoneally with EP at 40 mg/kg b.w. The piglets in FM + *G. parasuis* group were injected intramuscularly with FM at 2 mg/kg b.w. In baicalin + *G. parasuis* groups, sodium baicalin dissolved in saline was administered intramuscularly at 25, 50, and 100 mg/kg b.w., respectively. After 30 min of the drug treatment, all the piglets except those in control group were challenged intraperitoneally with 1×10^9 CFU of the *G. parasuis* strain (SH0165) in 2 mL of normal saline. The piglets in the control group were injected intraperitoneally with an equivalent volume of saline. Dosing of EP, FM, and baicalin were performed twice daily with an interval of 6 h until the day of post-mortem examination.

4.4. Experimental Sample Collection

On the 8th day after *G. parasuis* challenge, the living piglets were humanely euthanized by intravenous injection of sodium pentobarbital, followed by exsanguination. Peritoneum tissue samples were collected, stored at −80°C for further experiment processing detection or fixed in 4% paraformaldehyde for pathological examination.

4.5. RNA Extraction and RT-PCR

The total RNA was isolated from peritoneum homogenates using RNA prep pure Cell/Bacteria Kit following the manufacturer's instructions (Tiangen, Beijing, China). The RNA was reverse transcribed into cDNA using the Reverse Transcription Kit following the manufacturer's instructions (Takara Biotechnology, Kusatsu, Japan). Specific expression primers for Claudin-1, JAM-1, ZO-1, Occludin and β-actin were designed using Primer 6.0 (Premier, West Toronto, ON, Canada). The primers used for RT-PCR are listed in Table 1. PCR was performed according to the following conditions: 95 °C for 5 min followed by 32 cycles of amplification at 95 °C for 30 s, Tm temperature for 32 s and 72 °C for 30 s, then a final extension at 72 °C for 5 min. The densities of each band were quantified using a gel imaging system (Tanon 4100, Tanon, Shanghai, China) and a ratio was calculated using β-actin as a control. The quantitative results for fluorescence were calculated by $2^{-\Delta\Delta Ct}$ using the normalization method.

Table 1. Primer sequences for Q-RT PCR.

Gene		Nucleotide Sequences (5'–3')	T_m (°C)	Length (bp)
β-actin	Forward	TGCGGGACATCAAGGAGAAG	57.4	216
	Reverse	AGTTGAAGGTGGTCTCGTGG	57.4	
Claudin-1	Forward	CCTTGCTGAATCTGAACAC	49.5	135
	Reverse	GCACCTCATCATCTTCCAT	50.0	
JAM-1	Forward	TGACAGAACAGGCGAATG	50.1	167
	Reverse	GCAGCATAGGCAGGAATT	50.1	
ZO-1	Forward	GAAGATGATGAAGATGAGGATG	50.3	184
	Reverse	GGAGGATGCTGTTGTCTC	49.9	
Occludin	Forward	GAGTGATTCGGATTCTGTCT	50.3	181
	Reverse	TAGCCATAACCATAGCCATAG	50.2	

4.6. Immunofluorescence Microscopy

Immunofluorescence was carried out to detect the distribution patterns of claudin-1, occludin, ZO-1 and JAM-1 proteins in the peritoneum. Thin sections (3 mm) of paraffin-embedded sections of peritoneum were prepared and mounted into adhesive microscopic glass slides. After dewaxing, the sections were permeabilized with citrate buffer for 15 min in microwave, washed 3 times with phosphate buffered saline (PBS) and then blocked with 5% GSA (diluted in PBS) for 1.0 h at RT. The sections were incubated overnight with rabbit anti-occludin, anti-ZO-1, anti-claudin-1, and anti-JAM-1 antibody, respectively, at a 1:100 dilution at 4 °C, then incubated with Cy3-labeled goat anti rabbit (Beyotime, Shanghai, China) at a dilution of 1:100 for 1 h at RT. Fluorescence images were captured using a confocal microscope. The Image J software 1.8.0 (National Institutes of Health, Bethesda, MD, USA) was used to evaluate the amounts of each protein present at the intercellular junctions by semi-quantitatively measuring fluorescence density in the selected areas.

4.7. Western Blotting Analysis

The peritoneum samples of the piglets were collected, dissociated by RIPA lysis buffer supplemented with protease inhibitor mixture and centrifuged at 12,000 g for 15 min at 4 °C. The total protein was measured with BCA protein extraction kit (Beyotime). Subsequently, samples with the same amount of protein (80 μg) were fractionated using 10% SDS-PAGE and then transferred onto polyvinylidene fluoride (PVDF) membranes. After blocked with 5% skimmed milk for 3 h, the PVDF membranes were incubated with special primary antibody (containing 5% BSA TBS-T solution, 1:1000 dilution, rabbit anti-β-actin, anti-PKC-α, anti-p-PKC-α, Cell Signaling, Danvers, MA, USA; anti-MLCK, anti-MLC-2 and anti-p-MLC-2, Abcam, Shanghai, China) at 4 °C overnight, and then incubated with the corresponding HRP labeled secondary antibodies (1:4000 dilution) at 37 °C for 3 h. Protein level was determined using the enhanced chemiluminescent (ECL) reagent (Beyotime) and the images were captured with a ChemiDoc MP Imaging System (Bio-Rad, Hercules, CA, USA). Quantitative analysis was carried out using FluorChem FC2 (Alpha Innotech, San Leandro, CA, USA). The β-actin was used as the inner loading control. Gray value was analyzed and the relative expression level of protein was obtained.

4.8. Histopathology

Peritoneum histopathology was evaluated via haematoxylin and eosin (H&E) staining. Peritoneum were fixed in 10% neutral-buffered formalin, and embedded in paraffin. The sections (4 μm) were stained with H&E with the standard method and observed with a light microscope.

4.9. Statistical Analysis

SPSS Statistics version 17.0 (IBM, Armonk, NY, USA) was used for statistical analysis. The data were shown as the mean ± standard deviation (SD). The differences between the data sets were assessed by one-way analysis of variance (ANOVA) and multiple comparisons between the groups were performed using LSD method. Probability value of $p < 0.05$ was considered significant.

5. Conclusions

In conclusion, our results provide novel evidence to support the notion that *G. parasuis* can downregulate peritoneal tight junction gene expressions and disrupt the distribution of tight junction proteins. Baicalin has the capacity to protect peritoneal tight junctions from *G. parasuis*-induced injuries. The protective mechanisms of baicalin could be associated with the inhibition of the activation of the PKC and MLCK/MLC signaling pathways. The pharmacological features of baicalin thus make it a promising natural antimicrobial compound for prevention and treating of Glässer's disease.

Author Contributions: Conceptualization, Y.Q. and Y.L.; methodology, J.Z. and Z.Z.; software, J.X.; validation, J.X. and C.Y.; formal analysis, C.-A.A.H.; investigation, S.F.; resources, Z.Z.; data curation, C.Y.; writing—original draft preparation, J.Z.; writing—review and editing, Z.Z. and Y.L.; visualization, C.Y. and J.X.; supervision, Y.Q.; project administration, Y.Q. and Y.L.; funding acquisition, Y.L. All authors have read and agreed to the published version of the manuscript.

Funding: This research was funded by the National Natural Science Foundation of China, grant number 31672607.

Institutional Review Board Statement: The study was conducted according to the guidelines of the Declaration of Helsinki, and approved by the Institutional Ethics Committee of Wuhan Polytechnic University Laboratory Animals Welfare and Animal Experimental Ethical Inspection (reference number WP20100501).

Informed Consent Statement: Not applicable.

Data Availability Statement: All relevant data have been presented as an integral part of this manuscript.

Acknowledgments: The authors are grateful to Ping Zhou and his team for the care of the animals.

Conflicts of Interest: The authors declare no conflict of interest.

Sample Availability: Samples of the compounds may be available from the authors.

References

1. Dickerman, A.; Bandara, A.B.; Inzana, T.J. Phylogenomic analysis of *Haemophilus parasuis* and proposed reclassification to *Glaesserella parasuis*, gen. nov., comb. nov. *Int. J. Syst. Evol. Microbiol.* **2020**, *70*, 180–186. [CrossRef]
2. Macedo, N.; Rovira, A.; Torremorell, M. *Haemophilus parasuis*: Infection, immunity and enrofloxacin. *Vet. Res.* **2015**, *46*, 128. [CrossRef]
3. Ni, H.B.; Gong, Q.L.; Zhao, Q.; Li, X.Y.; Zhang, X.X. Prevalence of *Haemophilus parasuis* "*Glaesserella parasuis*" in pigs in China: A systematic review and meta-analysis. *Prev. Vet. Med.* **2020**, *182*, 105083. [CrossRef]
4. Costa-Hurtado, M.; Barba-Vidal, E.; Maldonado, J.; Aragon, V. Update on Glässer's disease: How to control the disease under restrictive use of antimicrobials. *Vet. Microbiol.* **2020**, *242*, 108595. [CrossRef]

5. Awad, W.A.; Hess, C.; Hess, M. Enteric pathogens and their toxin-induced disruption of the intestinal barrier through alteration of tight junctions in chickens. *Toxins* **2017**, *9*, 60. [CrossRef]
6. Blackburn, S.C.; Stanton, M.P. Anatomy and physiology of the peritoneum. *Semin. Pediatr. Surg.* **2014**, *23*, 326–330. [CrossRef]
7. Markov, A.G.; Amasheh, S. Tight junction physiology of pleural mesothelium. *Front. Physiol.* **2014**, *5*, 221. [CrossRef] [PubMed]
8. Bhat, A.A.; Uppada, S.; Achkar, I.W.; Hashem, S.; Yadav, S.K.; Shanmugakonar, M.; Al-Naemi, H.A.; Haris, M.; Uddin, S. Tight Junction proteins and signaling pathways in cancer and inflammation: A functional crosstalk. *Front. Physiol.* **2019**, *9*, 1942. [CrossRef]
9. Cereijido, M.; Contreras, R.G.; Shoshani, L.; Flores-Benitez, D.; Larre, I. Tight junction and polarity interaction in the transporting epithelial phenotype. *Biochim. Biophys. Acta.* **2008**, *1778*, 770–793. [CrossRef] [PubMed]
10. Lu, R.Y.; Yang, W.X.; Hu, Y.J. The role of epithelial tight junctions involved in pathogen infections. *Mol. Biol. Rep.* **2014**, *41*, 6591–6610. [CrossRef] [PubMed]
11. Ulluwishewa, D.; Anderson, R.C.; McNabb, W.C.; Moughan, P.J.; Wells, J.M.; Roy, N.C. Regulation of tight junction permeability by intestinal bacteria and dietary components. *J. Nutr.* **2011**, *141*, 769–776. [CrossRef] [PubMed]
12. Clarke, H.; Marano, C.W.; Soler, A.P.; Mullin, J.M. Modification of tight junction function by protein kinase C isoforms. *Adv. Drug Deliv. Rev.* **2000**, *41*, 283–301. [CrossRef]
13. Cheng, X.; Wang, X.; Wan, Y.; Zhou, Q.; Zhu, H.; Wang, Y. Myosin light chain kinase inhibitor ML7 improves vascular endothelial dysfunction via tight junction regulation in a rabbit model of atherosclerosis. *Mol. Med. Rep.* **2015**, *12*, 4109–4116. [CrossRef] [PubMed]
14. Zhou, H.Y.; Zhu, H.; Yao, X.M.; Qian, J.P.; Yang, J.; Pan, X.D.; Chen, X.D. Metformin regulates tight junction of intestinal epithelial cells via MLCK-MLC signaling pathway. *Eur. Rev. Med. Pharmacol. Sci.* **2017**, *21*, 5239–5246. [CrossRef]
15. Pan, M.H.; Lai, C.S.; Ho, C.T. Anti-inflammatory activity of natural dietary flavonoids. *Food Funct.* **2010**, *1*, 15–31. [CrossRef]
16. Maleki, S.J.; Crespo, J.F.; Cabanillas, B. Anti-inflammatory effects of flavonoids. *Food Chem.* **2019**, *299*, 125124. [CrossRef] [PubMed]
17. Chen, J.; Zhang, R.; Wang, J.; Yu, P.; Liu, Q.; Zeng, D.; Song, H.; Kuang, Z. Protective effects of baicalin on LPS-induced injury in intestinal epithelial cells and intercellular tight junctions. *Can. J. Physiol. Pharmacol.* **2015**, *93*, 233–237. [CrossRef] [PubMed]
18. Nakashima, M.; Hisada, M.; Goda, N.; Tenno, T.; Kotake, A.; Inotsume, Y.; Kameoka, I.; Hiroaki, H. Opposing effect of naringenin and quercetin on the junctional compartment of MDCK II cells to modulate the tight junction. *Nutrients* **2020**, *12*, 3285. [CrossRef]
19. Suzuki, T.; Hara, H. Role of flavonoids in intestinal tight junction regulation. *J. Nutr. Biochem.* **2011**, *22*, 401–408. [CrossRef]
20. Sharma, S.; Tripathi, P.; Sharma, J.; Dixit, A. Flavonoids modulate tight junction barrier functions in hyperglycemic human intestinal Caco-2 cells. *Nutrition* **2020**, *78*, 110792. [CrossRef]
21. Peng, L.Y.; Yuan, M.; Wu, Z.M.; Song, K.; Zhang, C.L.; An, Q.; Xia, F.; Yu, J.L.; Yi, P.F.; Fu, B.D.; et al. Anti-bacterial activity of baicalin against APEC through inhibition of quorum sensing and inflammatory responses. *Sci. Rep.* **2019**, *9*, 4063. [CrossRef]
22. Lee, W.; Ku, S.K.; Bae, J.S. Anti-inflammatory effects of Baicalin, Baicalein, and Wogonin in vitro and in vivo. *Inflammation* **2015**, *38*, 110–125. [CrossRef]
23. Orzechowska, B.U.; Wróbel, G.; Turlej, E.; Jatczak, B.; Sochocka, M.; Chaber, R. Antitumor effect of baicalin from the Scutellaria baicalensis radix extract in B-acute lymphoblastic leukemia with different chromosomal rearrangements. *Int. Immunopharmacol.* **2020**, *79*, 106114. [CrossRef] [PubMed]
24. Paudel, K.R.; Kim, D.W. Microparticles-mediated vascular inflammation and its amelioration by antioxidant activity of Baicalin. *Antioxidants* **2020**, *9*, 890. [CrossRef] [PubMed]
25. Fu, S.; Liu, H.; Chen, X.; Qiu, Y.; Ye, C.; Liu, Y.; Wu, Z.; Guo, L.; Hou, Y.; Hu, C.A. Baicalin inhibits *Haemophilus parasuis*-induced high-mobility group box 1 release during inflammation. *Int. J. Mol. Sci.* **2018**, *19*, 1307. [CrossRef]
26. Fu, S.; Liu, H.; Xu, L.; Qiu, Y.; Liu, Y.; Wu, Z.; Ye, C.; Hou, Y.; Hu, C.A. Baicalin modulates NF-κB and NLRP3 inflammasome signaling in porcine aortic vascular endothelial cells infected by *Haemophilus parasuis* causing Glässer's disease. *Sci. Rep.* **2018**, *8*, 807. [CrossRef]
27. Ye, C.; Li, R.; Xu, L.; Qiu, Y.; Fu, S.; Liu, Y.; Wu, Z.; Hou, Y.; Hu, C.A. Effects of Baicalin on piglet monocytes involving PKC-MAPK signaling pathways induced by *Haemophilus parasuis*. *BMC Vet. Res.* **2019**, *15*, 98. [CrossRef]
28. Fu, S.; Yin, R.; Zuo, S.; Liu, J.; Zhang, Y.; Guo, L.; Qiu, Y.; Ye, C.; Liu, Y.; Wu, Z.; et al. The effects of Baicalin on piglets challenged with *Glaesserella parasuis*. *Vet. Res.* **2020**, *51*, 102. [CrossRef] [PubMed]
29. Zhu, H.; Wang, Z.; Xing, Y.; Gao, Y.; Ma, T.; Lou, L.; Lou, J.; Gao, Y.; Wang, S.; Wang, Y. Baicalin reduces the permeability of the blood-brain barrier during hypoxia in vitro by increasing the expression of tight junction proteins in brain microvascular endothelial cells. *J. Ethnopharmacol.* **2012**, *141*, 714–720. [CrossRef] [PubMed]
30. Wang, L.; Zhang, R.; Chen, J.; Wu, Q.; Kuang, Z. Baicalin protects against TNF-α-induced injury by down-regulating miR-191a that targets the tight junction protein ZO-1 in IEC-6 Cells. *Biol. Pharm. Bull.* **2017**, *40*, 435–443. [CrossRef]
31. Hisada, M.; Hiranuma, M.; Nakashima, M.; Goda, N.; Tenno, T.; Hiroaki, H. High dose of Baicalin or baicalein can reduce tight junction integrity by partly targeting the first PDZ domain of zonula occludens-1 (ZO-1). *Eur. J. Pharmacol.* **2020**, *887*, 173436. [CrossRef]
32. Zihni, C.; Mills, C.; Matter, K.; Balda, M.S. Tight junctions: From simple barriers to multifunctional molecular gates. *Nat. Rev. Mol. Cell Biol.* **2016**, *17*, 564–580. [CrossRef] [PubMed]
33. Förster, C. Tight junctions and the modulation of barrier function in disease. *Histochem. Cell Biol.* **2008**, *130*, 55–70. [CrossRef]

34. Buschmann, M.M.; Shen, L.; Rajapakse, H.; Raleigh, D.R.; Wang, Y.; Wang, Y.; Lingaraju, A.; Zha, J.; Abbott, E.; McAuley, E.M.; et al. Occludin OCEL-domain interactions are required for maintenance and regulation of the tight junction barrier to macromolecular flux. *Mol. Biol. Cell* **2013**, *24*, 3056–3068. [CrossRef]
35. Saitou, M.; Furuse, M.; Sasaki, H.; Schulzke, J.D.; Fromm, M.; Takano, H.; Noda, T.; Tsukita, S. Complex phenotype of mice lacking occludin, a component of tight junction strands. *Mol. Biol. Cell* **2000**, *11*, 4131–4142. [CrossRef] [PubMed]
36. Yamamoto-Furusho, J.K.; Mendivil, E.J.; Fonseca-Camarillo, G. Differential expression of occludin in patients with ulcerative colitis and healthy controls. *Inflamm. Bowel. Dis.* **2012**, *18*, E1999. [CrossRef] [PubMed]
37. Stuart, R.O.; Nigam, S.K. Regulated assembly of tight junctions by protein kinase C. *Proc. Natl. Acad. Sci. USA* **1995**, *92*, 6072–6076. [CrossRef] [PubMed]
38. Ogasawara, N.; Kojima, T.; Go, M.; Ohkuni, T.; Koizumi, J.; Kamekura, R.; Masaki, T.; Murata, M.; Tanaka, S.; Fuchimoto, J.; et al. PPARgamma agonists upregulate the barrier function of tight junctions via a PKC pathway in human nasal epithelial cells. *Pharmacol. Res.* **2010**, *61*, 489–498. [CrossRef] [PubMed]
39. Mullin, J.M.; Laughlin, K.V.; Ginanni, N.; Marano, C.W.; Clarke, H.M.; Soler, A.P. Increased tight junction permeability can result from protein kinase C activation/translocation and act as a tumor promotional event in epithelial cancers. *Ann. N. Y. Acad. Sci.* **2000**, *915*, 231–236. [CrossRef]
40. Jo, H.; Hwang, D.; Kim, J.K.; Lim, Y.H. Oxyresveratrol improves tight junction integrity through the PKC and MAPK signaling pathways in Caco-2 cells. *Food Chem. Toxicol.* **2017**, *108*, 203–213. [CrossRef]
41. Andreeva, A.Y.; Krause, E.; Müller, E.C.; Blasig, I.E.; Utepbergenov, D.I. Protein kinase C regulates the phosphorylation and cellular localization of occludin. *J. Biol. Chem.* **2001**, *276*, 38480–38486. [CrossRef]
42. Chai, J.; Long, B.; Liu, X.; Li, Y.; Han, N.; Zhao, P.; Chen, W. Effects of sevoflurane on tight junction protein expression and PKC-α translocation after pulmonary ischemia-reperfusion injury. *Exp. Mol. Med.* **2015**, *47*, e167. [CrossRef]
43. Avila-Flores, A.; Rendón-Huerta, E.; Moreno, J.; Islas, S.; Betanzos, A.; Robles-Flores, M.; González-Mariscal, L. Tight-junction protein zonula occludens 2 is a target of phosphorylation by protein kinase C. *Biochem. J.* **2001**, *360*, 295–304. [CrossRef] [PubMed]
44. Amaya, E.; Alarcón, L.; Martín-Tapia, D.; Cuellar-Pérez, F.; Cano-Cortina, M.; Ortega-Olvera, J.M.; Cisneros, B.; Rodriguez, A.J.; Gamba, G.; González-Mariscal, L. Activation of the Ca^{2+} sensing receptor and the PKC/WNK$_4$ downstream signaling cascade induces incorporation of ZO-2 to tight junctions and its separation from 14-3-3. *Mol. Biol. Cell.* **2019**, *30*, 2377–2398. [CrossRef] [PubMed]
45. Shi, L.; Hao, Z.; Zhang, S.; Wei, M.; Lu, B.; Wang, Z.; Ji, L. Baicalein and Baicalin alleviate acetaminophen-induced liver injury by activating Nrf2 antioxidative pathway: The involvement of ERK1/2 and PKC. *Biochem. Pharmacol.* **2018**, *150*, 9–23. [CrossRef]
46. Wang, Q.; Xu, H.; Zhao, X. Baicalin inhibits human cervical cancer cells by suppressing protein kinase C/signal transducer and activator of transcription (PKC/STAT3) signaling pathway. *Med. Sci. Monit.* **2018**, *24*, 1955–1961. [CrossRef] [PubMed]
47. Shou, X.; Wang, B.; Zhou, R.; Wang, L.; Ren, A.; Xin, S.; Zhu, L. Protective effects of Baicalin on oxygen/glucose deprivation- and NMDA-induced injuries in rat hippocampal slices. *J. Pharm. Pharmacol.* **2005**, *57*, 1019–1026. [CrossRef]
48. Rossi, J.L.; Ranaivo, R.H.; Patel, F.; Chrzaszcz, M.; Venkatesan, C.; Wainwright, M.S. Albumin causes increased myosin light chain kinase expression in astrocytes via p38 mitogen-activated protein kinase. *J. Neurosci. Res.* **2011**, *89*, 852–861. [CrossRef]
49. Cunningham, K.E.; Turner, J.R. Myosin light chain kinase: Pulling the strings of epithelial tight junction function. *Ann. N. Y. Acad. Sci.* **2012**, *1258*, 34–42. [CrossRef] [PubMed]
50. Zhu, H.Q.; Zhou, Q.; Jiang, Z.K.; Gui, S.Y.; Wang, Y. Association of aorta intima permeability with myosin light chain kinase expression in hypercholesterolemic rabbits. *Mol. Cell. Biochem.* **2011**, *347*, 209–215. [CrossRef] [PubMed]
51. Qasim, M.; Rahman, H.; Ahmed, R.; Oellerich, M.; Asif, A.R. Mycophenolic acid mediated disruption of the intestinal epithelial tight junctions. *Exp. Cell Res.* **2014**, *322*, 277–289. [CrossRef] [PubMed]
52. Liu, Y.; Zhao, W.; Xu, J.; Yu, X.; Ye, C.; Fu, S.; Qiu, Y. Pharmacokinetics of sodium baicalin following intravenous and intramuscular administration to piglets. *J. Vet. Pharmacol. Ther.* **2019**, *42*, 580–584. [CrossRef] [PubMed]

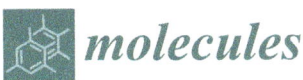

Article

Sulforaphane Inhibits Osteoclastogenesis via Suppression of the Autophagic Pathway

Tingting Luo [1], Xiazhou Fu [1], Yaoli Liu [1], Yaoting Ji [1,*] and Zhengjun Shang [1,2,*]

[1] The State Key Laboratory Breeding Base of Basic Science of Stomatology (Hubei-MOST) & Key Laboratory of Oral Biomedicine Ministry of Education, School & Hospital of Stomatology, Wuhan University, Wuhan 430000, China; luotingting@whu.edu.cn (T.L.); fuxiazhou@whu.edu.cn (X.F.); liuyaoli2017@whu.edu.cn (Y.L.)

[2] Department of Oral and Maxillofacial-Head and Neck Oncology, School and Hospital of Stomatology, Wuhan University, Wuhan 430000, China

* Correspondence: yaotingji@whu.edu.cn (Y.J.); shangzhengjun@whu.edu.cn (Z.S.); Tel.: +86-138-8607-0344 (Y.J.); +86-27-8768-6129 (Z.S.)

Abstract: Previous studies have demonstrated that sulforaphane (SFN) is a promising agent against osteoclastic bone destruction. However, the mechanism underlying its anti-osteoclastogenic activity is still unclear. Herein, for the first time, we explored the potential role of autophagy in SFN-mediated anti-osteoclastogenesis in vitro and in vivo. We established an osteoclastogenesis model using receptor activator of nuclear factor kappa-β ligand (RANKL)-induced RAW264.7 cells and bone marrow macrophages (BMMs). Tartrate-resistant acid phosphatase (TRAP) staining showed the formation of osteoclasts. We observed autophagosomes by transmission electron microscopy (TEM). In vitro, we found that SFN inhibited osteoclastogenesis (number of osteoclasts: 22.67 ± 0.88 in the SFN (0) group vs. 20.33 ± 1.45 in the SFN (1 μM) group vs. 13.00 ± 1.00 in the SFN (2.5 μM) group vs. 6.66 ± 1.20 in the SFN (2.5 μM) group), decreased the number of autophagosomes, and suppressed the accumulation of several autophagic proteins in osteoclast precursors. The activation of autophagy by rapamycin (RAP) almost reversed the SFN-elicited anti-osteoclastogenesis (number of osteoclasts: 22.67 ± 0.88 in the control group vs. 13.00 ± 1.00 in the SFN group vs. 17.33 ± 0.33 in the SFN+RAP group). Furthermore, Western blot (WB) analysis revealed that SFN inhibited the phosphorylation of c-Jun N-terminal kinase (JNK). The JNK activator anisomycin significantly promoted autophagy, whereas the inhibitor SP600125 markedly suppressed autophagic activation in pre-osteoclasts. Microcomputed tomography (CT), immunohistochemistry (IHC), and immunofluorescence (IF) were used to analyze the results in vivo. Consistent with the in vitro results, we found that the administration of SFN could decrease the number of osteoclasts and the expression of autophagic light chain 3 (LC3) and protect against lipopolysaccharide (LPS)-induced calvarial erosion. Our findings highlight autophagy as a crucial mechanism of SFN-mediated anti-osteoclastogenesis and show that the JNK signaling pathway participates in this process.

Keywords: sulforaphane; osteoclastogenesis; autophagy; JNK signaling pathway

Citation: Luo, T.; Fu, X.; Liu, Y.; Ji, Y.; Shang, Z. Sulforaphane Inhibits Osteoclastogenesis via Suppression of the Autophagic Pathway. *Molecules* **2021**, *26*, 347. https://doi.org/10.3390/molecules26020347

Academic Editors: Francesco Maione and Gerd Bendas

Received: 11 December 2020
Accepted: 3 January 2021
Published: 12 January 2021

Publisher's Note: MDPI stays neutral with regard to jurisdictional claims in published maps and institutional affiliations.

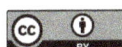

Copyright: © 2021 by the authors. Licensee MDPI, Basel, Switzerland. This article is an open access article distributed under the terms and conditions of the Creative Commons Attribution (CC BY) license (https://creativecommons.org/licenses/by/4.0/).

1. Introduction

Throughout life, bone remodeling is precisely regulated by the balance between osteoblastic bone formation and osteoclastic bone resorption. This balance is often disturbed by diseases associated with excessive bone resorption, such as osteoporosis, rheumatoid arthritis (RA), periodontitis, and bone metastasis [1–3]. Osteoclasts, multinucleated cells that derive from the monocyte–macrophage lineage of hematopoietic stem cells, are responsible for bone destruction in these diseases. Therefore, osteoclasts are crucial targets in the treatment of such diseases.

Sulforaphane (SFN), a sulfur-containing compound, is derived from cruciferous vegetables like broccoli sprouts [4]. The properties of SFN that have been mostly studied include anti-tumor, anti-inflammatory, and anti-oxidative activities [5]. Furthermore, SFN is reported to have potential beneficial effects in the treatment of diabetes, RA, and osteosarcoma, possibly by activating the antioxidant response and inhibiting inflammatory responses [6–8]. Recently, SFN was found to exhibit bone anabolic effects resulting from anti-osteoclastogenic and osteoblastic stimulatory effects [9]. Therefore, SFN shows promising efficacy as a potential therapy against excessive bone resorption-related pathologies. Takagi et al. suggested that SFN inhibits osteoclastic differentiation and cell fusion [10]. However, the underlying mechanisms are still unknown.

Autophagy, a conserved lysosome degradation pathway, plays an adaptive role in cellular survival, differentiation, and homeostasis [11]. Autophagy is associated with various diseases, including cancers and infection. Recent studies have implicated changes in autophagy in osteoclast-related diseases such as osteoporosis and RA [12,13]. Therefore, the pharmacological regulation of autophagy could be helpful in treating these diseases. For instance, rapamycin (RAP), a classical autophagy inducer, can efficiently decrease osteolysis associated with bone metastases in breast cancer [14]. Moreover, autophagy-related genes (Atgs) and Beclin1, the necessary molecules for autophagy, play pivotal roles in osteoclastogenesis. Carl et al. suggested that the Atg5–Atg12 complex is also crucial for osteoclastic lysosome localization and bone resorption and that its deficiency could impair the formation of osteoclasts' ruffled border, resulting in osteopetrosis [15]. Beclin1 can be activated as early as 2 h after receptor activator of nuclear factor kappa-β ligand (RANKL) treatment, and bone marrow macrophages (BMMs) from Beclin1 conditional deletion mice exhibit suppression of osteoclastogenesis [16]. Therefore, autophagy is believed to be a critical participant in osteoclastogenesis. Notably, SFN exhibits a modulatory role of autophagy which has been implicated in neurodegenerative diseases, tumor therapy, and diabetic kidney disease. It was reported that SFN could induce autophagy in neuron cells and breast cancer cells, while it plays a negative role in renal tubule cells and esophageal cancer [17–20]. However, whether autophagy plays a significant role in anti-osteoclastogenesis mediated by SFN remains unclear.

Herein, the potential role of autophagy in SFN-mediated anti-osteoclastogenesis was explored for the first time. We demonstrate the effects of SFN on bone resorption in mice with lipopolysaccharide (LPS)-induced erosion of the calvarial bone and we investigated the alterations of autophagy in this process.

2. Results

2.1. SFN Inhibited Osteoclastogenesis in a Dose-Dependent Manner

To explore the effect of SFN on the proliferative activity of pre-osteoclasts, we performed a Cell Counting Kit-8 (CCK-8) assay. We found that cell viability decreased along a gradient by treating RAW264.7 cells and BMMs with various concentration SFN (0, 0.5, 1, 2.5, 5, 10, 20 μM, Figure 1a). We cultured RAW264.7 cells and BMMs with RANKL (50 ng/mL) and treated them with various concentrations of SFN (0, 1, 2.5, 5 μM) for 5 days. Tartrate-resistant acid phosphatase (TRAP) staining showed that SFN decreased the number of osteoclasts in a dose-dependent manner (RAW264.7 cells: 22.67 ± 0.88 in the SFN (0) group vs. 20.33 ± 1.45 in the SFN (1 μM) group vs. 13.00 ± 1.00 in the SFN (2.5 μM) group vs. 6.66 ± 1.20 in the SFN (2.5 μM) group; BMMs: 23.67 ± 0.33 in the SFN (0) group vs. 20.67 ± 1.45 in the SFN (1 μM) group vs. 16.67 ± 0.88 in the SFN (2.5 μM) group vs. 7.67 ± 0.88 in the SFN (2.5 μM) group) (Figure 1b,c). Given the cytotoxicity of SFN, SFN at 2.5 μM, which has no obvious cytotoxicity, completely inhibited osteoclastogenesis. In addition, quantitative reverse-transcription polymerase chain reaction (qRT-PCR) and Western blot (WB) analyses showed that SFN suppressed the expression of both cathepsin K (CTSK) and matrix metalloproteinase 9 (MMP9) induced by RANKL (Figure 1d,e).

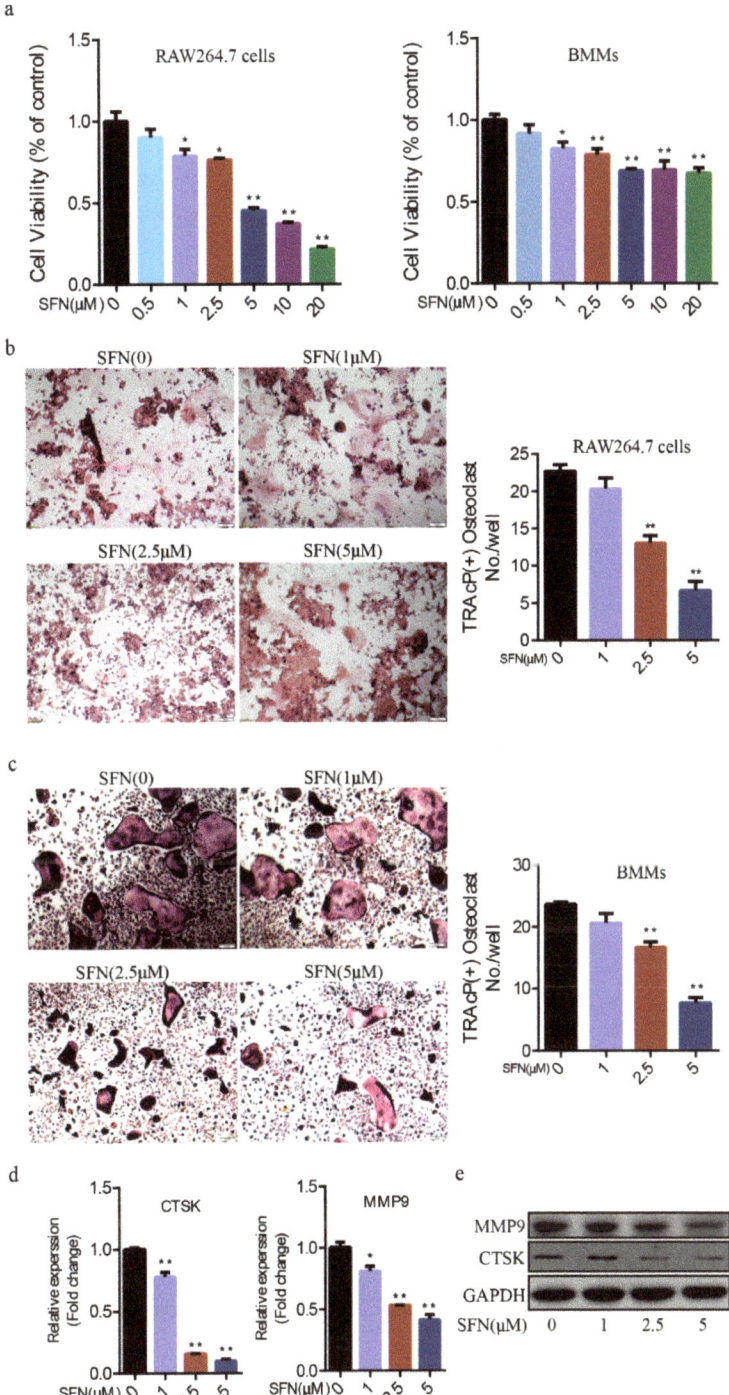

Figure 1. Sulforaphane (SFN) inhibited osteoclastogenesis in a dose-dependent manner. (**a**) The proliferative activity of RAW264.7 cells and bone marrow macrophages (BMMs) was detected by Cell Counting Kit-8 (CCK-8) assay after 24 h in the presence of the indicated concentration of SFN.

For the osteoclastogenesis assay, RAW264.7 cells and BMMs were cultured with receptor activator of nuclear factor kappa-β ligand (RANKL, 50 ng/mL) and treated with varying concentrations of SFN (0, 1, 2.5, 5 μM) for 5 days. Representative images of osteoclasts differentiated from RAW264.7 cells (**b**) and BMMs (**c**) in each group and corresponding statistics. (**d**,**e**) Representative qRT-PCR and WB results showing the effects of SFN on osteoclastic matrix metalloproteinase 9 (MMP9) and cathepsin K (CTSK) expression. Values are mean ± SEM of three independent experiments; * $p < 0.05$, ** $p < 0.01$.

2.2. SFN Treatment Blocked the Autophagic Pathway in Pre-Osteoclasts

Subsequently, we investigated the precise mechanisms underlying SFN-mediated anti-osteoclastogenesis. Recent studies have shown that the activation of autophagy plays a vital role in osteoclast differentiation. Notably, obvious accumulation of light chain 3 (LC3)-II and Beclin1 indicated by punctuated fluorescence within osteoclasts was suppressed by SFN treatment (Figure 2a,b). To explore the stage at which SFN mainly inhibited osteoclastogenesis, we exposed pre-osteoclasts to SFN at different time points (days 0, 1, 2 and 3). RAW264.7 cells were cultured with 50 ng/mL RANKL plus 2.5 μM SFN at the indicated time points. The results demonstrated that SFN treatment on day 0 efficiently inhibited osteoclastogenesis, whereas at later stages the inhibitory effect was limited (number of osteoclasts/well: 20.33 ± 1.45 in control group vs. 10.67 ± 0.88 on Day 0 group vs. 12.33 ± 0.88 in Day 1 group vs. 15.33 ± 0.88 on Day 2 group vs. 19.00 ± 1.00 on Day 3 group, Figure 3a). To explore the effect of SFN on autophagy in pre-osteoclasts, we stimulated RAW 264.7 cells with SFN for 2 h and then treated them with 50 ng/mL RANKL for 24 h. Compared with the control group, transmission electron microscopy (TEM) analysis showed a significant reduction in autophagosomes in the SFN (2.5 μM) group (Figure 3b). As shown in Figure 3c,d, SFN treatment significantly attenuated the transcriptional and translational levels of the autophagy markers LC3-II, Beclin1, and Atg5–Atg12.

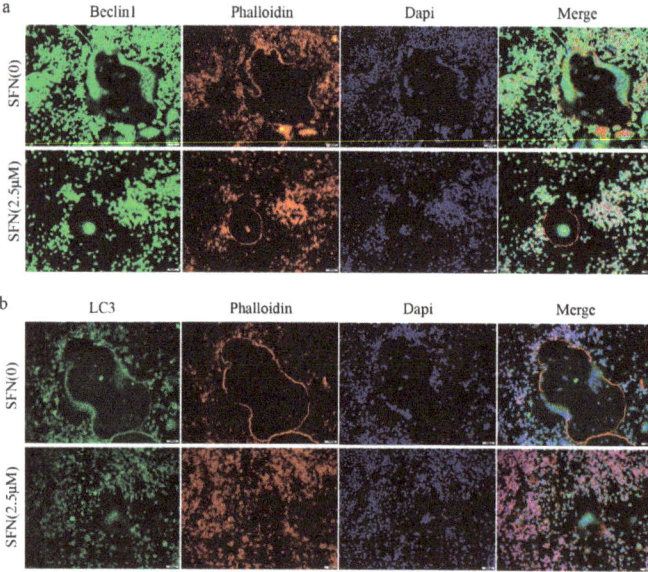

Figure 2. SFN inhibited the accumulation of autophagic light chain 3 (LC3) and Beclin1 within osteoclasts. RAW264.7 cells were induced by 50 ng/mL of RANKL for 5 days, and immunofluorescence (IF) analysis was performed. (**a**) Representative IF images locating LC3 (green) within the osteoclasts. (**b**) Representative IF images locating Beclin1 (green) within the osteoclasts. F-actin was stained with phalloidin (red). DAPI (blue) was used to visualize the nuclei.

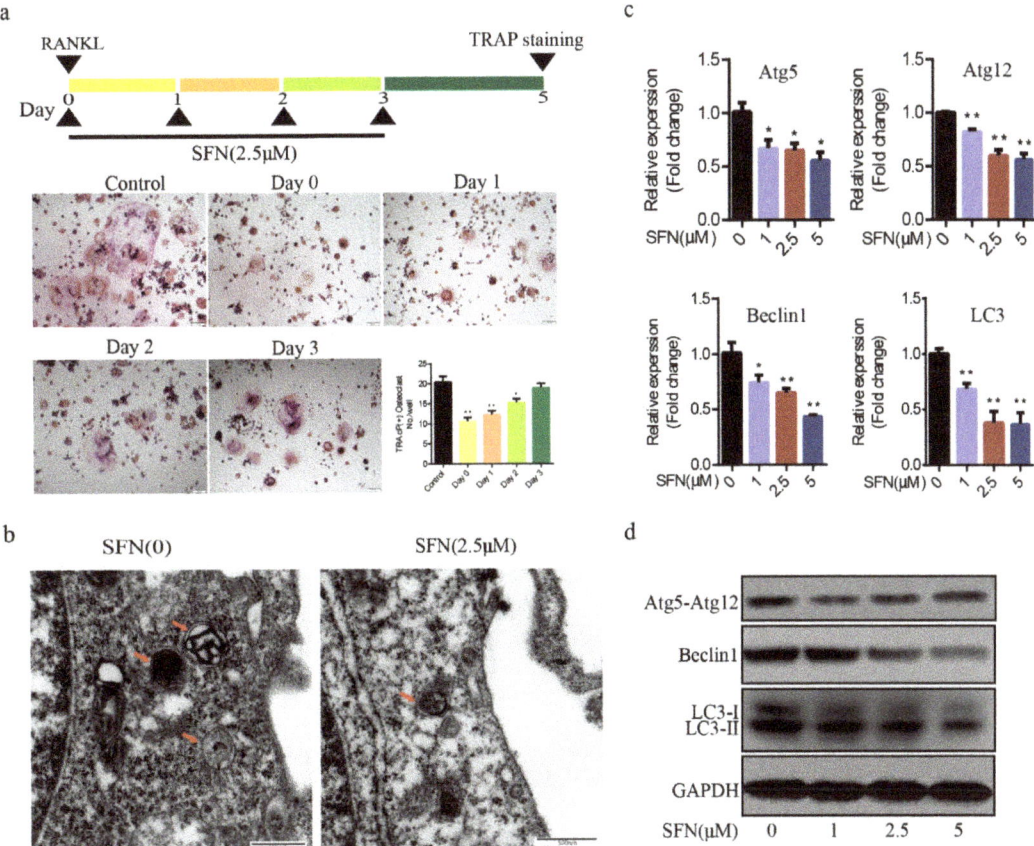

Figure 3. SFN treatment blocked the autophagic pathway in pre-osteoclasts. RAW264.7 cells were cultured with 50 ng/mL of RANKL for 5 days plus 2.5 μM SFN at the indicated time points. (**a**) Representative images showing osteoclastogenesis in each group and corresponding statistics. To explore the effect of SFN on autophagy in pre-osteoclasts, we stimulated RAW 264.7 cells with SFN for 2 h and then treated them with 50 ng/mL of RANKL for 24 h. (**b**) Representative images of autophagosomes (red arrow) as observed by TEM. (**c**,**d**) Representative qRT-PCR and WB results showing the effects of SFN on autophagic molecules (Atg5, Atg12, Beclin1, and LC3) expression. Values are mean ± SEM of three independent experiments; * $p < 0.05$, ** $p < 0.01$.

2.3. Rapamycin Reversed SFN-Mediated Anti-Osteoclatogenic Effects

To investigate whether autophagy was involved in SFN-mediated anti-osteoclastogenesis, we used RAP to active autophagy in RAW264.7 cells. The cells were cultured with 50 ng/mL of RANKL in the absence or presence of 2.5 μM SFN and 10 μM RAP for 5 days. We found that RAP rescued the transcription of Beclin1, Atg5, Atg12, and LC3, which was inhibited by SFN (Figure 4a). RAP stimulation reversed SFN inhibition of osteoclastogenesis (number of osteoclasts/well: 22.67 ± 0.88 in the control group vs. 13.00 ± 1.00 in the SFN group vs. 17.33 ± 0.33 in the SFN+RAP group, Figure 4a). Similarly, SFN reduced the size of F-actin rings, whereas RAP reversed this reduction (Figure 4b). As expected, the expression of MMP9 and CTSK at the transcriptional and translational levels exhibited similar changes (Figure 4c,d). These results indicated that autophagy could be involved in SFN-mediated anti-osteoclastogenesis in vitro.

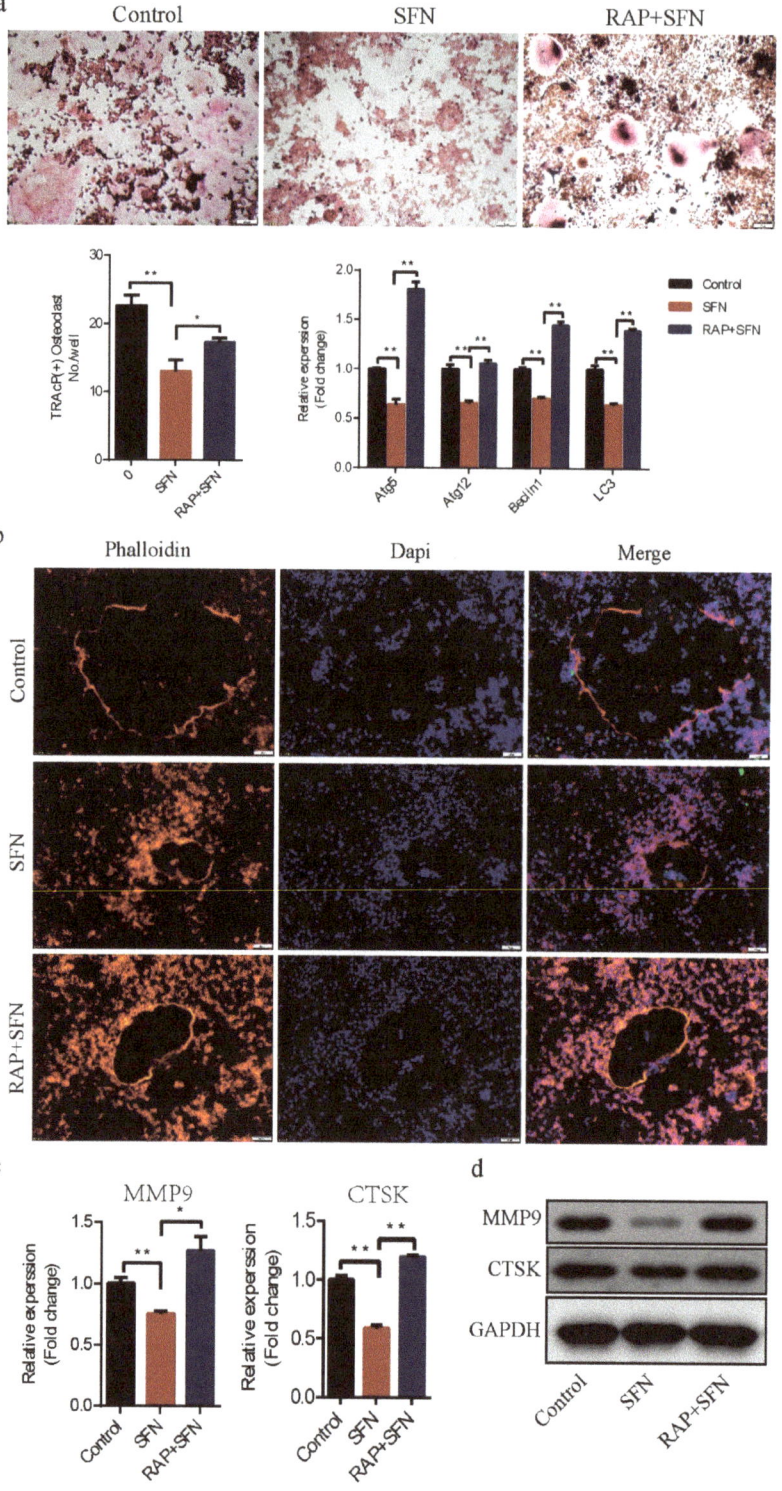

Figure 4. Cont.

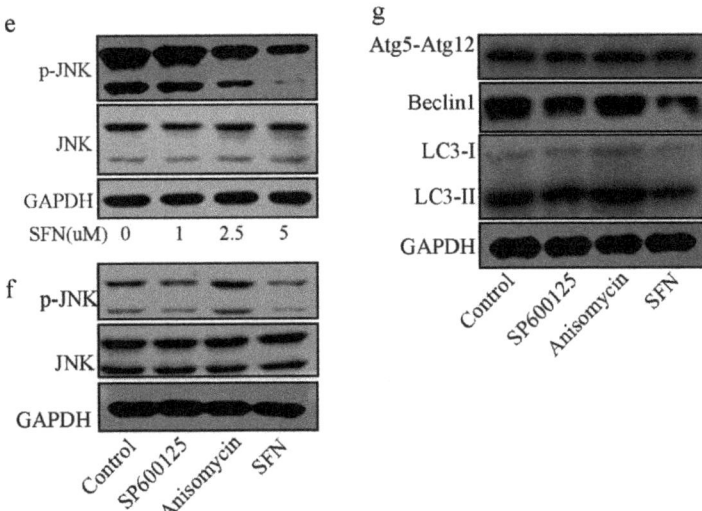

Figure 4. RAP reversed SFN-mediated anti-osteoclatogenic effects. Raw264.7 cells were cultured with 50 ng/mL of RANKL in the absence or presence of 2.5 μM SFN and 10 μM RAP for 5 days. (**a**) Representative images showing osteoclastogenesis in each group and corresponding statistics. (**b**) Representative images showing F-actin stained with phalloidin (red). DAPI (blue) was used to visualize the nuclei. (**c,d**) Representative qRT-PCR and WB results showing MMP9 and CTSK expression. To detect JNK signaling, RAW 264.7 cells were stimulated with SP600125. Anisomycin, or SFN for 2 h and then treated with 50 ng/mL of RANKL for 30 min. (**e**) WB results showing the activation level of JNK signaling after treatment with varying concentrations of SFN. (**f**) WB results showing the activation level of JNK signaling. To explore the role of JNK signaling in SFN-mediated inhibition of autophagy, we stimulated RAW 264.7 cells with SP600125, anisomycin, or SFN for 2 h and then treated them with 50 ng/mL of RANKL for 24 h. (**g**) WB results showing protein levels of autophagic molecules (Atg5, Atg12, Beclin1, and LC3). Values are mean ± SEM of three independent experiments; * $p < 0.05$, ** $p < 0.01$.

2.4. c-Jun N-Terminal Kinase (JNK) Signaling Pathway Appeared to Participate in SFN-Mediated Autophagy Inhibition in the Early Period of Osteoclastogenesis

To explore the role of JNK signaling in SFN-mediated autophagy inhibition in the early period of osteoclastogenesis, we stimulated RAW 264.7 cells with SP600125, anisomycin, or SFN for 2 h and then treated them with 50 ng/mL of RANKL for 30 min. As shown in Figure 4e, SFN suppressed the phosphorylation of JNK in a dose-dependent manner. To demonstrate the role of JNK signaling in autophagy during osteoclasogenesis, we treated RAW 264.7 cells with anisomycin, a JNK signaling activator, and SP600125, a JNK signaling inhibitor. WB results showed that anisomycin increased JNK phosphorylation, and SP600125 exerted a negative effect (Figure 4f). After stimulation with SFN for 2 h, RAW 264.7 cells were treated with 50 ng/mL of RANKL for 24 h. We found that the protein levels of LC3-II and Beclin1 were augmented after treatment with anisomycin, whereas SP600125 markedly decreased the expression of these proteins at the translational level (Figure 4g). Considering the suppression of autophagy in SFN-mediated anti-osteoclastogenesis, we suggest that SFN could inhibit autophagy via the suppression of JNK phosphorylation in the early period of osteoclastogenesis.

2.5. SFN Protected Against LPS-Induced Calvarial Bone Destruction in Mice

Mouse calvarial models were established to assess how well SFN could prevent pathological erosion. Microcomputed-tomography (CT) scanning and three-dimensional (3D) reconstruction revealed that LPS-injected calvarias had obvious surface erosion, while the simultaneous administration of SFN showed limited calvarial destruction (Figure 5a). Consistent with the microCT analysis, hematoxylin-and-eosin (HE) staining revealed the interruption of bone continuity in the LPS group, while the administration of SFN inhibited this effect. Therefore, we suggest that SFN could protect bone against destruction (Figure 5b). Trabecular bone volume (BV) /total volume (TV) and number (Tb.N) were higher in the SFN than in the LPS group, while trabecular separation (Tb.Sp) was clearly lower in the SFN group (Figure 5c). In addition, LPS-stimulated calvarias showed an increase in osteoclasts, while SFN significantly decreased the number of osteoclasts induced by LPS (Figure 5d). We also analyzed by immunohistochemistry (IHC) and immunofluorescence (IF) the expression of CTSK, an osteoclastic marker protein. CTSK staining was distributed at a higher intensity in the LPS group and was weakened in the SFN group. These results revealed that SFN could suppress osteoclastogenesis to prevent calvarial bone erosion.

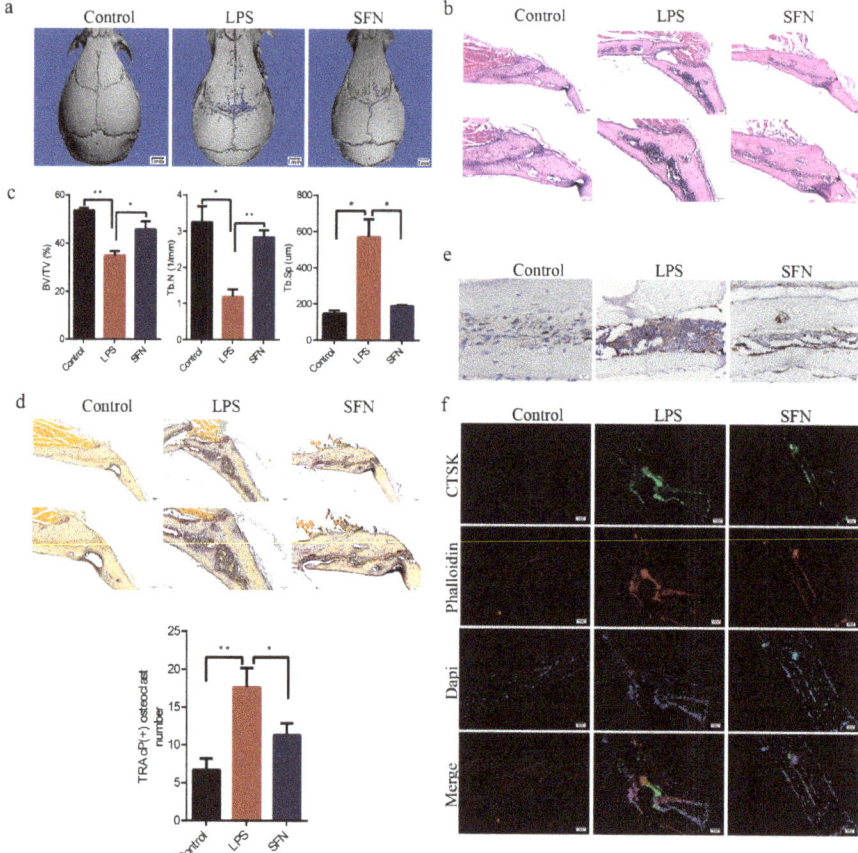

Figure 5. SFN protected against lipopolysaccharide (LPS)-induced calvarial bone destruction in mice. (**a**) Micro computed-tomography (CT) 3D reconstructed images. Calvarias were fixed, decalcified, dehydrated, embedded, and sectioned. (**b**) Representative hematoxylin-and-eosin (HE) staining images. (**c**) Microarchitectural parameter analysis: trabecular bone volume/total volume (BV/TV), trabecular number (Tb.N), and trabecular separation (Tb.Sp). (**d**) Representative tartrate-resistant acid phosphatase (TRAP) staining images showing osteoclastogenesis in each sample and corresponding statistics. (**e**) Representative IHC images locating CTSK. (**f**) Representative IF images of the distribution of CTSK (green). Phalloidin (red) indicates cytoskeleton and bone. DAPI (blue) was used to counterstain the nuclei. Values are mean ± SEM of three independent experiments; * $p < 0.05$, ** $p < 0.01$.

Subsequently, we examined the expression level of LC3 in vivo. As shown in Figure 6a, IHC analysis indicated that the expression of LC3 was induced in the LPS group compared with the control group in mice calvaria, while SFN suppressed this effect. IF analysis showed similar results (Figure 6b).

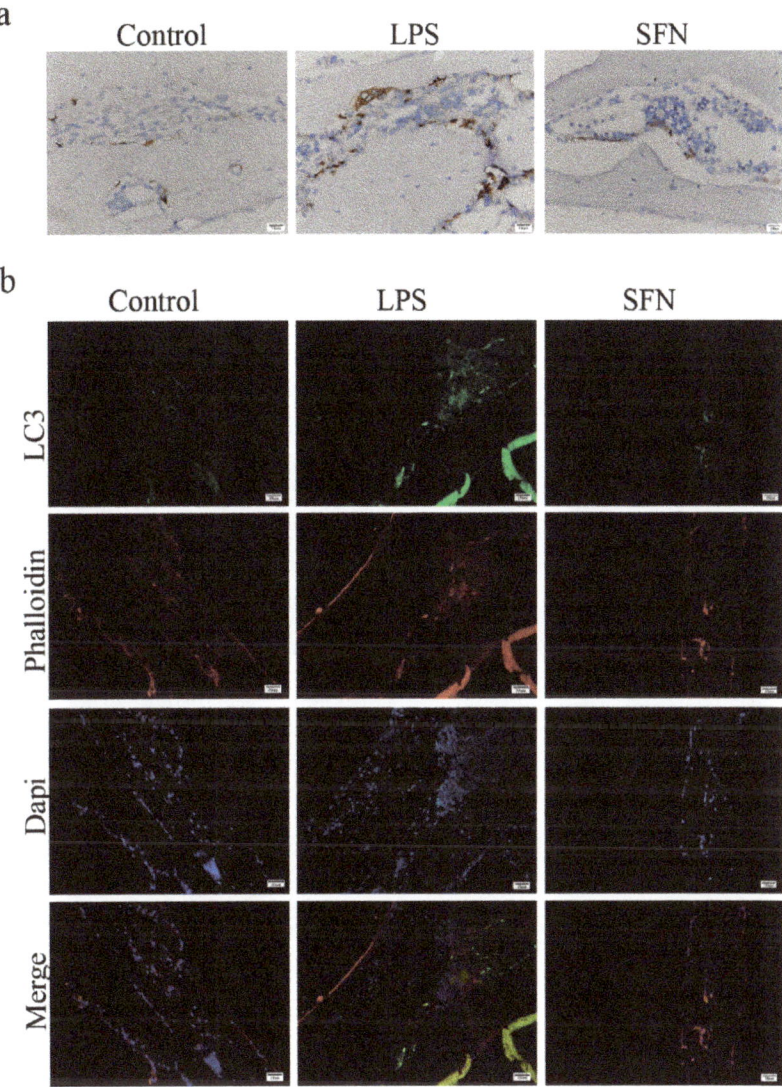

Figure 6. The administration of SFN attenuated autophagic LC3 expression in an LPS-induced mouse calvaria model. Calvarias were fixed, decalcified, dehydrated, embedded, and sectioned. (**a**) Representative IHC images locating LC3. (**b**) Representative IF images of the distribution of LC3 (green). Phalloidin (red) indicates cytoskeleton and bone. DAPI (blue) was used to counterstain the nuclei.

3. Discussion

SFN is an isothiocyanate derived from cruciferous vegetables. Over recent decades, extensive studies have focused on its antitumor activity at different tumor stages, from tumorigenesis to progression. As a pleiotropic compound, SFN is known to protect cells from deoxyribonucleic acid (DNA) damage and to modulate cell proliferation, apoptosis, angiogenesis, invasion, and metastasis in cancer [21–24]. Recently, it was reported that SFN could also be used to treat diseases associated with pathological bone resorption, such as bone metastasis in breast cancer, osteoporosis, and osteoarthritis [25–27]. In addition, Tomohiro Takagi et al. suggested that SFN plays a negative role in RANKL-induced osteoclastogenesis, but the underlying mechanisms need to be further investigated [10,28]. Autophagy is required during osteoclastogenesis and could be modulated by SFN. In this study, for the first time, we demonstrated that the suppression of the autophagy pathway is a significant mechanism by which SFN negatively regulated osteoclastogenesis.

SFN, a multipotent compound, has been reported to mediate autophagy in esophageal squamous cell carcinoma, pancreatic cancer, and neuronal cells [20,29,30]. SFN could inhibit autophagy in esophageal squamous cell carcinoma and renal tubule cells, while it promoted autophagy in neuronal cells [17–20]. As is well known, the level of autophagy varies in different cell types. We first investigated the effect of SFN on autophagy in pre-osteoclasts. Autophagy is characterized by three distinct stages: phagophore, autophagosome, and autolysosome. This process is regulated and executed by autophagy-related proteins such as the Atg system [31]. Beclin1 (Atg6) is responsible for forming an initial autophagosome complex; LC3 (Atg8), recruited by the Atg5–Atg12 complex, is essential for the formation and maturation of autophagosomes [32,33]. Herein, our data showed that SFN largely decreased the expression of these markers in RANKL-induced RAW264.7 cells, indicating that it interrupted autophagy. In addition, TEM observation showed that SFN also reduced the number of double-membraned autophagosomes. This confirmed that SFN could significantly inhibit autophagy in pre-osteoclasts.

Autophagy, which is involved in various biological cell processes such as proliferation, differentiation, and survival, principally plays an adaptive role in order to maintain organismal homeostasis [34–36]. Emerging evidence shows that autophagy might be a potential target for regulating osteoclastic differentiation. Particular conditions, such as starvation and high-glucose inflammation, could alter autophagy in pre-osteoclasts and influence osteoclastogenesis, leading to pathological changes [37–39]. Fortunately, autophagy can be pharmacologically regulated by certain agents. For instance, RAP, an inhibitor of mammalian target of rapamycin (mTOR) which negatively regulates autophagy, can induce autophagy [40]. Our data showed that SFN attenuated LC3-II accumulation in pre-osteoclasts, while RAP almost reversed this effect, thereby contributing to the recovery of osteoclastogenesis and the expression of osteoclast-related proteins (MMP9 and CTSK). Collectively, our data highlight the suppression of autophagy as a significant mechanism in SFN-mediated anti-osteoclastogenesis.

Mitogen-activated protein kinase (MAPK) signaling (involving JNK, p38, and extracellular signal-regulated kinase [ERK]) induced by RANKL is required for osteoclastic differentiation [41]. p38/ERK signaling is reported to play a dual role in the regulation of autophagy, acting as an activator or an inhibitor depending on the cellular context and particular conditions [42–44]. JNK signaling can induce autophagy and consequently contributes to cell survival, indicating a positive correlation between JNK signaling and autophagy [45]. Therefore, in this study, we focused on the role of the JNK signaling pathway in SFN-mediated anti-osteoclastogenesis. Our results showed that SFN treatment decreased JNK phosphorylation during osteoclastic differentiation. In addition, the activation of JNK signaling promoted the expression of autophagic proteins, while the inhibition of JNK phosphorylation suppressed such expression, which indicated that JNK signaling participated in the activation of autophagy during osteoclastogenesis. Considering the role of autophagy in SFN-mediated anti-osteoclastogenesis, we suggest that SFN could inhibit osteoclastogenesis by suppressing autophagy through the disruption of the JNK signaling pathway.

LPS can induce osteoclastic bone erosion by mediating the production of inflammatory factors such as interleukin-1 (IL-1) and tumor necrosis factor (TNF) [46,47]. In our study, we established a bone erosion model by subcutaneously injecting LPS into the center of mouse calvarias. Our results showed that SFN suppressed LPS-induced local calvarial erosion in vivo, supporting the possible application of SFN against diseases that feature inflammatory bone destruction. In addition, the number of osteoclasts was significantly reduced after treatment with SFN, indicating that osteoclasts were a target in SFN-mediated prevention of bone destruction. Furthermore, our data showed accumulation of LC3-II in LPS-stimulated calvarias.

Taken together, our results reveal for the first time that SFN inhibits RANKL-induced osteoclastogenesis in vitro and LPS-mediated bone erosion in vivo by suppressing autophagy. Furthermore, we demonstrated that the JNK signaling pathway participated in the activation of autophagy and SFN inhibited the phosphorylation of JNK in osteoclastogenesis. Taken together, we suggest that SFN could inhibit osteoclastogenesis by suppressing autophagy through the disruption of the JNK signaling pathway. Therefore, this study highlights SFN as a potent drug candidate for the prevention and treatment of bone loss-related diseases and shows that autophagy is a promising important mechanism of SFN-dependent anti-osteoclastogenic effect.

4. Materials and Methods

4.1. Reagents and Mice

RAW 264.7 cells were obtained from the China Center for Type Culture Collection (Shanghai, China). RANKL and M-CSF were purchased from R&D Systems (Minneapolis, MN, USA); α-modified Eagle's medium (MEM) was from Hyclone (UT, USA). Fetal bovine serum (FBS) was obtained from Gibco (Gaithersburg, MD, USA). SFN (Cat. No. S4441) was purchased from Sigma-Aldrich (St. Louis, MO, USA). The primary antibodies to Atg12–Atg5 (Cat.No. 4180), Beclin-1 (Cat.No. 3495), LC3 (Cat.No. 3868), phospho-JNK (Cat.No. 9255), and JNK (Cat.No. 9252) were obtained from Cell Signaling Technology (MA, USA). The primary antibody for MMP9 (Cat.No. 10375-2-AP) was from Proteintech (Hubei, China). The primary antibody for CTSK (Cat.No. AP7381) was obtained from Abcepta (Jiangsu, China). GAPDH Mouse Monoclonal Antibody (2B8) HRP-conjugated (Cat.No. PMK053) and (FITC)-conjugated secondary antibodies (Cat.No. PMK-014-093) were obtained from Bioprimacy (Hubei, China). C57/BL6 mice (female; 8-week-old) were purchased from Beijing Vital River Laboratory Animal Technology (Beijing, China). TRAP staining kit, LPS, and rapamycin were purchased from Sigma-Aldrich (MO, USA). BCA protein assay kit was from Thermo Fisher Scientific (Rockford, IL, USA). PCR-related agents were from Takara (Tokyo, Japan).

4.2. Preparation of Bone Marrow Macrophages (BMMs)

Fresh BMMs were flushed from the femur and tibia marrow of 5-week-old C57/BL6 female mice with α-MEM. The cells were slowly layered on a Ficoll-Hypaque gradient and then centrifuged at 440 g for 30 min at 4 °C. Cells at the gradient interface were classified as BMMs. BMMs were cultured in α-MEM containing 10% FBS and 30 ng/mL of M-CSF at 37 °C in a humidified atmosphere with 5% CO_2.

4.3. Proliferation Viability Assay

RAW 264.7 cells and BMMs (10^3 cells/well) were plated in 96-well plates in α-MEM with the indicated concentration (0, 0.5, 1, 2.5, 5, 10, 20 µM) of SFN. After 24 h of incubation, cell viability was measured using the CCK-8 assay according to the manufacturer's instructions. Absorbance was measured at 450 nm. Cell viability was expressed as a percentage of the control.

4.4. Osteoclast Differentiation Assay and Fibrous Actin (F-actin) Ring Observation

RAW264.7 cells (10^4/mL) and BMMs (10^5/mL) were plated in 96-well plate with α-MEM containing 10% FBS, 50 ng/mL RANKL, and varying concentrations of SFN. M-CSF (30 ng/mL) was used for BMMs growth. Every 2 days, the medium was removed and substituted with fresh medium supplemented with the appropriate treatment reagents.

Osteoclasts were observed after 5 days. Then, the cells were fixed with 4% PFA for 10 min and stained with the TRAP kit according to manufacturer's instructions. TRAP-positive cells with >3 nuclei/cell were counted as osteoclasts under a light microscope.

After induction for 5 days, osteoclasts were fixed with 4% PFA for 10 min, permeabilized with 0.5% Triton X-100 for 5 min, and incubated with TRITC–phalloidin for 30 min at room temperature. After washing with PBS thrice, the cells were stained with DAPI for 30 s and washed again, and images were captured under an inverted fluorescence microscope.

4.5. Immunofluorescence Analysis

Appropriately treated cells were fixed with 4% paraformaldehyde, permeabilized with 0.5% Triton X-100 for 5 min, and blocked in 2.5% BSA for 1 h at room temperature. Then, the cells were incubated with a primary antibody (CTSK and LC3) at 4 °C overnight, washed twice with PBS, and then incubated with FITC-conjugated anti-goat IgG (1:100) for 1 h at room temperature. After washing with PBS thrice, the cells were incubated with TRITC–phalloidin for 30 min, and the nuclei were stained with DAPI for 30 s at room temperature. Then, the cells were observed and photographed under a fluorescence microscope.

4.6. Transmission Electron Microscopy (TEM)

The autophagosomes were observed by TEM (HT7700, Japan). Briefly, appropriately treated cells were collected, centrifuged, washed, and fixed with 2.5% glutaraldehyde in 0.1 M phosphate buffer. After dehydration with an ethanol gradient, the cells were embedded in resin and sectioned. Ultrathin sections were stained with saturated solutions of uranyl acetate and observed by TEM.

4.7. Quantitative Real-Time PCR (qRT-PCR) Analysis

Total cellular RNA was extracted by Trizol reagent. Then, mRNA was reverse-transcribed with the PrimeScriptTMRT reagent Kit with gDNA Eraser. qRT-PCR was conducted with SYBR Premix Ex Taq™ II. The primer sequences were designed (Table 1). Glyceraldehyde-3-phosphate dehydrogenase (GAPDH) was used to normalize the data and compared them to control values.

Table 1. Sequences of quantitative PCR primers.

Genes	Forward Primer	Reverse Primer
MMP9	CAAAGACCTGAAAACCTCCAAC	GACTGCTTCTCTCCCATCATC
CTSK	GCTTGGCATCTTTCCAGTTTTA	CAACACTGCATGGTTCACATTA
Atg5	AGTCAAGTGATCAACGAAATGC	TATTCCATGAGTTTCCGGTTGA
Atg12	GCCTCGGAACAGTTGTTTATTT	CAGTTTACCATCACTGCCAAAA
Beclin1	TAATAGCTTCACTCTGATCGGG	CAAACAGCGTTTGTAGTTCTGA
LC3	CTGTCCTGGATAAGACCAAGTT	GTCTTCATCCTTCTCCTGTTCA
GAPDH	GAPDH primer F and R were purchased from Sangon Biotech (Shanghai, China)	

4.8. Western Blot Assay

Total proteins were extracted by radioimmunoprecipitation lysis buffer containing protease and phosphatase inhibitor, and the concentration was measured by the BCA assay. Western blot analyses were conducted after performing 10% SDS-PAGE, using 0.45 μM polyvinylidene fluoride membranes. Briefly, 30 μg of proteins were electrophoresed (60 V, 30 min; 110 V, 1 h) and subsequently transferred to the membranes (100 V, 53 min). After blocking with 5% BSA for 1 h at room temperature, the membranes were incubated with primary antibodies overnight at 4 °C. Following washing and incubating with horseradish peroxidase-conjugated anti-mouse/rabbit IgG for 1 h, the signals were detected by chemiluminescence (Bio-Rad, Singapore). The resulting protein levels were normalized to GAPDH level.

4.9. LPS-Mediated Calvarial Bone Erosion Experiment

The study was approved by the Ethics Committee of the Hospital of Stomatology at Wuhan University (approval numbers: S07918110A). All mice were raised in an SPF animal laboratory. C57/BL6 mice were divided into three groups (n = 3/group): control group, LPS group, and LPS plus SFN group. Mice were intraperitoneally injected with PBS or SFN (10 mg/kg body weight) the day before LPS treatment. Then, PBS or SFN was intraperitoneally injected 30 min before the daily LPS injection every other day for 6 days. LPS (10 mg/kg body weight) was injected at the midline of the calvaria located between the eyes and ears. All mice were sacrificed, and their calvarias were removed and fixed with 4% polyformaldehyde.

4.10. MicroCT Scanning and Analysis

Calvarias were scanned with a Skyscan 1176 microCT instrument (Broker, Kontich, Belgium) at a voxel size of 9 µM. The images were then reconstructed for the analysis. Bone histomorphometry analyses were performed with a microCT-associated software (Version 6.1, Scanco Medical AG, Wangen-Brüttisellen, Switzerland).

4.11. Bone Histological Analysis

After microCT, calvarias were sectioned for HE and TRAP staining. Briefly, calvarias were decalcified in 10% ethylenediaminetetraacetic acid, dehydrated in an alcohol gradient, embedded in paraffin, and sectioned. HE staining was conducted to show the erosion of bone. Then, parameters were evaluated including bone volume/total volume (BV/TV), trabecular number (Tb.N), trabecular thickness (Tb.Th), and trabecular separation (Tb.Sp). TRAP staining was performed according to manufacturer's instructions to identify osteoclasts on the bone surface.

4.12. Immunohistochemical and Immunofluorescence Analysis

After deparaffinization in xylene, rehydration, antigen retrieval with a gastric enzyme, and block of endogenous peroxidase activity with 3% hydrogen peroxide, the sections were blocked with bovine serum albumin for 1 h and subsequently incubated with primary antibodies against CTSK or LC3 overnight at 4 °C. Subsequently, the sections were incubated with the Polink-2 plus polymer HRP detection system (immunohistochemical) or (FITC)-conjugated secondary antibodies (immunofluorescent analysis) for 1 h at room temperature. After washing with PBS thrice, the sections were observed and photographed under a microscope.

4.13. Statistical Analysis

Each independent experiment included three separate replicates. All quantitative values were expressed as mean ± SEM. All statistical data were analyzed with SPSS software (Chicago, IL, USA). Statistical comparisons were performed by one-way ANOVA followed by the Student–Newman–Keul test. Values with * $p < 0.05$ or ** $p < 0.01$ were considered statistically significance.

5. Conclusions

SFN could inhibit osteoclastogenesis by suppressing autophagy through the disruption of the JNK signaling pathway. (Figure 7). Therefore, SFN has great potential for the prevention and treatment of excessive osteoclastic bone destruction due to its ability to suppress this pathway. SFN administration might therefore be a new strategy for preventing and treating bone loss-related diseases.

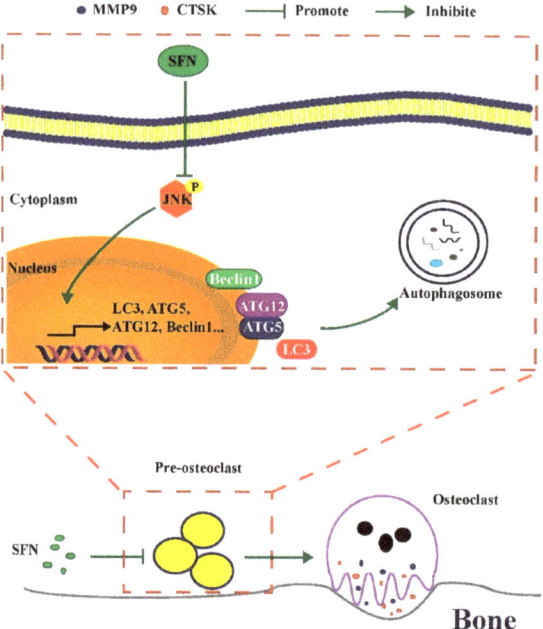

Figure 7. Schematic model of SFN-mediated anti-osteoclastogenesis. SFN inhibits the phosphorylation of JNK, decreasing the expression levels of autophagic proteins (Atg5, Atg12, Beclin1, and LC3). Subsequently, the level of osteoclastic autophagy is attenuated, which consequently suppresses osteoclastogenesis and bone erosion.

Author Contributions: Conceptualization, Y.J. and Z.S., Methodology, T.L., X.F., Y.L., Y.J., and Z.S.; data curation, T.L., X.F., Y.L. and Y.J.; formal analysis, T.L., X.F., Y.L., Y.J., and Z.S.; writing—original draft preparation, T.L., Y.L. and Y.J.; writing—review and editing, X.F., Y.J. and Z.S. All authors have read and agreed to the published version of the manuscript.

Funding: This research was funded by the National Natural Science Foundation of China (No. 81700772, No. 81672666, No. 81900987).

Institutional Review Board Statement: The study was conducted according to the guidelines of the Declaration of Helsinki, and approved by the Ethics Committee of the Hospital of Stomatology at Wuhan University (protocol code: S07918110A 201812).

Informed Consent Statement: Not applicable.

Data Availability Statement: The data presented in this study are available manuscript.

Conflicts of Interest: The authors declare no conflict of interest.

References

1. Inoue, K.; Hu, X.; Zhao, B. Regulatory network mediated by RBP-J/NFATc1-miR182 controls inflammatory bone resorption. *FASEB J. Off. Publ. Fed. Am. Soc. Exp. Biol.* **2020**, *34*, 2392–2407. [CrossRef] [PubMed]
2. Kittaka, M.; Yoshimoto, T.; Schlosser, C.; Rottapel, R.; Kajiya, M.; Kurihara, H.; Reichenberger, E.J.; Ueki, Y. Alveolar Bone Protection by Targeting the SH3BP2-SYK Axis in Osteoclasts. *J. Bone Miner. Res. Off. J. Am. Soc. Bone Miner. Res.* **2020**, *35*, 382–395. [CrossRef] [PubMed]
3. Zhang, X. Interactions between cancer cells and bone microenvironment promote bone metastasis in prostate cancer. *Cancer Commun.* **2019**, *39*, 76. [CrossRef] [PubMed]
4. Zhang, Y.; Talalay, P.; Cho, C.G.; Posner, G.H. A major inducer of anticarcinogenic protective enzymes from broccoli: Isolation and elucidation of structure. *Proc. Natl. Acad. Sci. USA* **1992**, *89*, 2399–2403. [CrossRef] [PubMed]
5. Houghton, C.A.; Fassett, R.G.; Coombes, J.S. Sulforaphane: Translational research from laboratory bench to clinic. *Nutr. Rev.* **2013**, *71*, 709–726. [CrossRef]

6. Ko, J.Y.; Choi, Y.J.; Jeong, G.J.; Im, G.I. Sulforaphane-PLGA microspheres for the intra-articular treatment of osteoarthritis. *Biomaterials* **2013**, *34*, 5359–5368. [CrossRef]
7. Patel, B.; Mann, G.E.; Chapple, S.J. Concerted redox modulation by sulforaphane alleviates diabetes and cardiometabolic syndrome. *Free Radic. Biol. Med.* **2018**, *122*, 150–160. [CrossRef]
8. Matsui, T.A.; Sowa, Y.; Yoshida, T.; Murata, H.; Horinaka, M.; Wakada, M.; Nakanishi, R.; Sakabe, T.; Kubo, T.; Sakai, T. Sulforaphane enhances TRAIL-induced apoptosis through the induction of DR5 expression in human osteosarcoma cells. *Carcinogenesis* **2006**, *27*, 1768–1777. [CrossRef]
9. Thaler, R.; Maurizi, A.; Roschger, P.; Sturmlechner, I.; Khani, F.; Spitzer, S.; Rumpler, M.; Zwerina, J.; Karlic, H.; Dudakovic, A.; et al. Anabolic and Antiresorptive Modulation of Bone Homeostasis by the Epigenetic Modulator Sulforaphane, a Naturally Occurring Isothiocyanate. *J. Biol. Chem.* **2016**, *291*, 6754–6771. [CrossRef]
10. Takagi, T.; Inoue, H.; Takahashi, N.; Katsumata-Tsuboi, R.; Uehara, M. Sulforaphane inhibits osteoclast differentiation by suppressing the cell-cell fusion molecules DC-STAMP and OC-STAMP. *Biochem. Biophys. Res. Commun.* **2017**, *483*, 718–724. [CrossRef]
11. Levine, B.; Kroemer, G. Autophagy in the pathogenesis of disease. *Cell* **2008**, *132*, 27–42. [CrossRef] [PubMed]
12. Dai, Y.; Hu, S. Recent insights into the role of autophagy in the pathogenesis of rheumatoid arthritis. *Rheumatology* **2016**, *55*, 403–410. [CrossRef] [PubMed]
13. Shen, G.; Ren, H.; Shang, Q.; Qiu, T.; Yu, X.; Zhang, Z.; Huang, J.; Zhao, W.; Zhang, Y.; Liang, D.; et al. Autophagy as a target for glucocorticoid-induced osteoporosis therapy. *Cell. Mol. Life Sci. CMLS* **2018**, *75*, 2683–2693. [CrossRef]
14. Abdelaziz, D.M.; Stone, L.S.; Komarova, S.V. Osteolysis and pain due to experimental bone metastases are improved by treatment with rapamycin. *Breast Cancer Res. Treat.* **2014**, *143*, 227–237. [CrossRef] [PubMed]
15. DeSelm, C.J.; Miller, B.C.; Zou, W.; Beatty, W.L.; van Meel, E.; Takahata, Y.; Klumperman, J.; Tooze, S.A.; Teitelbaum, S.L.; Virgin, H.W. Autophagy proteins regulate the secretory component of osteoclastic bone resorption. *Dev. Cell* **2011**, *21*, 966–974. [CrossRef]
16. Arai, A.; Kim, S.; Goldshteyn, V.; Kim, T.; Park, N.H.; Wang, C.Y.; Kim, R.H. Beclin1 Modulates Bone Homeostasis by Regulating Osteoclast and Chondrocyte Differentiation. *J. Bone Miner. Res. Off. J. Am. Soc. Bone Miner. Res.* **2019**, *34*, 1753–1766. [CrossRef]
17. Lee, J.H.; Jeong, J.K.; Park, S.Y. Sulforaphane-induced autophagy flux prevents prion protein-mediated neurotoxicity through AMPK pathway. *Neuroscience* **2014**, *278*, 31–39. [CrossRef]
18. Yang, F.; Wang, F.; Liu, Y.; Wang, S.; Li, X.; Huang, Y.; Xia, Y.; Cao, C. Sulforaphane induces autophagy by inhibition of HDAC6-mediated PTEN activation in triple negative breast cancer cells. *Life Sci.* **2018**, *213*, 149–157. [CrossRef]
19. Kim, J.H.; Kim, K.M.; Jeong, J.U.; Shin, J.H.; Shin, J.M.; Bang, K.T. Nrf2-heme oxygenase-1 modulates autophagy and inhibits apoptosis triggered by elevated glucose levels in renal tubule cells. *Kidney Res. Clin. Pract.* **2019**, *38*, 318–325. [CrossRef]
20. Zheng, K.; Ma, J.; Wang, Y.; He, Z.; Deng, K. Sulforaphane inhibits autophagy and induces exosome-mediated paracrine senescence via regulating mtor/tfe3. *Mol. Nutr. Food Res.* **2020**, *64*, e1901231. [CrossRef]
21. Tope, A.M.; Rogers, P.F. Evaluation of protective effects of sulforaphane on DNA damage caused by exposure to low levels of pesticide mixture using comet assay. *J. Environ. Sci. Health Part B Pestic. Food Contam. Agric. Wastes* **2009**, *44*, 657–662. [CrossRef] [PubMed]
22. Shan, Y.; Wang, X.; Wang, W.; He, C.; Bao, Y. p38 MAPK plays a distinct role in sulforaphane-induced up-regulation of ARE-dependent enzymes and down-regulation of COX-2 in human bladder cancer cells. *Oncol. Rep.* **2010**, *23*, 1133–1138. [CrossRef]
23. Lan, F.; Pan, Q.; Yu, H.; Yue, X. Sulforaphane enhances temozolomide-induced apoptosis because of down-regulation of miR-21 via Wnt/beta-catenin signaling in glioblastoma. *J. Neurochem.* **2015**, *134*, 811–818. [CrossRef] [PubMed]
24. Bertl, E.; Bartsch, H.; Gerhauser, C. Inhibition of angiogenesis and endothelial cell functions are novel sulforaphane-mediated mechanisms in chemoprevention. *Mol. Cancer Ther.* **2006**, *5*, 575–585. [CrossRef] [PubMed]
25. Pore, S.K.; Hahm, E.R.; Kim, S.H.; Singh, K.B.; Nyiranshuti, L.; Latoche, J.D.; Anderson, C.J.; Adamik, J.; Galson, D.L.; Weiss, K.R.; et al. A Novel Sulforaphane-Regulated Gene Network in Suppression of Breast Cancer-Induced Osteolytic Bone Resorption. *Mol. Cancer Ther.* **2020**, *19*, 420–431. [CrossRef] [PubMed]
26. Lin, H.; Wei, B.; Li, G.; Zheng, J.; Sun, J.; Chu, J.; Zeng, R.; Niu, Y. Sulforaphane reverses glucocorticoid-induced apoptosis in osteoblastic cells through regulation of the Nrf2 pathway. *Drug Design Dev. Ther.* **2014**, *8*, 973–982. [CrossRef]
27. Javaheri, B.; Poulet, B.; Aljazzar, A.; de Souza, R.; Piles, M.; Hopkinson, M.; Shervill, E.; Pollard, A.; Chan, B.; Chang, Y.M.; et al. Stable sulforaphane protects against gait anomalies and modifies bone microarchitecture in the spontaneous STR/Ort model of osteoarthritis. *Bone* **2017**, *103*, 308–317. [CrossRef]
28. Xue, P.; Hu, X.; Powers, J.; Nay, N.; Chang, E.; Kwon, J.; Wong, S.W.; Han, L.; Wu, T.H.; Lee, D.J.; et al. CDDO-Me, Sulforaphane and tBHQ attenuate the RANKL-induced osteoclast differentiation via activating the NRF2-mediated antioxidant response. *Biochem. Biophys. Res. Commun.* **2019**, *511*, 637–643. [CrossRef]
29. Naumann, P.; Fortunato, F.; Zentgraf, H.; Buchler, M.W.; Herr, I.; Werner, J. Autophagy and cell death signaling following dietary sulforaphane act independently of each other and require oxidative stress in pancreatic cancer. *Int. J. Oncol.* **2011**, *39*, 101–109. [CrossRef]
30. Jo, C.; Kim, S.; Cho, S.J.; Choi, K.J.; Yun, S.M.; Koh, Y.H.; Johnson, G.V.; Park, S.I. Sulforaphane induces autophagy through ERK activation in neuronal cells. *FEBS Lett.* **2014**, *588*, 3081–3088. [CrossRef]

31. Van Limbergen, J.; Stevens, C.; Nimmo, E.R.; Wilson, D.C.; Satsangi, J. Autophagy: From basic science to clinical application. *Mucosal Immunol.* **2009**, *2*, 315–330. [CrossRef] [PubMed]
32. Wirawan, E.; Lippens, S.; Vanden Berghe, T.; Romagnoli, A.; Fimia, G.M.; Piacentini, M.; Vandenabeele, P. Beclin1: A role in membrane dynamics and beyond. *Autophagy* **2012**, *8*, 6–17. [CrossRef] [PubMed]
33. Itoh, T.; Fujita, N.; Kanno, E.; Yamamoto, A.; Yoshimori, T.; Fukuda, M. Golgi-resident small GTPase Rab33B interacts with Atg16L and modulates autophagosome formation. *Mol. Biol. Cell* **2008**, *19*, 2916–2925. [CrossRef] [PubMed]
34. Mizushima, N.; Levine, B.; Cuervo, A.M.; Klionsky, D.J. Autophagy fights disease through cellular self-digestion. *Nature* **2008**, *451*, 1069–1075. [CrossRef] [PubMed]
35. Liu, K.; Ren, T.; Huang, Y.; Sun, K.; Bao, X.; Wang, S.; Zheng, B.; Guo, W. Apatinib promotes autophagy and apoptosis through VEGFR2/STAT3/BCL-2 signaling in osteosarcoma. *Cell Death Dis.* **2017**, *8*, e3015. [CrossRef]
36. Mizushima, N.; Levine, B. Autophagy in mammalian development and differentiation. *Nat. Cell Biol.* **2010**, *12*, 823–830. [CrossRef] [PubMed]
37. Zhao, S.J.; Kong, F.Q.; Cai, W.; Xu, T.; Zhou, Z.M.; Wang, Z.B.; Xu, A.D.; Yang, Y.Q.; Chen, J.; Tang, P.Y.; et al. GIT1 contributes to autophagy in osteoclast through disruption of the binding of Beclin1 and Bcl2 under starvation condition. *Cell Death Dis.* **2018**, *9*, 1195. [CrossRef] [PubMed]
38. Cai, Z.Y.; Yang, B.; Shi, Y.X.; Zhang, W.L.; Liu, F.; Zhao, W.; Yang, M.W. High glucose downregulates the effects of autophagy on osteoclastogenesis via the AMPK/mTOR/ULK1 pathway. *Biochem. Biophys. Res. Commun.* **2018**, *503*, 428–435. [CrossRef]
39. Ke, D.; Fu, X.; Xue, Y.; Wu, H.; Zhang, Y.; Chen, X.; Hou, J. IL-17A regulates the autophagic activity of osteoclast precursors through RANKL-JNK1 signaling during osteoclastogenesis in vitro. *Biochem. Biophys. Res. Commun.* **2018**, *497*, 890–896. [CrossRef]
40. Rubinsztein, D.C.; Gestwicki, J.E.; Murphy, L.O.; Klionsky, D.J. Potential therapeutic applications of autophagy. *Nat. Rev. Drug Discov.* **2007**, *6*, 304–312. [CrossRef]
41. Lee, K.; Chung, Y.H.; Ahn, H.; Kim, H.; Rho, J.; Jeong, D. Selective Regulation of MAPK Signaling Mediates RANKL-dependent Osteoclast Differentiation. *Int. J. Biol. Sci.* **2016**, *12*, 235–245. [CrossRef]
42. Zhou, J.; Fan, Y.; Zhong, J.; Huang, Z.; Huang, T.; Lin, S.; Chen, H. TAK1 mediates excessive autophagy via p38 and ERK in cisplatin-induced acute kidney injury. *J. Cell. Mol. Med.* **2018**, *22*, 2908–2921. [CrossRef] [PubMed]
43. He, Y.; She, H.; Zhang, T.; Xu, H.; Cheng, L.; Yepes, M.; Zhao, Y.; Mao, Z. p38 MAPK inhibits autophagy and promotes microglial inflammatory responses by phosphorylating ULK1. *J. Cell Biol.* **2018**, *217*, 315–328. [CrossRef] [PubMed]
44. Bryant, K.L.; Stalnecker, C.A.; Zeitouni, D.; Klomp, J.E.; Peng, S.; Tikunov, A.P.; Gunda, V.; Pierobon, M.; Waters, A.M.; George, S.D.; et al. Combination of ERK and autophagy inhibition as a treatment approach for pancreatic cancer. *Nat. Med.* **2019**, *25*, 628–640. [CrossRef]
45. Liu, G.Y.; Jiang, X.X.; Zhu, X.; He, W.Y.; Kuang, Y.L.; Ren, K.; Lin, Y.; Gou, X. ROS activates JNK-mediated autophagy to counteract apoptosis in mouse mesenchymal stem cells in vitro. *Acta Pharmacol. Sin.* **2015**, *36*, 1473–1479. [CrossRef]
46. Suda, K.; Woo, J.T.; Takami, M.; Sexton, P.M.; Nagai, K. Lipopolysaccharide supports survival and fusion of preosteoclasts independent of TNF-alpha, IL-1, and RANKL. *J. Cell. Physiol.* **2002**, *190*, 101–108. [CrossRef]
47. Wu, H.; Hu, B.; Zhou, X.; Zhou, C.; Meng, J.; Yang, Y.; Zhao, X.; Shi, Z.; Yan, S. Artemether attenuates LPS-induced inflammatory bone loss by inhibiting osteoclastogenesis and bone resorption via suppression of MAPK signaling pathway. *Cell Death Dis.* **2018**, *9*, 498. [CrossRef]

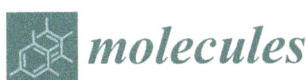

Article

Alginic Acid from *Padina boryana* Abate Particulate Matter-Induced Inflammatory Responses in Keratinocytes and Dermal Fibroblasts

Thilina U. Jayawardena [1], K. K. Asanka Sanjeewa [1], Lei Wang [1,2], Won-Suk Kim [3], Tae-Ki Lee [4], Yong-Tae Kim [5,*] and You-Jin Jeon [1,2,*]

1. Department of Marine Life Sciences, Jeju National University, Jeju 690-756, Korea; tuduwaka@gmail.com (T.U.J.); asanka.sanjeewa001@gmail.com (K.K.A.S.); comeonleiwang@163.com (L.W.)
2. Marine Science Institute, Jeju National University, Jeju Self-Governing Province 63333, Korea
3. Department of Pharmaceutical Engineering, Silla University, Busan 46958, Korea; wskim@silla.ac.kr
4. Department of Hotel Cuisine & Baking, Jeonnam State University, Jeonnam 57337, Korea; tglee@dorip.ac.kr
5. Department of Food Science and Biotechnology, Kunsan National University, Gunsan 54150, Korea
* Correspondence: kimyt@kunsan.ac.kr (Y.-T.K.); youjin2014@gmail.com (Y.-J.J.); Tel.: +82-064-754-3475 (Y.-J.J.)

Academic Editor: Francesco Maione
Received: 2 November 2020; Accepted: 4 December 2020; Published: 5 December 2020

Abstract: Particulate matter (PM) is a significant participant in air pollution and is hence an inducer of serious health issues. This study aimed to evaluate the dust protective effects of alginate from *Padina boryana* (PBA) via inflammatory-associated pathways to develop anti-fine dust skincare products. In between the external and internal environments, the skin is considered to be more than a physical barrier. It was observed that PM stimulates inflammation in the skin via activating NF-κB and MAPK pathways. The potential of PBA to inhibit the studied pathways were evident. The metal ion content of PM was considerably reduced by PBA and thus attributed to its chelation ability. Current research demonstrated the potential of *P. boryana* alginates to be implemented as a protective barrier against inflammation imposed with heavy metal and bacterial-derived endotoxin bound to the surface of the PM. Concisely, the results suggest that the bioactive components derived from the brown algae *Padina boryana* increased the cellular resistance to PM-stimulated inflammation-driven skin damage.

Keywords: *Padina boryana*; alginic acid; particulate matter; skin; inflammation; chelation

1. Introduction

Air pollution is supported via particulate matter (PM) and is comprised of a heterogeneous mixture of components. These include volatile particles, organic matter, metals, and ionic material [1]. The composition of the mixture varies depending on the source of generation. Both anthropogenic and natural sources contribute to this phenomenon. The PM could cause health issues due to its accumulation in the atmosphere. Pulmonary toxicity, as well as skin irritations, are possible considering their constituents. Several studies have been conducted regarding PMs' effect on the respiratory system. Fernando et al. (2017) report on the influence of ERM-CZ100 (organic constituent fine dust) and ERM-CZ120 (inorganic constituents) on RAW macrophages and inflammation induction [2]. RAW macrophages were further assessed against CRM No.28, considering pulmonary issues and taking it as a model by Jayawardena et al. (2018) [3].

When considering the literature, two distinct sources of PM in the induction of inflammation are emphasized. Several reports account for the source to be the transition metal ion content which influences the inflammation via an oxidative stress pathway. The oxidative stress arises due to the Fenton chemistry pathway-implicated radicals and are made responsible by some authors [4,5]. The oxidative mechanism is most applicable to the smaller sized PM, in which it possesses a higher surface area and a large number of particles. These have been evident to be higher in toxicity compared to their larger counterparts [6]. The second suggestion is the bacteria-derived endotoxin bound to the surface of the particle causing the inflammation stimulation [7,8].

The skin is the outermost barrier of the body and is susceptible to alien factors and these could cause inflammatory disorders. For this reason, anti-inflammatory agents applicable to the skin are important. A distinct role of the skin is to provide immunity against foreign matter and to become a critical point between the external and internal environments. Even though it can individually act as an immunological organ, its effective function is observed with the resources supported by the immune system. A major component of the skin is its outermost keratinocyte layer. It performs immune function via the production of cytokines and by responding to cytokines. The dermal component of the skin contains fibroblasts. This is traditionally not considered a component of the immune system. But recent research suggests the crosstalk between the keratinocytes and the fibroblasts significantly contributes to maintaining the homeostasis of the skin immune system [9]. These generate secondary cytokines such as IL-6. It was reported during wound healing that the dermal fibroblasts contribute as a major source of keratinocyte growth factor (KGF) [10].

The present study was conducted focusing on the effect of PM (CRM no. 28) on the skin cells. Selectively, the keratinocytes and the inner layer fibroblasts extracted alginic acid from *P. boryana* to inhibit the inflammation-induced via PM. Marine algal polysaccharides have received much attention due to their high availability and ability in sustainable use as well as their biocompatibility. Alginate, which is a polymer comprised mainly of β-D-mannuronic acid and α-L-guluronic acid, forms hydrogels, chelate metals and performs anti-inflammatory, anti-oxidant properties [11,12]. In this study, researchers believe that the effect of transition metal ions and bacteria-derived endotoxin bound to the surface of the PM causes inflammation. Therefore, it aims to evaluate the potential of *P. boryana*-derived alginate to counteract the effect caused by PM. This could open up the sustainable usage of naturally derived phytochemicals as candidates for formulating skin care products against PM-induced skin damage.

2. Results

2.1. Proximate Composition and Chemical Composition

The proximate composition results provide a better understanding of the nutritional components of the selected seaweed. Accordingly, *P boryana* consists of a higher amount of crude polysaccharides (57.87 ± 0.63). Crude proteins are also present in the sample (16.36 ± 0.32). The ash content was reported as 14.14 ± 0.72, symbolizing higher mineral content due to its natural habitat. The moisture content was 6.2 ± 0.54, while the lipid content was reported as the lowest (1.03 ± 0.25). Table 1 indicates the chemical composition of the purified alginate (PBA).

Table 1. Chemical composition of purified alginic acid from *P. boryana*.

Composition	Content (%)
Polysaccharide	79.84 ± 1.32
Ash	3.42 ± 0.56
Protein	1.22 ± 0.18
Polyphenol	2.17 ± 0.69
Yield	16.85 ± 0.32

All results expressed as means ± SE, based on triplicated trials.

2.2. Structural Characterization of PBA

The structure of the PBA was characterized by FTIR analysis (Figure 1d). Distinct peak patterns were referred to with the commercial sodium alginate available. The prominent peaks were also referred to with the early reports published. It was confirmed that PBA well aligns with the commercial level alginic acid. O-H stretching vibrations were observed in the range of 3425 cm^{-1}. Carboxylic group stretching vibrations were visible in 1680 cm^{-1} and 1420 cm^{-1} [13]. Furthermore, these data were referred to with the pre-defined spectral features obtained via computational quantum chemistry calculations. The constructed disaccharides were analyzed via Gaussian software to generate Cartesian coordinates. These were optimized using semi-empirical methods. This was subjected to the harmonic vibrational calculations with time-dependent density functional quantum chemical (DFT) theory using the B3LYP level, 6–31G (d,p) basis set. Figure 1a–c indicate the resulting structure geometry of dimers constructed, their free energies calculated and the vibrational spectroscopy obtained.

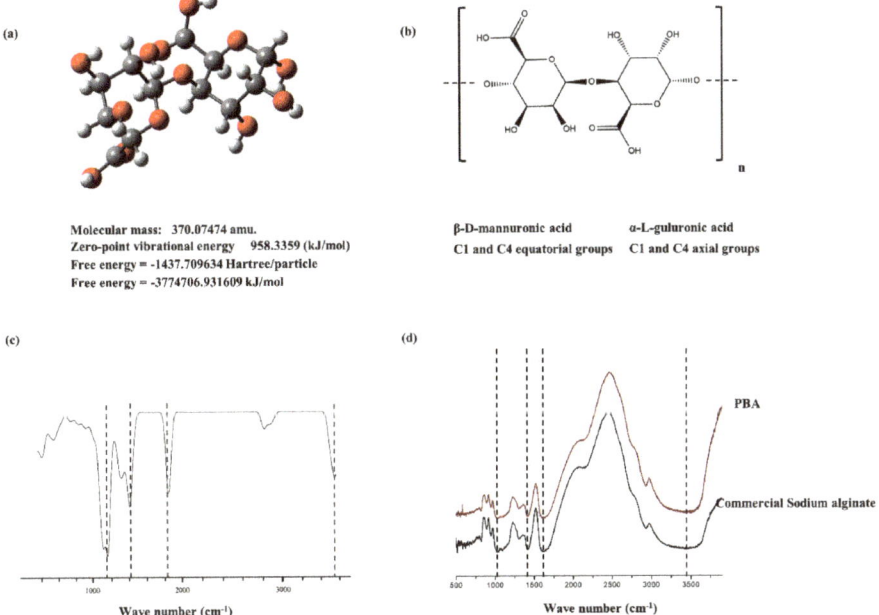

Figure 1. Characterization of alginic acid. (**a**) Structure of constructed dimeric unit of alginic acid 3D, (**b**) Skeletal formula of the alginic acid dimer with its monomeric units representing stereochemistry in 2D, (**c**) Vibrational spectra of alginic acid dimer calculated and constructed with density functional quantum chemical (DFT) calculations using B3LYP level, 6–31G (d,p) basis set, (**d**) FTIR spectroscopic analysis of PBA compared with commercial sodium alginate.

2.3. Potential of PBA to Reduce PM-Stimulated Inflammatory Responses in Keratinocytes and Fibroblasts

The treatment of PBA resulted in the recovery of the cell viability, which was downregulated due to the stimulation of PM in keratinocytes and fibroblasts. ROS level in PM-stimulated keratinocytes was significantly declined in the 50, 100, 200 µg/mL concentrations where 25 µg/mL of PBA was not effective (Figure 2b). The cell viability was significantly affected due to PM stimulation and was successfully restored by the PBA treatment (Figure 2a). Fibroblasts expressed a similar trend (Figure 2c,d). Accordingly, with the results, concentrations except for 25 µg/mL were selected for subsequent experiments. NO levels or iNOS production was not evident during the study. A significant upregulation of the pro-inflammatory mediators including PGE$_2$ (Figure 3d) and its modulator COX-2 was observed with the treatment against PM (Figure 4e,f). This was successfully downregulated via the treatment of PBA in keratinocytes. A similar trend was evident with the pro-inflammatory cytokines IL-1β and IL-6 (Figure 3a–c).

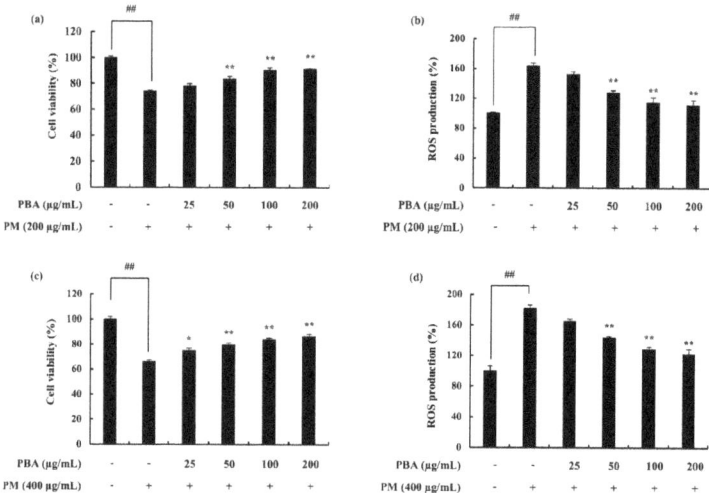

Figure 2. (a) PBA cytoprotective effect evaluation, (b) ROS production inhibition effect of PBA, in PM-induced keratinocytes, (c) Cytoprotective ability of PBA, (d) ROS production inhibition effect of PBA, in PM-induced HDF. Triplicated experiments were used to evaluate the data. Results are represented as mean ± SD; * $p < 0.05$, ** $p < 0.01$. (# denotes significance compared to control while * represents significance compared to the PM-treated group).

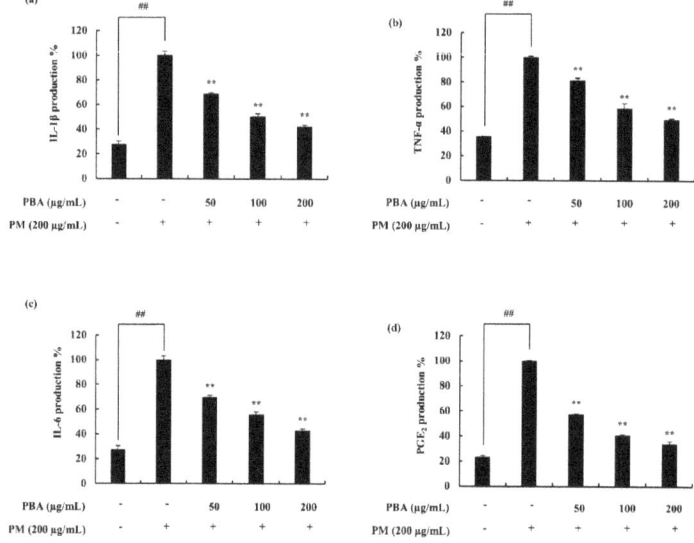

Figure 3. Effect of PBA on the keratinocytes and its production of inflammatory mediators (PGE2) including cytokines (IL-1β, IL-6, and TNF-α). Culture supernatants of RAW 264.7 cells after successful treatment of PM were used to quantify the inflammatory cytokines and PGE2. Triplicated experiments were used to evaluate the data and the mean value is expressed with ± SD. ** $p < 0.01$. (# denotes significance compared to control while * represents significance compared to PM treated group).

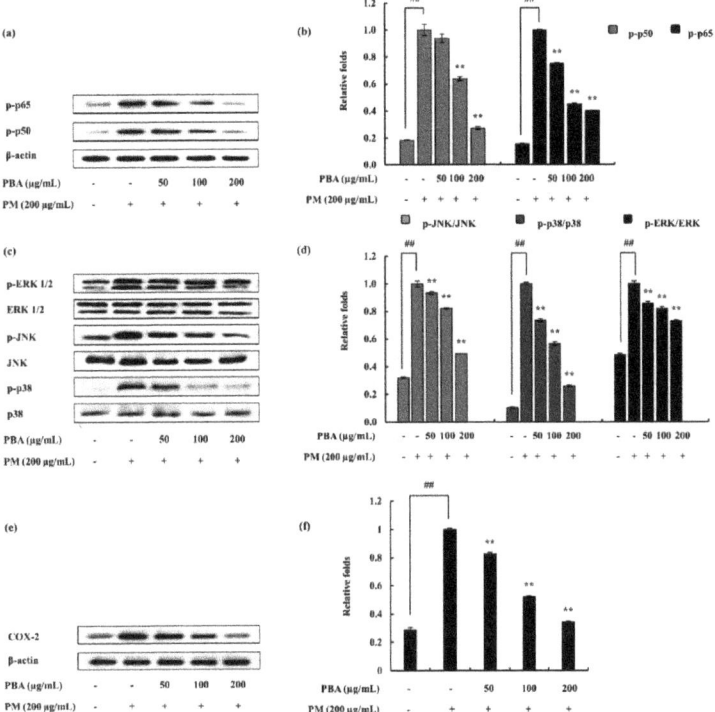

Figure 4. Effect of PBA on keratinocytes to inhibit NF-κB-associated signals, MAPK pathway molecules, and COX-2. (**a**) p50 and p65 in the cytosol, (**c**) p38, JNK and ERK, (**e**) COX-2 data determined using Western blotting. Quantitative data were analyzed using ImageJ software (**b**,**d**,**f**). Results are expressed as the mean ± SD of three separate experiments. ** $p < 0.01$. (# denotes significance compared to control while * represents significance compared to the PM-treated group).

2.4. Potential of PBA to Abate PM-Induced Inflammatory Responses via NF-κB and MAPK Pathways in Keratinocytes

In the process of evaluating the activity of PBA as an anti-inflammatory agent, this research subsequently assessed whether or not the inhibition of inflammation responses are mediated via the NF-κB and MAPK pathways. The PM-induced phosphorylation of p38, ERK1/2, and JNK MAPKs in keratinocytes were considered via Western blotting. As illustrated (Figure 4a–d), PM encouraged the phosphorylation of NF-κB and MAPK mediators. PBA treatment (50, 100, and 200 μg/mL) gradually down-regulated the phosphorylation of p38, ERK1/2, and JNK. The results suggesting that PBA acts effectively upon p38 though all the MAPKs were significantly inhibited. Cytosolic p-50 and p-65 mediators were observed to be phosphorylated against PM induction and were successfully downregulated via the PBA treatment.

2.5. Effect of PBA on PM-Induced NF-κB and MAPK Proteins in Fibroblasts

As illustrated in Figure 5a,b, cytosolic p50 and p65 phosphorylation were stimulated by PM. This was effectively and dose-dependently reduced by the PBA treatment. To determine fibroblasts, PM-induced inflammation is mediated via the MAPK pathway and to evaluate the effect of PBA, pathway proteins were assessed via Western blotting. Phosphorylation of JNK, p38, and ERK1/2 was upregulated via PM stimulation. However, PBA (50, 100, 200 μg/mL) reduced MAPKs in PM activated fibroblasts. Comparatively, PBA to act upon JNK was observed among the PBA's significant potential.

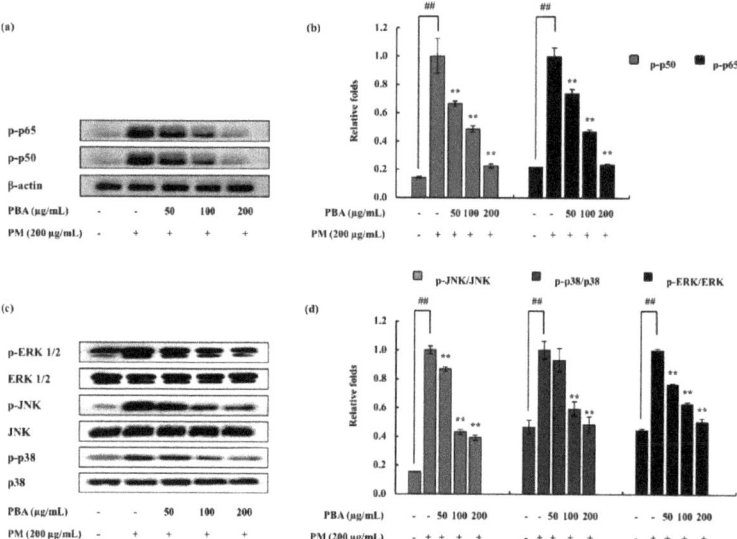

Figure 5. PM-induced HDF cells and co-treatment with PBA. (**a**) p50 and p65 in the cytosol, (**c**) p38, JNK, and ERK, data determined using Western blotting. Quantitative data were analyzed using ImageJ software (**b**,**d**). Results are expressed as the mean ± SD of three separate experiments. ** $p < 0.01$. (# denotes significance compared to control while * represents significance compared to PM treated group).

2.6. Keratinocytes Stimulated with PM and Treated with PBA; Compositional Analysis

To analyze the metal ion composition of the samples which were treated with PBA following stimulation of keratinocytes with PM, ICP-OES was used. Several metal ions including Mg, Al, K, Ca, Fe, Mn, Cu, Sr, Ba, and Pb were observed to be significantly increased in the PM-treated group (Table 2). The record highest was Pb, while Cu remained the lowest. Our experiment suggested that, with the treatment of PBA, the metal concentrations downregulated dose-dependently. Substantial cutbacks were observed in Pb and Cu, followed by Sr, Ba, and Mg.

Table 2. Metal composition analysis.

	Control	PM	PM + PBA (50)	PM + PBA (100)	PM + PBA (200)
Mg	54.67 ± 1.47	128.53 ± 2.51	137.44 ± 4.97	101.46 ± 6.14	84.95 ± 2.11
Al	0.91	125.08 ± 9.1	119.33 ± 8.21	79.31 ± 5.12	56.92 ± 3.52
K	452.98 ± 14.56	437.37 ± 18.47	522.65 ± 20.22	504.28 ± 31.58	466.12 ± 19.68
Ca	224.44 ± 12.56	344.37 ± 10.45	385.24 ± 9.56	321.07 ± 5.36	256.44 ± 7.48
Fe	ND	174.50 ± 4.57	163.62 ± 6.89	106.52 ± 7.58	77.27 ± 5.23
Mn	ND	80.2 ± 2.47	68.4 ± 3.93	45.2 ± 2.42	32.1 ± 2.9
Cu	ND	20.1 ± 1.44	10.84 ± 1.89	6.53 ± 2.01	ND
Sr	0.71	42.18 ± 1.32	31.94 ± 2.58	21.37 ± 1.22	11.86 ± 1.09
Ba	ND	92.92 ± 6.33	72.56 ± 4.39	51.99 ± 3.15	20.41 ± 1.02
Pb	ND	241.74 ± 12.46	168.41 ± 14.15	102.47 ± 6.27	58.96 ± 3.68

All results expressed as means ± SE, based on triplicated trials. ND—Not detected. Mg; Magnesium, Al; Aluminium, K; Potassium, Ca; Calcium, Fe; Iron, Mn; Manganese, Cu; Copper, Sr; Strontium, Ba; Barium, Pb; Lead.

3. Discussion

Air pollution due to particulate matter has become a major concern in recent years. The East Asian region is reported to be highly affected. Contemporary publications suggest that particulate matter exposure is related to respiratory complications, allergic reactions, and inflammatory skin conditions.

This is a complex mixture of different components. It includes various dust types such as tobacco smoke, pollen, and exhaust gas from traffic emissions [14].

The present study evaluated the physical parameters of the PM via the SEM and continued on inflammatory effects in keratinocytes and fibroblasts. Alginic acid was purified from *P. boryana* and its ability to inhibit PM-stimulated inflammation was evaluated. As indicated in Table 1, the purified alginate (PBA) consisted of a comparatively high amount of polysaccharide and traceable amounts of proteins and polyphenols. This supports the efficient purification of alginate. Initially, the *P. boryana* powder was depigmented using both hexane and 95% ethanol. This ensures the removal of lipids, pigments both non-polar and polar, as well as polyphenols reasonably. It is rather difficult to remove the effect of polyphenolic compounds due to their strong dipolar moments between polysaccharides. The usage of 10% formaldehyde in ethanol facilitates the formation of a phenolic polymer which in result lowers the solubility of phenolic substances and hence could be removed from the sample [15]. The alginic acid is presented in brown seaweed, prominently as calcium salt, but other forms such as magnesium, potassium, and sodium salts are also available in minute amounts. In this particular method, the alginates in the seaweed are converted into soluble alginate via alkaline treatment. Before this step to increase the extraction efficacy, the sample is acid washed with dilute mineral acid (HCl). The calcium ions are exchanged with the protons and at the same time, mineral acid removes the acid-soluble phenolic compounds. The following filtration step guarantees the removal of insoluble seaweed residues and the subsequent continuation of the sodium alginate solution. Recovering sodium alginate from this solution is not practical via evaporation due to its low concentration. Hence, the alginates can be precipitated as its calcium salt through the addition of $CaCl_2$. The recovered alginates in the form of calcium alginates are then converted into alginic acid by the addition of dilute mineral acid. Finally, the alginic acid is further converted into sodium alginate using NaOH and the pH is uplifted to a neutral value [16]. The dialysis process removes excess ions. Alginic acid is mainly based on two monomeric units. B-D-mannuronic acid and α-L-guluronic acid, which are respectively designated as M and G blocks. The polymer is formed via joining the monomers at C-1 and C-4 positions. The polymer chain consists of three kinds of molecules: M blocks based entirely on β-D-mannuronic acid, G blocks derived from α-L-guluronic acid, and MG blocks including interchanging units of the two acids. The proportion of the three types of blocks determine the physical properties of alginates [17–19]. Donati et al. (2003) reported that the monomer sequence is possible to differ not only among different species but also in variable tissues in the same species [20].

The chemical characterization of PBA is in good argument with the sodium alginate commercial sample. The study referred to several previously published data along with the analyzed data of this research. The broad peak at the 3425 cm^{-1} indicates the O-H stretching vibrations of the hydrogen bonds. The asymmetric O-C-O stretching vibrations of the carboxylate groups are represented via the 1680 cm^{-1} intense peak, while symmetric vibrations are indicated via the 1420 cm^{-1} intense band. Furthermore, a weak band at the 1035 cm^{-1} assigns C-O and C-C stretching vibrations in the pyranose ring. The anomeric carbons are represented in the 750–950 cm^{-1} region [13]. The interaction between metal ions and carboxylate groups in alginates in FTIR representation is further discussed in the report published by Papageorgiou et al. (2010) [21]

In between the external and internal environments, the skin is considered to be more than a physical barrier. A crucial role of the skin is to provide immune functions. It is suggested to function as a semiautonomous immunological organ. As the keratinocytes are the outermost layer of the skin, it is regularly used to assess the effect of the irritants in the dermatology. These cells participate in immune responses via the production of cytokines against the inflammatory events. This function widely contributes to the skin's function as an immune organ. Keratinocytes can transfer stimuli into signals and successively to the other members of the skin immune system [9].

Heavy metal contamination is associated with biosorption, accumulation and toxicity; thus it has become a major concern that causes both environmental and health issues. The metal ion concentrations (Pb, Ca, Sr, Ba, and Mg) were significantly down-regulated dose-dependently via the treatment of

PBA. Earlier reports by Schaumann et al. (2004) indicate that transition metal ions (Zn, Cu, and Cd) are responsible for the cause of inflammation via inducing oxidant generation. The report further illustrates that the increased concentrations of metal ions in the particulate matter contributes to the oxidative stress and hence promotes the activation of several transcription factors leading to discharge of pro-inflammatory mediators [22]. Heavy metals can be removed from a system using vivid methods according to Wang et al. (2011), one of them being the chemical precipitation of metal ions using potassium/sodiumthiocarbonate, sodium-dimethyl dithiocarbamate, and tri mercapto triazine. Some other methods are sulfide precipitation, adsorption, filtration using membranes, and ion exchange. Furthermore, the chelation of heavy metals using biopolymers now receiving much attention among the scientific community [23,24]. This follows the formation of complexes between the biopolymers and the metal ions. The affinity is influenced by several factors including the structure of the polymer and ionic charge, electronic configuration, and the coordination number of the metal ion [25]. Alginic acid as well as its derivatives are considered as capable polysaccharides in metal chelation [26]. As alginic acid contains carboxylic groups, metal carboxylate coordination can take place. Four distinct metal-carboxylate coordination types are described by Papageorgiou et al. (2010): ionic uncoordinated, unidentate coordination, bidentate chelating coordination, and bidentate bridging [21]. The structure of the alginic acid consists of M and G blocks and this influences the metal ion chelation. The "egg-box" model proposed by Grant et al. (1973) describes alginates as preferring to bind with divalent cations [27,28].

The inflammation process is regulated via complex signaling pathways. The process possibly initiated and developed involving several pro-inflammatory cytokines. The cytokines addressed in this research were downregulated upon the PBA treatment. Among them, IL-6 indicated significant downregulation compared to others. Furthermore, PGE_2, another inflammatory mediator, was also declined. The COX-2 downregulation supported the PGE_2 decrement as it is an enzyme involved in the generation of PGE_2 via the arachidonic pathway. Downstream signals in the NF-κB and MAPK pathways were also investigated. Kim et al. (2014) address these signals as important regulators in inflammation studies focusing on cytokine-induced keratinocytes and skin. It reports the inhibition of JAK/STAT, NF-κB, and PI3K/Akt signaling to result in pro-inflammatory mediator, enzyme, cytokine, and chemokine inhibition [29]. The NF-κB dimers residing in the cytoplasm interact with the inhibitory proteins, IκBs. With the stimulation mainly due to pro-inflammatory cytokines, the IκB kinase (IKK) is activated and phosphorylation is initiated (p50 and p65). Hence, these are translocated to the nucleus to activate gene transcription. IKK is a complex formed from three distinct subunits with different functions: IKKα, IKKβ, and IKKγ. Among these, IKKβ is essential in NF-κB activation while IKKα is involved in the signal development process [30]. The present study indicated a significant downstream in the NF-κB-associated signals, confirming the effect of PBA against the stimulation of PM. Similarly, MAPK signals were also down-regulated, convincing the potential of PBA against the PM. MAPKs play an important role in inflammation via activating pro-inflammatory cytokines and chemokines [31,32]. These are a family of serine/threonine protein kinases that mediate biological processes in response to external stress signals. Out of the three main MAPKs (p38, JNK, and ERK), p38 MAPK signals are especially involved in the regulation of the synthesis of inflammatory regulators. These factors make MAPKs a potential target in anti-inflammatory therapeutics [33].

The study enhances the understanding of cellular mechanisms related to PM-induced inflammation that could result in effective drug development. PBA could be used as a potential candidate for the treatment of PM-stimulated skin damage. This simple model is applicable to evaluate the further effects of PM in the skin, such as intracellular and intercellular molecular cascades that lead to skin damage. As the skin is comprised of multiple layers of cellular components, the impact of the inflammation of the outermost layer can be assessed on other layers. Current research demonstrated the potential of *P. boryana* alginates to be implemented as a protective barrier against inflammation imposed with heavy metal and bacterial-derived endotoxins bound to the surface of the PM. Furthermore, in vivo studies could provide information concerning application methods, frequency of usage, and complex biological attributes accompanied.

4. Materials and Methods

4.1. Materials

The certified reference material, CRM No. 28 (Urban aerosols), was purchased from the Centre for Environmental Measurement and Analysis, National Institute for Environmental Studies, Ibaraki, Japan. The cell lines required for the experiments, HaCaT cells, and the human dermal fibroblast (HDF) were purchased from the Korean Cell line Bank (KCLB, Seoul, Korea). Dulbecco's modified Eagle's medium (DMEM), fetal bovine serum (FBS), and antibiotics (penicillin and streptomycin) for growth medium were purchased from the GIBCO Inc. (Grand Island, NY, USA). 3-(4,5-dimethylthiazol-2-yl)-2,5-diphenyltetrazolium bromide (MTT) was obtained from Sigma-Aldrich (St. Louis, MO, USA). Antibodies used in the Western blot analysis were from Santa Cruz Biotechnology (Santa Cruz, CA, USA). The cytokine kits used in the experiments were purchased from eBioscience (San Diego, CA, USA), R&D Systems (Minneapolis, MN, USA), BD Opteia (San Diego, CA, USA), and Invitrogen (Carlsbad, CA, USA). All the organic solvents used in the experiments were of analytical grade unless specified and were purchased from Sigma-Aldrich.

4.2. Alginic Acid Purification from P. boryana

P. boryana samples were collected from the coastal areas of Fulhadhoo Island, the Maldives. Samples were immediately washed with running water to remove salts and debris. The sample identification was assisted by Jeju Biodiversity Research Institute. Sample repositories were kept in the Laboratory of Marine Bioresource Technology at Jeju National University. Samples were then lyophilized and ground into a fine powder. Alginic acid extraction followed the method described by Fernando et al. (2018) with some minor modifications [28]. An initial depigmentation was carried out, first with hexane, and was followed by 95% ethanol. This was then soaked in 10% formaldehyde (in ethanol) for 10 h, filtered, and thoroughly washed with 95% ethanol to remove residual formaldehyde. The powder was air-dried and lyophilized. This was immersed in distilled water and the pH was adjusted to 4.0 using diluted HCl. The pH of the suspension was maintained at 4.0 during the whole step. The mixture was agitated at 30 °C for 24 h and was filtered and washed with distilled water. The sample was then soaked in 5% Na_2CO_3 (w/v) and agitated at 30 °C for 24 h. The resulting extract was filtered and the debris was clarified through centrifugation (10,000× g, 4 °C for 10 min). The recovered supernatant pH was adjusted to 6.0 by the addition of diluted HCl. This was treated with a saturated $CaCl_2$ solution and alginic acid was precipitated as calcium alginate. The pellet was recovered via centrifugation and suspended in 10% HCl for 2 h (acid wash, 6×). Centrifugation was repeated to recover the pellet. Finally, the suspension was washed with distilled water and was neutralized using NaOH. The resulting alginate solution was extensively dialyzed and lyophilized to obtain P. boryana alginate powder (PBA).

4.3. Analysis of the Proximate Composition of P. boryana

The assessment included moisture, ash, protein, lipid, and polysaccharide contents. Moisture by drying at 100 °C, ashing in a furnace at 600 °C for 5 h, protein content via Kjeldahl digestion, soxhlet method for lipids and polysaccharides by phenol sulphuric method. The Association of Official Analytical Chemists standard methods (AOAC 1990), were implemented in analyzing the above of P. boryana.

4.4. Evaluation of Chemical Composition of PBA

Chemical composition evaluation of an extract is an essential step before proceeding to further biological and physical properties. This includes the assessment of polysaccharide, protein, and polyphenol content.

The polysaccharide content was evaluated via the phenol sulfuric method as described by DuBois et al. (1956) [34], with minor modifications. The method, in brief, including a calibration standard curve was plotted using d-glucose 0 to 0.1 mg/mL. Sample concentrations were maintained at 0.1 mg/mL. Phenol (80%), 25 µL, was treated into each tube. This was followed by the addition of 2.5 mL of conc. sulfuric acid and vortexed. The tubes were kept in the dark at an ambient temperature for 30 min. A volume of 200 µL from each tube was transferred to a 96 well plate and the absorbance was measured at 480 nm.

The polyphenol content was measured accordingly with the method described by Chandler and Dodds [35], with minor modifications. Gallic acid was used as the standard and a calibration curve was plotted (0 to 0.1 mg/mL). Samples were prepared to be 0.1 mg/mL. Each test tube was introduced with 1 mL of 95% ethanol, and was followed by 5 mL of distilled water and 0.5 mL of 50% (1N) Folin-Ciocalteau reagent. Tubes were vortexed and incubated for 1 h in a dark environment. Subsequently, a volume of 200 µL was transferred to a 96 well plate and the absorbance was measured at 700 nm.

Protein percentages were quantified using Pierce™ BCA Protein Assay Kit and bovine serum albumin used as the standard.

4.5. Functional Group Analysis of PBA Using FTIR

The powder method was used to analyze the functional groups via FTIR. Fourier-transform infrared spectroscopic (FTIR) analysis of the alginate was performed with a Thermo Scientific NicoletTM 6700 FTIR spectrometer (Thermo Fisher Scientific, Waltham, MA, USA). Potassium bromide (KBr) pellets were cast by combining a 5 mg sample with 5 g KBr powder. A fine powder was generated using a mortar and pestle. KBr pellets were cast by applying pressure to the mold (5000–10,000 psi). The pellets were then placed in the sample holder and scans (32) were collected within the range of 500–4000 cm^{-1} wavenumber having a resolution of 4 cm^{-1}. A background scan was collected initially. The results were analyzed using the "Origin pro-2015" software package.

4.6. FTIR Spectra Interpretation Using Computational Calculations

Gaussian view molecular modeling software was used to develop the Cartesian coordinates for the Gaussian calculations. Initial energy calculations: geometry optimization of the molecule was performed using B3LYP quantum mechanical methods. The molecule was optimized finely and the harmonic vibrational frequencies were performed by ab initio time-dependent density functional theory (DFT) calculations at B3LYP level using the 6–31G (d,p) basis set as described by Cardenas-Jiron et al. (2011) [36] A scaling factor of 0.9645 was added to the calculated vibrational spectra.

4.7. Maintenance of Cell Lines

HaCaT cell line was maintained in the DMEM medium, which was supplemented with 10% FBS and 1% antibiotics. DMEM medium supplemented with F12 (25%), FBS (10%) and 1% antibiotics were used to maintain the human dermal fibroblast (HDF) cell line. The cells were maintained under controlled conditions at 5% CO_2 level and 37 °C temperature. The cells were periodically subcultured and were used for experiments in their exponential growth phase.

4.8. Analysis of Cell Viability and Intracellular ROS

The cytotoxicity was evaluated using the MTT assay in PM-induced HaCaT and HDF cells. An MTT colorimetric assay was performed following the method described by Mosmann et al. (1983) with slight modifications [37]. The cells were seeded with a concentration of 1×10^5 cells mL^{-1}, in 24 well plates. After a 24 h incubation period, PBA with different concentrations was treated. The growth media DMEM was used to suspend the PM achieving a stock concentration. To obtain the treatment concentrations, a serial dilution was performed. PM was treated and given a 1 h incubation. Following a 24 h incubation period, MTT (2 mg/mL in PBS) was added and incubated for another 3 h. Then the medium was aspirated and the formazan crystals were dissolved in DMSO. The absorbance reading was taken at 540 nm. The optimum PM treatment concentration was selected via this method.

The intracellular ROS levels were evaluated using the DCF-DA assay. The cells were seeded, samples were treated, and following a 1 h incubation period, the cells were treated with a DCF-DA reagent. This was incubated for 10 min and the fluorescence intensity was determined at an excitation wavelength of 485 nm and an emission wavelength of 535 nm [38].

4.9. PGE$_2$ and Pro-Inflammatory Cytokine Production Level Assessment

To obtain the cell culture media for the assessment of cytokine experiments, the cells were seeded in a similar manner described in the above experiments. HaCaT cells were seeded and incubated for 24 h. Samples were treated and after 1 h, PM was treated. After 23 h incubation, the media were retrieved for cytokine analysis. The culture media were collected separately and the expression levels of prostaglandin E2 (PGE$_2$), tumor necrosis factor α (TNF-α), interleukin (IL)-1β, and IL-6 were measured. The process was assisted with commercially available cytokine assessing kits and the test was performed following the given instructions by manufacturers.

4.10. Western Blot Analysis

To identify several key molecular mediators, Western blot analysis was performed. The cells which were induced with PM were harvested within 30 min to analyze the upstream molecules in the MAPK and NF-κB pathway. A further 24 h incubation was continued to evaluate the COX-2 levels [28]. Ice-cold PBS was used to wash the harvested cells and was lysed using a nuclear and cytoplasmic protein extraction kit (NE-PER®, Thermo Scientific, Rockford, IL, USA). Each extract protein level was measured using a BCA protein assay kit and was standardized (Bio-Rad, Irvine, CA, USA). Electrophoresis was carried out using sodium sulfate-polyacrylamide gels (12%). Subsequently, transferred onto nitrocellulose membranes. The membranes were blocked with skim milk and were incubated overnight with relevant primary antibodies: β-actin, COX-2, p38, p-p38, ERK1/2, p-ERK1/2, JNK, p-JNK, p50, p-p50, p65, and p-p65 (Santa Cruz Biotechnology). After the incubation period, primary antibodies were removed and the HRP-conjugated secondary antibodies (anti-mouse IgG, Santa Cruz Biotechnology) were added. Then, signals were developed using the chemiluminescent substrate (Cyanagen Srl, Bologna, Italy). Membranes were photographed (FUSION SOLO Vilber Lourmat system) and the ImageJ program was assisted in the quantification of the band intensities [39].

4.11. Spectroscopic Analysis (ICP-OES)

Similarly, HaCaT cells were seeded and samples were treated. PM was treated following an incubation period. After the procedure, the cells were harvested and collected into pre-weighed tubes. Cells were dried, and the final weight was taken. This was digested in concentrated HNO$_3$ using thermal energy (10% H$_2$O$_2$ was added). The acid digests were diluted in 3% HNO3 acid. The metal ions were analyzed by inductively coupled plasma optical emission spectrometry (ICP-OES) system (PerkinElmer OPTIMA 7300DV, Inc., Waltham, MA, USA). The calibration curves were plotted using a multi-element standard (PerkinElmer N9300233) including 10 ppm (10 µg/mL) of each element (Mg, Al, K, Ca, Fe, Mn, Cu, Sr, Ba, Pb). The elements were detected by non-overlapping wavelengths (≥2) [11].

Ultrapure deionized water was used in each step of the experiment. The final concentrations of the samples were calculated concerning the calibration plots.

4.12. Statistical Analysis

Based on triplicated experiments, data are expressed as means ± SD. One-way ANOVA and Turkey's test was used to determine the significant differences among data values. A $p < 0.05$ was considered statistically significant. * $p < 0.05$ and ** $p < 0.01$. (# denotes significance compared to control while * represents significance compared to PM-treated group).

5. Conclusions

The anti-inflammatory effects of alginic acid purified from *P. boryana* are evident in this research. Particulate matter induced inflammation in keratinocytes, as well as fibroblasts, were inhibited via the activity of PBA. Even though it requires further experimental confirmation, the researchers believe the inflammation was highly encouraged due to the effects of heavy metal content in the PM. Hence, PBA successfully chelated the metal ions, reducing their concentrations in the cell digests. Thus, PBA, a natural bioactive, is applicable as a source of skin cosmetics to abate PM-induced inflammation.

Author Contributions: Conceptualization, Y.-J.J. and T.U.J.; methodology, T.U.J.; software, T.U.J., K.K.A.S.; validation, T.U.J.; formal analysis, T.U.J.; investigation, T.U.J.; resources, K.K.A.S., L.W., W.-S.K., T.-K.L.; data curation, Y.-T.K.; writing—original draft preparation, T.U.J.; writing—review and editing, T.U.J. and Y.-J.J.; supervision, Y.-J.J.; project administration, Y.-J.J.; funding acquisition, Y.-J.J. All authors have read and agreed to the published version of the manuscript.

Funding: This research was financially supported by a grant from the "Marine Biotechnology program—20170488", funded by the Ministry of Oceans and Fisheries, Korea.

Conflicts of Interest: The authors declare to possess no competing interests.

References

1. Turnbull, A.B.; Harrison, R.M. Major component contributions to PM10 composition in the UK atmosphere. *Atmos. Environ.* **2000**, *34*, 3129–3137. [CrossRef]
2. Fernando, I.P.S.; Kim, H.-S.; Sanjeewa, K.K.A.; Oh, J.-Y.; Jeon, Y.-J.; Lee, W.W. Inhibition of inflammatory responses elicited by urban fine dust particles in keratinocytes and macrophages by diphlorethohydroxycarmalol isolated from a brown alga Ishige okamurae. *Algae* **2017**, *32*, 261–273. [CrossRef]
3. Jayawardena, T.U.; Asanka Sanjeewa, K.K.; Shanura Fernando, I.P.; Ryu, B.M.; Kang, M.C.; Jee, Y.; Lee, W.W.; Jeon, Y.J. Sargassum horneri (Turner) C. Agardh ethanol extract inhibits the fine dust inflammation response via activating Nrf2/HO-1 signaling in RAW 264.7 cells. *BMC Complement. Altern. Med.* **2018**, *18*, 249. [CrossRef] [PubMed]
4. Gilmour, P.S.; Brown, D.M.; Lindsay, T.G.; Beswick, P.H.; MacNee, W.; Donaldson, K. Adverse health effects of PM10 particles: Involvement of iron in generation of hydroxyl radical. *Occup. Environ. Med.* **1996**, *53*, 817–822. [CrossRef] [PubMed]
5. Knaapen, A.M.; Shi, T.; Borm, P.J.A.; Schins, R.P.F. Soluble metals as well as the insoluble particle fraction are involved in cellular DNA damage induced by particulate matter. In *Oxygen/Nitrogen Radicals: Cell Injury and Disease*; Vallyathan, V., Shi, X., Castranova, V., Eds.; Springer US: Boston, MA, USA, 2002; pp. 317–326. [CrossRef]
6. Brown, D.M.; Wilson, M.R.; MacNee, W.; Stone, V.; Donaldson, K. Size-dependent proinflammatory effects of ultrafine polystyrene particles: A role for surface area and oxidative stress in the enhanced activity of ultrafines. *Toxicol. Appl. Pharmacol.* **2001**, *175*, 191–199. [CrossRef] [PubMed]
7. Becker, S.; Soukup, J.M.; Gilmour, M.I.; Devlin, R.B. Stimulation of human and rat alveolar macrophages by urban air particulates: Effects on oxidant radical generation and cytokine production. *Toxicol. Appl. Pharmacol.* **1996**, *141*, 637–648. [CrossRef]
8. Schins, R.P.; Lightbody, J.H.; Borm, P.J.; Shi, T.; Donaldson, K.; Stone, V. Inflammatory effects of coarse and fine particulate matter in relation to chemical and biological constituents. *Toxicol. Appl. Pharmacol.* **2004**, *195*, 1–11. [CrossRef]

9. Williams, I.R.; Kupper, T.S. Immunity at the surface: Homeostatic mechanisms of the skin immune system. *Life Sci.* **1996**, *58*, 1485–1507. [CrossRef]
10. Werner, S.; Peters, K.G.; Longaker, M.T.; Fuller-Pace, F.; Banda, M.J.; Williams, L.T. Large induction of keratinocyte growth factor expression in the dermis during wound healing. *Proc. Natl. Acad. Sci. USA* **1992**, *89*, 6896–6900. [CrossRef]
11. Fernando, I.P.S.; Sanjeewa, K.K.A.; Kim, S.Y.; Lee, J.S.; Jeon, Y.J. Reduction of heavy metal (Pb2+) biosorption in zebrafish model using alginic acid purified from Ecklonia cava and two of its synthetic derivatives. *Int. J. Biol. Macromol.* **2018**, *106*, 330–337. [CrossRef]
12. Sarithakumari, C.H.; Renju, G.L.; Kurup, G.M. Anti-inflammatory and antioxidant potential of alginic acid isolated from the marine algae, Sargassum wightii on adjuvant-induced arthritic rats. *Inflammopharmacology* **2013**, *21*, 261–268. [CrossRef] [PubMed]
13. Fertah, M.; Belfkira, A.; Dahmane, E.M.; Taourirte, M.; Brouillette, F. Extraction and characterization of sodium alginate from Moroccan Laminaria digitata brown seaweed. *Arab. J. Chem.* **2017**, *10*, S3707–S3714. [CrossRef]
14. Kim, K.E.; Cho, D.; Park, H.J. Air pollution and skin diseases: Adverse effects of airborne particulate matter on various skin diseases. *Life Sci.* **2016**, *152*, 126–134. [CrossRef] [PubMed]
15. Hahn, T.; Lang, S.; Ulber, R.; Muffler, K. Novel procedures for the extraction of fucoidan from brown algae. *Process. Biochem.* **2012**, *47*, 1691–1698. [CrossRef]
16. McHugh, D.J. Production, properties and uses of alginates. *Prod. Util. Prod. Commer. Seaweeds. FAO Fish. Tech. Pap.* **1987**, *288*, 58–115.
17. Smidsrod, O.; Haug, A. Dependence upon the gel-sol state of the ion-exchange properties of alginates. *Acta Chem. Scand.* **1972**, *26*, 2063–2074. [CrossRef]
18. Penman, A.; Sanderson, G.R. A method for the determination of uronic acid sequence in alginates. *Carbohydr. Res.* **1972**, *25*, 273–282. [CrossRef]
19. Haug, A.; Larsen, B.; Smidsrod, O. Uronic Acid Sequence in Alginate from Different Sources. *Carbohydr. Res.* **1974**, *32*, 217–225. [CrossRef]
20. Donati, I.; Vetere, A.; Gamini, A.; Skjak-Braek, G.; Coslovi, A.; Campa, C.; Paoletti, S. Galactose-substituted alginate: Preliminary characterization and study of gelling properties. *Biomacromolecules* **2003**, *4*, 624–631. [CrossRef]
21. Papageorgiou, S.K.; Kouvelos, E.P.; Favvas, E.P.; Sapalidis, A.A.; Romanos, G.E.; Katsaros, F.K. Metal-carboxylate interactions in metal-alginate complexes studied with FTIR spectroscopy. *Carbohydr. Res.* **2010**, *345*, 469–473. [CrossRef]
22. Schaumann, F.; Borm, P.J.; Herbrich, A.; Knoch, J.; Pitz, M.; Schins, R.P.; Luettig, B.; Hohlfeld, J.M.; Heinrich, J.; Krug, N. Metal-rich ambient particles (particulate matter 2.5) cause airway inflammation in healthy subjects. *Am. J. Respir. Crit. Care Med.* **2004**, *170*, 898–903. [CrossRef] [PubMed]
23. Fu, F.; Wang, Q. Removal of heavy metal ions from wastewaters: A review. *J. Environ. Manag.* **2011**, *92*, 407–418. [CrossRef] [PubMed]
24. Blue, L.Y.; Van Aelstyn, M.A.; Matlock, M.; Atwood, D.A. Low-level mercury removal from groundwater using a synthetic chelating ligand. *Water Res.* **2008**, *42*, 2025–2028. [CrossRef] [PubMed]
25. King, R.B. Coordination number, electronic configuration, and ionic charge as discrete variables in coordination chemistry. *Adv. Chem. Ser.* **1967**, *62*, 203–220. [CrossRef]
26. Jeon, C.; Park, J.Y.; Yoo, Y.J. Novel immobilization of alginic acid for heavy metal removal. *Biochem. Eng. J.* **2002**, *11*, 159–166. [CrossRef]
27. Grant, G.T.; Morris, E.R.; Rees, D.A.; Smith, P.J.C.; Thom, D. Biological interactions between polysaccharides and divalent cations: The egg-box model. *FEBS Lett.* **1973**, *32*, 195–198. [CrossRef]
28. Fernando, I.P.S.; Jayawardena, T.U.; Sanjeewa, K.K.A.; Wang, L.; Jeon, Y.J.; Lee, W.W. Anti-inflammatory potential of alginic acid from Sargassum horneri against urban aerosol-induced inflammatory responses in keratinocytes and macrophages. *Ecotoxicol. Environ. Saf.* **2018**, *160*, 24–31. [CrossRef]
29. Kim, B.H.; Oh, I.; Kim, J.H.; Jeon, J.E.; Jeon, B.; Shin, J.; Kim, T.Y. Anti-inflammatory activity of compounds isolated from Astragalus sinicus L. in cytokine-induced keratinocytes and skin. *Exp. Mol. Med.* **2014**, *46*, e87. [CrossRef]
30. Karin, M.; Delhase, M. The I kappa B kinase (IKK) and NF-kappa B: Key elements of proinflammatory signalling. *Semin. Immunol.* **2000**, *12*, 85–98. [CrossRef]
31. Sanjeewa, K.K.A.; Jayawardena, T.U.; Kim, H.-S.; Kim, S.-Y.; Ahn, G.; Kim, H.-J.; Fu, X.; Jee, Y.; Jeon, Y.-J. Ethanol extract separated from Sargassum horneri (Turner) abate LPS-induced inflammation in RAW 264.7 macrophages. *Fish. Aquat. Sci.* **2019**, *22*, 6. [CrossRef]

32. Akira, S. Toll-like Receptors and Innate Immunity. In *Advances in Immunology*; Dixon, F.J., Ed.; Academic Press: Cambridge, MA, USA, 2001; Volume 78, pp. 1–56.
33. Kaminska, B. MAPK signalling pathways as molecular targets for anti-inflammatory therapy—From molecular mechanisms to therapeutic benefits. *Biochim. Biophys. Acta (BBA) Proteins Proteom.* **2005**, *1754*, 253–262. [CrossRef] [PubMed]
34. Dubois, M.; Gilles, K.A.; Hamilton, J.K.; Rebers, P.T.; Smith, F. Colorimetric method for determination of sugars and related substances. *Anal. Chem.* **1956**, *28*, 350–356. [CrossRef]
35. Chandler, S.F.; Dodds, J.H. The effect of phosphate, nitrogen and sucrose on the production of phenolics and solasodine in callus cultures of solanum laciniatum. *Plant Cell Rep.* **1983**, *2*, 205–208. [CrossRef] [PubMed]
36. Cardenas-Jiron, G.; Leal, D.; Matsuhiro, B.; Osorio-Roman, I.O. Vibrational spectroscopy and density functional theory calculations of poly-D-mannuronate and heteropolymeric fractions from sodium alginate. *J. Raman Spectrosc.* **2011**, *42*, 870–878. [CrossRef]
37. Mosmann, T. Rapid colorimetric assay for cellular growth and survival: Application to proliferation and cytotoxicity assays. *J. Immunol. Methods* **1983**, *65*, 55–63. [CrossRef]
38. Wang, L.; Ryu, B.; Kim, W.S.; Kim, G.H.; Jeon, Y.J. Protective effect of gallic acid derivatives from the freshwater green alga Spirogyra sp against ultraviolet B-induced apoptosis through reactive oxygen species clearance in human keratinocytes and zebrafish. *Algae* **2017**, *32*, 379–388. [CrossRef]
39. Jayawardena, T.U.; Kim, H.-S.; Sanjeewa, K.K.A.; Kim, S.-Y.; Rho, J.-R.; Jee, Y.; Ahn, G.; Jeon, Y.-J. Sargassum horneri and isolated 6-hydroxy-4,4,7a-trimethyl-5,6,7,7a-tetrahydrobenzofuran-2(4H)-one (HTT); LPS-induced inflammation attenuation via suppressing NF-κB, MAPK and oxidative stress through Nrf2/HO-1 pathways in RAW 264.7 macrophages. *Algal Res.* **2019**, *40*, 101513. [CrossRef]

Publisher's Note: MDPI stays neutral with regard to jurisdictional claims in published maps and institutional affiliations.

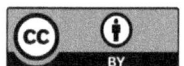

© 2020 by the authors. Licensee MDPI, Basel, Switzerland. This article is an open access article distributed under the terms and conditions of the Creative Commons Attribution (CC BY) license (http://creativecommons.org/licenses/by/4.0/).

MDPI
St. Alban-Anlage 66
4052 Basel
Switzerland
Tel. +41 61 683 77 34
Fax +41 61 302 89 18
www.mdpi.com

Molecules Editorial Office
E-mail: molecules@mdpi.com
www.mdpi.com/journal/molecules

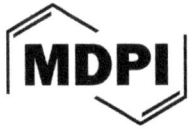

www.ingramcontent.com/pod-product-compliance
Lightning Source LLC
LaVergne TN
LVHW070630100526
838202LV00012B/769